《(英汉对照)精编实用中医文库》

编纂委员会

编译委员会

《中药学》

主编 郭 忻

编委 金素安 何世民 袁 颖

主译 徐 瑶

An Intensively Compiled Practical English-Chinese Library of Traditional Chinese Medicine

(英汉对照)精编实用中医文库

Chief General Compilers CHEN Kaixian LI Qizhong(Executive) HE Xinghai

总主编 陈凯先 李其忠(执行) 何星海

Chief General Translators SHI Jianrong HU Hongyi XU Yao(Executive)

总主译 施建蓉 胡鸿毅 徐 瑶(执行)

Chinese Materia Medica

中 药 学

Chief Compiler GUO Xin

Chief Translator XU Yao

主编 郭 忻

主译 徐 瑶

上海浦江教育出版社(原上海中医药大学出版社)

Shanghai Pujiang Education Press (Former Shanghai University of TCM Press)

An Intensively Compiled Practical English-Chinese Library of Traditional Chinese Medicine

Compilation Board of the Library

Chief General Compilers CHEN Kaixian LI Qizhong(Executive) HE Xinghai

Members(Listed in the order of the number of strokes in the Chinese names)

MA Lieguang	HE Jiancheng	YU Xiaoping	SHEN Xueyong
ZHANG Tingting	CHEN Hongfeng	CHEN Dexing	ZHAO Yi
GUO Xin	HUANG Ping	YU Jian'er	ZHAN Hongsheng
MIAO Wanhong			

Compilation and Translation Committee of the Library

Chief General Translators SHI Jianrong HU Hongyi XU Yao(Executive)

Translations(Listed in the order of the number of strokes in the Chinese names)

ZHU Aixiu	YANG Yu	XIAO Yuanchun	ZHANG Yiping
ZHU Jianmin	HUANG Guoqi	DONG Jing	HAN Chouping

Chinese Materia Medica

Chief Editor GUO Xin

Editing Members JIN Su'an HE Shimin YUAN Ying

Chief Translator XU Yao

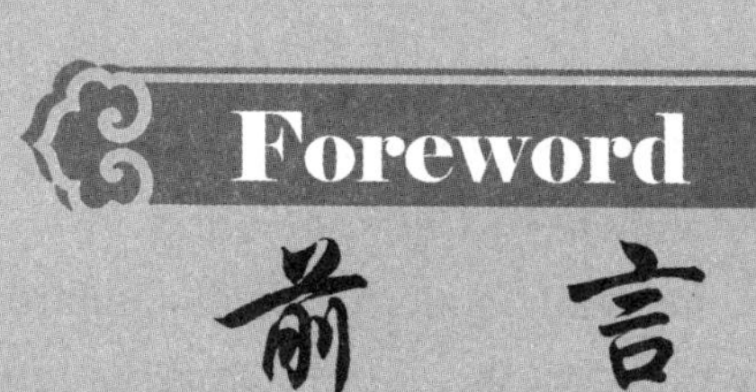

Foreword
前　言

With the traditional medical philosophy and clinical experience as the principal body, the science of Traditional Chinese Medicine (TCM) is a comprehensive subject to study the rules of life activities and the disease prevention, diagnosis, treatment, rehabilitation as well as healthcare. The science of TCM has a long history of development and belongs to a summary of experiences that Chinese nation has fought against diseases for over several thousand years, is also an important component part of Chinese outstanding traditional culture and has contributed greatly to the health-care undertaking and development of Chinese nation.

By increasing enhancement of modern living standard, change of living modes and acceleration of ageing process, the chronic diseases represented by tumors, cardiovascular diseases and diabetes become gradually the important factors in impacting the health of mankind, but TCM presents the better therapeutic effects. Nowadays, the modern medical mode of "society-psychology-biology" has been advocated in medical science, changing from the medical idea of "disease treatment" to "health promotion". The more and more patients in China and abroad have chosen natural and low side-effect Chinese herbal medicine for their problems. With the changes in medicine modes and in spectrum of diseases in the recent several dozens of years, TCM has increasingly been concerned by the medical experts and ordinary people in China and abroad, and the global " TCM upsurge" keeps rising. In order to meet the growing needs of the domestic and international professionals in learning the knowledge of TCM, we have edited particularly the series books of *An Intensively Compiled Practical English-Chinese Library of Traditional Chinese Medicine*.

The scientific, systematic and practical features have been emphasized in the series books. Based upon the full absorption of new progress in teaching and research achievements of TCM , the series books highlight the academic essentials of TCM, with precise exposition of medical philosophy and down-to-earth clinical practice, to introduce the "original and authentic" TCM to the readers. The series books introduce the commonly used therapeutic methods and clinical skills in Chinese medicine, by the clinically encountered and frequently seen diseases and the relevant ailments predominantly effective by Chinese medical therapies.By studying the series books, the readers can learn the knowledge and techniques of TCM on gradual progress and become proficient gradually in TCM.

The series books highlight "the precise features in three aspects"—capable in authors, refined in contents and accurate in translation. The majority of the authors of the series books are senior experts from the related faculties of Shanghai University of Traditional Chinese Medicine. The translator team is composed of the senior teachers with plentiful expertise in translation of TCM from international education college and foreign language center of Shanghai University of Traditional Chinese Medicine. In order to meet the needs of the readers in China and abroad, the basic and clinical core contents are selected and the latest research achievements are consulted based upon the principle "to seek its essentials but its completion" in the series books.

The series books can satisfy the beginners with certain knowledge of English language in studying TCM systematically and can also be used as the textbooks for education of TCM and pharmacy for foreign students. We sincerely hope the publication of the series books plays its promoting role for TCM going to the world.

Editors

June, 2017

中医学是以传统医学理论与实践经验为主体，研究人体生命活动规律和疾病预防、诊断、治疗、康复以及保健的一门综合性学科。中医学历史悠久，源远流长，是中华民族几千年来同疾病作斗争的经验总结，也是中国传统文化的重要组成部分，长期以来为中国人民的健康保健事业和民族繁衍作出了巨大的贡献。

随着现代生活水平的不断提高、生活方式的改变以及老龄化进程的加快，以肿瘤、心血管疾病和糖尿病等为代表的慢性病日渐成为影响人类健康的重要因素，而中医药显示了良好的治疗效果。当今的医学倡导“社会—心理—生物”的现代医学模式，医学理念从“疾病治疗”向“健康促进”转变，国内外越来越多的患者选择天然、毒副作用低的中医药治疗疾病。近几十年来，随着医学模式的转变和疾病谱的改变，中医学日益引起越来越多的海内外医学专家和普通民众的关注，全球性的“中医热”正在持续升温。为了满足海内外人士日益高涨的学习中医学知识的需求，我们特地编撰了《(英汉对照)精编实用中医文库》丛书。

本丛书注重“三性”——科学性、系统性、实用性。丛书在充分吸取近年中医教学、科研进展的基础上，突出中医学术精华，理论阐述准确、临床切合实际，向读者介绍“原汁原味”的中医学；丛书介绍中医学常用的治疗方法和临床技能，所涉及的病证均为临床常见病、多发病和中医优势病种。丛书的13个分册涵盖了中医基础与临床的主干课程，通过阅读本丛书，读者可以由浅入深、循序渐进地学习中医药知识和技能。

本丛书突出“三精”　　作者精干、内容精炼、翻译精准。丛书的中文作者绝大部分为上海中医药大学各相关教研室的资深专家，翻译团队由上海中医药大学国际教育学院和外语中心具有丰富的中医药学翻译经验的骨干教师组成。为了适合海内外读者的需求，丛书本着“求其精而不求其全”的原则，选取了基础和临床的核心内容，翻译上参考了最新的研究成果。

本丛书既可满足具有一定英语水平的初学中医者系统学习中医所用，也可供中医药留学生教育作为教材使用，衷心希望本丛书的出版在中医药走向海外进程中发挥应有的推动作用。

编者

2017年6月

Note for Compilation

编写说明

In the historical practice for thousands of years, the medicinal herbs have played the great role in preventing and treating diseases and in guaranteeing the human health. As a subject bridging the Basic Theory of Traditional Chinese Medicine and all the clinical departments, Chinese Materia Medica acts to illustrate the basic theory and clinical application of Chinese medicinal herbs. This book, under the guidance of the theories of traditional Chinese medicine and according to the practical and easily understanding principles, systematically introduces the basic theories and concrete application methods of Chinese Materia Medica.

The whole book consists of two parts of General Introduction and Specific Introduction.

General Introduction, consisting of three chapters, mainly introduces the natures and actions of Chinese medicinal herbs, including: four properties, five flavors, ascending, descending, floating and sinking actions, meridian tropism, and toxicity; the processing purpose and commonly-used processing methods of Chinese medicinal herbs; the application of Chinese medicinal herbs, including compatibilities, contraindications, dosages and administrations.

Specific Introduction, divided into eighteen chapters, collects and contains 260 commonly-used and practical herbs. It is introduced in each chapter the concept, action, classification, indications and notes for attention of this type of herbs. Each herb is illustrated according to the Pharmacopoeia of People's Republic of China 2015 in the order of formal name, source, property, flavor, meridian tropism, action, application, dosage, and administration. It is emphatically introduced the action features of each herb, for the purpose to easily understand. For some of the herbs, remarks are added to briefly illustrate the differences among the herbs with similar names or confusion, and the generalization and comparison of herbs with same sources but different parts, so as to increase the practicability and clinical application. There is a brief summary in the end of each chapter, which is to summarize the properties and actions of the sort of herbs in this chapter.

Index of herbs is added as the appendix.

在数千年的历史实践中，中医药在防治疾病、保障人类健康方面发挥了巨大的作用。中药学是阐述中药的基本理论和临床应用的一门学科，是中医药基础与临床各科之间的桥梁。本书以中医学理论为指导，遵循实用、易懂的原则，较为系统地介绍中药的基本理论和具体应用方法。

全书分总论和各论两大部分。

总论共有三章，主要介绍中药的性能，包括：四气、五味、升降浮沉、归经、有毒无毒等内容；中药炮制的目的和常用的炮制方法；中药的应用，包括配伍、用药禁忌、剂量、用法等。

各论按功效分列18章，共收载常用、实用的药物260味(含附药14味)。每章先简单叙述该章药物的概念、功效分类、适应证，以及使用注意等项。每味药以2015年版《中国药典》为依据，列药物正名、来源、性味归经、功效、应用、用量用法、使用注意等项，着重介绍每味药物的应用，阐述该药与应用相关的作用特性，以便于理解。在部分药物项下加设按语，简明扼要地对药名类似、作用有异、易混淆的药物加以区别；对来源相同、药用部位不同的药物作用进行归纳比较，以增加实用性，有利于临床应用。每章结束设小结，对章内药物性能功效加以归纳。

正文后附有中药药名中文名、拉丁名索引，以便于检索。

Contents

目　录

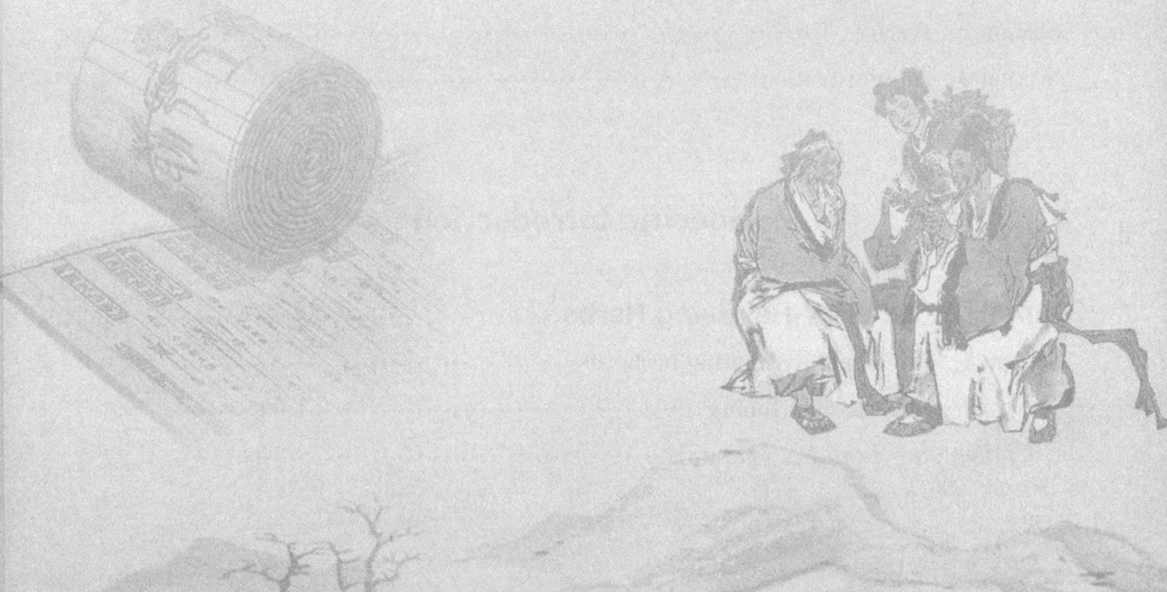

General Introduction

Specific Introduction

总　论

各　论

General Introduction

Chinese Materia Medica, based upon the theories of traditional Chinese medicine, implies the traditional Chinese medicinal herbs with unique theoretical guidance and application forms, playing an important role to guarantee the human health for thousands of years. The application of Chinese Materia Medica fully reflects the characteristics of the natural resources, history and culture in China, as one of the important component parts of "principle, method, formula and herb" used in treatment of diseases in traditional Chinese medicine.

中药是以中医学理论为基础，有着独特的理论指导和应用形式的中国传统药物。数千年来，中药为保障人类健康发挥了极大的作用。中药的应用充分反映了中国自然资源及历史、文化等方面的若干特点，是中医治病“理、法、方、药”的重要组成部分之一。

Chinese Materia Medica has many varieties and rich resources, involving the categories of plants, animals and minerals. Since most of the Chinese medicinal herbs are of the plants, Chinese Materia Medica is also called "herbal medicine", which can be found in many ancient classics of Chinese Materia Medica.

中药品种繁多，资源丰富，其来源涉及植物、动物、矿物等多种门类，其中以植物类药物居多，故又有“本草”之称。古代记载中药的专著常冠以“本草”之名。

Chinese Materia Medica is a science to study the basic theories, resources, collecting and processing, natures, actions and clinical application of Chinese medicinal herbs, emphasizing on the natures, actions and clinical application of Chinese medicinal herbs. Chinese Materia Medica, one of the important component parts of theoretical system of traditional Chinese medicine, closely related to the basics, diagnostics, formulas and various clinic departments of traditional Chinese medicine, and being the necessary measure of clinic practice.

中药学主要是研究中药的基本理论及其来源、采制、性能、功效及临床应用等知识的一门学科。其重点研究中药的性能、功效以及临床应用。中药学是中国传统医学理论体系中的一个重要组成部分，与中医学基础、诊断学、方剂学以及临床各科具有不可分割的密切关系，是临床应用的必备武器。

Chapter 1 Natures of Chinese Medicinal Herbs

第1章 中药的性能

The word "nature" refers to the property of Chinese medicinal herb and also the action of Chinese medicinal herb as well. The nature of Chinese medicinal herbs implies the high generalization of the basic nature and characteristics of Chinese medicinal herbs. The nature of Chinese medicinal herbs, the core of the theory of Chinese Materia Medica, includes four properties, five flavors, meridian tropism, ascending, descending, floating and sinking, and toxicity.

性，是指中药的性质；能，是指中药的作用。可以说，性能是中药作用的基本性质和特征的高度概括，又称药性。药性理论是中药理论的核心，主要包括四气、五味、归经、升降浮沉、毒性等。

Section 1 Four properties

第1节 四气

Four properties refer to the cold, hot, warm and cool properties of Chinese medicinal herbs. It is believed in traditional Chinese medicine that the cold or hot property of a disease is caused by the preponderance or weakness of yin or yang in the human body. The four properties imply that the Chinese medicinal herbs possess the acting tendency to the changes of yin and yang and of cold and heat in human body.

四气，是指药物寒、热、温、凉四种药性，又称四性。中医学认为，疾病的寒热性质是由于人体阴阳的偏盛、偏衰所导致的。药物的四气则表明了药物影响人体阴阳盛衰，寒热变化的作用倾向。

The cold and warm properties of Chinese me-

药性分寒温，最早记载

dicinal herbs were first mentioned in *Shen Nong's Herbal Canon* (Shen Nong Ben Cao Jing). In order to avoid the linguistic ambiguity of the word "property", some of the medical workers fells that "four properties" should be changed to "four natures". But the term "four properties" has been continued to use for a very long period of time. Anyway, no matter "four properties" or "four natures" refer to the cold, hot, warm and cool properties of Chinese medicinal herbs.

于《神农本草经》。为避免与药物的香臭之气相混淆，曾有医家主张将"四气"改为"四性"，然四气称谓沿用已久，故不论称四气，还是称四性，都是指寒、热、温、凉四种药性。

The four properties actually include two types of properties of cold-cool and warm-hot. In terms of attributions of yin and yang, warm and hot properties pertain to yang, while cold and cool properties pertain to yin. The warm and hot properties and the cold and cool properties are of same properties, but of different degrees. The hot property is stronger than the warm property, while the cold property is stronger than the cool property. In the classics of Chinese Materia Medica, there are more detailed descriptions, as heavy hot, heavy cold, light warm, light cold, etc., which are of the different degrees.

四气，实际包括寒凉与温热两类不同的性质。就阴阳属性而言，温与热的属性相同，均属阳；寒与凉的属性相同，均属阴。温与热、寒与凉在具有共同性质的同时，又有程度上的差异，如热较之温，温性更强些，寒较之凉，凉性更重些。在本草专著中，可以看到更为细化的四气描述，如有大热、大寒、微温、微寒等标注，对寒、热、温、凉的程度加以区分。

Besides the four properties of cold, hot, warm and cool, there are some other herbs which are not obviously cold or hot in properties, pertaining to the neutral property. Since the neutral property does not surpass the scope of the four properties of cold, hot, warm and cool, the properties of Chinese medicinal herbs are always called the four properties.

除了性质明确的寒、热、温、凉四种药性外，还有一些寒热偏性不甚明显的，称为平性。平性是相对寒热温凉四性而言的，未超出四性的范围，故习惯上还是称四气。

The cold, hot, warm and cool properties are generalized from the response of the body acted by the Chinese medicinal herbs, so they are corresponding to the cold or hot property diseases.

药性的寒热温凉，是从药物作用于机体所发生的反应概括出来的，是与所治疾病的寒热性质相对应的。

Generally speaking, the Chinese medicinal herbs with the actions of heat-clearing, fire-reducing, blood-cooling and toxin-relieving pertain to the cold and cool properties, used to treat the heat patterns. The Chinese medicinal herbs with the actions of fire-reinforcing, yang-strengthening, meridian-warming to dredge collateral and yang-enhancing to rescue from collapse pertain to the warm and hot properties, used to treat the cold patterns. So the therapeutic principles in the clinic application of the four property theory are "the heating method for cold and the cooling method for heat", i.e. it is advisable to apply the Chinese medicinal herbs of cold and cool properties to treat the yang and heat patterns, while the Chinese medicinal herbs of warm and hot properties to treat the yin and cold patterns. The application of the wrong herbs may cause harmful results.

一般来讲，具有清热泻火、凉血解毒等作用的药物，性属寒凉，主要用于热性病证。具有温里散寒、补火助阳、温经通络、回阳救逆等作用的药物，性属温热，主要用于寒性病证。故四气理论在临床应用时的原则是“寒者热之，热者寒之”。就是说阳热证用寒凉性药，阴寒证用温热性药。若用药错误则会造成不良后果。

In summary, the cold, hot, warm and cool properties of Chinese medicinal herbs act to work on the human body to influence the changes of yin and yang and of cold and heat, and to generalize the relevant changes, as the natures of the Chinese medicinal herbs. The cold and hot properties of the Chinese medicinal herbs are somewhat related to the actions, but only the general characters rather than all the actions and functions of each of the Chinese medicinal herbs. Therefore, it is necessary to integrate other theories to understand the Chinese medicinal herbs, so as to totally appreciate and master the natures and actions of the Chinese medicinal herbs.

总之，药物的寒、热、温、凉是药物作用于机体，影响人体的阴阳盛衰、寒热，并对相应变化所作的概括，仅限于药物的性质。药性的寒热性质虽与功效之间有一定的联系，但仅反映了一些共性，并不能反映每味药物的所有功效。所以，对药物的认识，还必须结合其他理论，方能全面地认识和掌握药物的药性和作用。

Section 2
Five flavors

第 2 节
五味

Five flavors refer to the pungent, sweet, sour, bitter and salty flavors of Chinese medicinal herbs. Besides the five basic flavors of pungent, sweet, sour, bitter and salty, there are also the flavors of bland and astringent. It holds that the astringent flavor is similar to the sour flavor, while the bland flavor falls under the sweet flavor category, so that the classification of five flavors is applied. In terms of the attributions of yin and yang, the pungent and sweet flavors pertain to yang, while the sour, bitter and salty flavors pertain to yin.

五味，是指辛、甘、酸、苦、咸五种滋味。辛、甘、酸、苦、咸是五种最基本的滋味，还有淡味和涩味等。因有酸、涩相似，淡附于甘之说，故习惯上还是称五味。五味的阴阳属性是辛、甘属阳，酸、苦、咸属阴。

The five flavors originate from the real tastes of Chinese medicinal herbs tasted by the tongue. Along with the development of medicine and herbs, the relations between the flavors and actions of the Chinese medicinal herbs were found. In the practical process of constant summarization and generalization, the flavors of the Chinese medicinal herbs are gradually integrated with the actions, so as to apply to guide the clinical practice. Simultaneously, along with the continuous enrichment of the human knowledge of medicinal herbs, the actions of some medicinal herbs cannot be illustrated by the flavors, so the inference method is applied to deduce the flavors based upon the actions, and it is believed that the flavor established by the action is more scientific than the flavor tasted by the tongue. It can be seen therefore that the establishment of the flavors is related to the original flavors of the Chinese medicinal herbs, and also to the actions of the Chinese medici-

五味最初来源于药物的真实滋味，通过口尝而得。随着医药的进步，人们在实践中发现了味与功效之间的关系，在不断总结归纳的过程中，逐步将味与功效结合并加以诠释，用于指导临床实践。同时，人们对药物作用的认识不断丰富，对于一些难以用味来解释的作用，采用了依据功效推定其味的方法，并认为以功效确定药味的方法比口尝更为科学。由此可知，味的确定与药物本身的滋味，以及药物的功效相关。

nal herbs as well.

The five flavors are the generalization of the different actions of Chinese medicinal herbs working on the human body. The five flavors possess the different actions and functions as follows:

五味是药物作用于人体所产生的不同效用的概括，五味的效用各异，概述如下。

1 Pungent

It acts to spread and to move, with the functions to disperse, to promote qi flow and blood flow. Generally, the Chinese medicinal herbs used to treat the exterior pattern, qi stagnation and blood stasis are of the pungent flavor, such as *Ephedrae Herba* (ma huang) used to make sweating to relieve the exterior, *Cyperi Rhizoma* (xiang fu) used to promote qi flow, *Chuanxiong Rhizoma* (chuan xiong) used to activate blood and dissolve stasis, etc.

1 辛

能散、能行，有发散、行气、行血等作用。一般治疗表证、气滞血瘀的药物，都有辛味。如发汗解表的麻黄，行气的香附，活血散瘀的川芎等。

2 Sweet

It acts to reinforce, to harmonize and to moderate, with the functions to reinforce and benefit, to harmonize the middle energizer, to modify other herb properties, and to relieve spasm and pain. Generally, most reinforcing herbs are sweet in flavor, such as *Ginseng Radix et Raizoma* (ren shen) to greatly reinforce the Yuan (Primary) Qi and *Rehmanniae Radix Praeparata* (shu di huang) to nourish and reinforce essence and blood, and the Chinese medicinal herbs, used to modify other herbs properties and to relieve spasm and pain, are of the sweet flavor, such as *Glycyrrhizae Radix et Rhizoma* (gan cao) used to modify all other herbs and to relieve spasm and pain. Besides, some Chinese medicinal herbs of sweet flavor act to relieve the toxicity in herbs and foods, such as gan cao, *Semen Phasoli Radiati* (lü dou), etc.

2 甘

能补、能和、能缓，有补益、和中、调和药性、缓急止痛的作用。一般补益类药大多有甘味，如大补元气的人参，滋补精血的熟地黄等。能调和药性、缓急止痛的药物亦具甘味，如既调和诸药，又缓急止痛的甘草。此外，某些甘味药能解药食中毒，如甘草、绿豆等。

3 Sour

It acts to inhibit and to restrain, with the functions to retrain, to astringe and to consolidate. Generally, the Chinese medicinal herbs, used to treat leakage and prolapse conditions as seminal emission, spermatorrhea, enuresis, frequency of urination, spontaneous sweating, nocturnal sweats, uterine bleeding, excessive leucorrhea, etc., are of sour flavor, such as *Schisandrae Chinensis Fructus* (wu wei zi) used to restrain the lung, stop sweating and restrain sperms, *Corni Fructus* (shan zhu yu) used to restrain and to consolidate, *Mume Fructus* (wu mei) used to restrain the intestines and to stop diarrhea, etc.

3 酸

能收、能涩,有收敛固涩作用。一般用于滑脱诸证,如治疗遗精滑精、遗尿尿频、自汗盗汗、崩漏带下等证的药物,都有酸味,如敛肺止汗、涩精的五味子,收敛固涩的山茱萸,涩肠止泻的乌梅等。

4 Bitter

It acts to reduce and to dry. To reduce has three implications: The first refers to the Chinese medicinal herbs used to dredge intestines and promote defecation, such as *Rhei Radix et Rhizoma* (da huang), bitter in flavor and cold in property, used to attack and purge to promote defecation. The second refers to the Chinese medicinal herbs used to subdue the lung qi, stop coughing and panting, subdue the stomach qi and stop vomiting, such as *Armeniacae Amarum Semen* (ku xing ren), bitter in flavor, used to subdue and reduce the lung qi to stop coughing and relieve panting, and *Haematitum* (zhe shi), bitter in flavor and cold in property, used to subdue the lung and stomach qi. The third refers to the Chinese medicinal herbs, used to clear and reduce the pathogenic heat, fire or toxin, such as *Gardeniae Fructus* (zhi zi), used to clear heat and reduce fire, etc. To dry implies to dry the

4 苦

能泄、能燥。泄的含义有:一指通泄,能通利排便的药物,如大黄苦寒,能攻下通便。二指降泄,能降肺气、止咳喘,降胃气、止呕吐的药物,如杏仁味苦,降泄肺气、止咳平喘;赭石苦寒,能降肺胃气逆。三指清泄,能清泄体内邪热火毒的药物,如清热泻火的栀子。燥即燥湿,用于湿证。湿证有寒湿、湿热的不同。味苦性温的药能温燥寒湿,如苍术、厚朴多用于寒湿病证。味苦性寒的药能清热燥湿,如黄连、黄柏多用于湿热证。

damp, used to treat the damp pattern. The damp pattern is divided into the cold-damp pattern and damp-heat pattern. The Chinese medicinal herbs, bitter in flavor and warm in property, act to warm and dry to treat the cold-damp pattern, such as *Atractylodis Rhizoma* (cang zhu) and *Magnoliae Officinalis Cortex* (hou po) are often used to treat the cold-damp pattern. The Chinese medicinal herbs, bitter in flavor and cold in property, act to clear the heat and dry the damp, such as *Coptidis Rhizoma* (huang lian) and *Phellodendri Cortex Chiensis* (huang bo) used to treat the damp-heat pattern.

5 Salty

It acts to soften and to purge, with the functions to soften the hard, to scatter the accumulation and to reduce and purge. Generally, the Chinese medicinal herbs, used to treat scrofula, simple goiter, globus hystericus and constipation, are of salty flavor, such as *Sargassum* (hai zao) and *Thallus Laminariae seu Eckloniae* (kun bu) used to soften the hard and scatter the accumulation to treat goiter and tumor, and *Natrii Sulfas* (mang xiao) used to soften the hard and moisturize the dry to treat constipation.

5 咸

能软、能下，有软坚散结和泻下作用。一般治疗瘰疬、瘿瘤、痰核以及便秘的药物，都有咸味。如软坚散结、消散瘿瘤的海藻、昆布，能软坚润燥通便的芒硝等。

6 Bland

It acts to remove and to promote, with the functions to remove the damp and promote urination. Generally, the Chinese medicinal herbs, used to treat edema dysuria, are of bland flavor, such as *Polyporus* (zhu ling), *Poria* (fu ling) and *Coicis Semen* (yi yi ren) used to promote urination and remove the damp.

6 淡

能渗、能利，有渗湿、利水作用。一般用于治疗水肿、小便不利等证的药物，具有淡味。如利水渗湿的猪苓、茯苓、薏苡仁等。

7 Astringent

Similar to the sour flavor, it acts to restrain, to

7 涩

能收敛固涩，与酸味作

astringe and to consolidate. Generally, the Chinese medicinal herbs, used to treat all types incontinence and prolapse, such as *Os Draconis* (long gu) used to restrain, astringe and consolidate, *Halloysitum Rubrum* (chi shi zhi) used to restrain the intestine to stop diarrhea, and *Endoconcha Sepiellae* (hai piao xiao) used to stanch bleeding, restrain sperms and decrease excessive leucorrhea.

用相似。一般用于滑脱诸证。如收敛固涩的龙骨，涩肠止泻的赤石脂，收敛止血、固精止带的海螵蛸等。

In the clinical application, it is advisable to integrate the property and flavor with the action of the Chinese medicinal herb for better understanding of the actions and functions of the Chinese medicinal herbs. There is some regulation of the relation between the property-flavor integration and the action. Generally, the Chinese medicinal herbs with same property or same flavor possess the partially same actions and functions. For example, *Perillae Folium* (zi su) and *Menthae Haplocalycis Herba* (bo he) are same in flavor but different in property, both are pungent in flavor, with the dispersing action. Zi su is warm in property, used to disperse the wind cold, while bo he is cool in property, used to disperse the wind-heat. *Scutellariae Radix* (huang qin) and bo he are same in property but different in flavor, both are cold-cool in property, with the heat-clearing function. Huang qin is bitter in flavor and cold in property, used to clear the heat and dry the damp, while bo he is pungent in flavor and cool in property, used to disperse the wind-heat. The Chinese medicinal herbs with same property and same flavor possess the quite similar actions and functions. For example, both *Coptidis Rhizoma* (huang lian) and *Phellodendri Cortex Chiensis* (huang bo) are bitter in flavor and cold in property,

临床应用时当性味合参，结合功效应用，才能较好地认识药物的作用和性能。性味合参与功效之间的关系有一定规律可循。一般来说，不同药物的气或味有一个方面相同者，则其功效有部分相同。例如，紫苏、薄荷味同性异，即皆有辛味，发散作用相同，但紫苏性温，发散风寒，薄荷性凉，发散风热；黄芩、薄荷性同味异，即皆为寒凉性，都有清热作用。然黄芩苦寒，能清热燥湿，薄荷辛凉，能发散风热。若不同药物的气味相同，则其功效相近，如黄连、黄柏均为苦寒之品，均能清热燥湿、泻火解毒。

so both of them act to clear the heat and dry the damp, and to reduce the fire and relieve the toxin.

Section 3 Ascending, descending, floating and sinking

第3节 升降浮沉

Ascending, descending, floating and sinking are the four action directions of the Chinese medicinal herbs inside the human body, as one of the concepts of the action natures of the Chinese medicinal herbs.

升降浮沉，即指药物在人体的作用趋向，是说明药物作用性质的概念之一。

The action directions of ascending, descending, floating and sinking are divided into two categories of ascending-floating and descending-sinking. The action direction of ascending-floating is toact upwards and outwards, while the action direction of descending-sinking is to act downwards and inwards. They are used to treat the diseases of different tendencies. If the qi activities of upflow, downflow, outflow and inflow are disturbed, there can be the diseases of different tendency directions. For example, if the disease direction tends to be upwards, there can be the symptoms as vomiting, coughing and panting, which can be treated by the Chinese medicinal herbs with the downward action direction. If the disease direction tends to be downwards, there can be the symptoms as diarrhea and proplapse of rectum, which can be treated by the Chinese medicinal herbs with the upward action direction. If the disease direction tends to be outwards, there can be the symptoms as spontaneous sweating and nocturnal sweats, which can be treated

升降浮沉的作用趋势可分为升浮和沉降两大类。升浮的作用趋势是向上、向外，沉降的作用是向下、向内，分别针对不同的疾病趋势。当人体气机升降出入发生障碍，可产生不同的病势趋向。如病势向上，出现如呕吐、喘咳，应选用作用趋势向下的药物；病势向下，出现泄泻、脱肛，应选用作用趋势向上的药物；病势向外，表现为自汗、盗汗，应选用趋势向内的药物；若病势向内，如表证不解，应选用作用趋势向外的药物。也就是说，药物的升降浮沉趋势与所疗疾病的趋势是相反的，应当正确选择不同作用趋势的药物。

by the Chinese medicinal herbs with the inward action direction. If the disease direction tends to be inwards, there can be the condition as the exterior pattern, which can be treated by the Chinese medicinal herbs with the outward action direction. In other words, the action directions of ascending, descending, floating and sinking of the Chinese medicinal herbs are opposite to the tendency directions of the diseases, so it is necessary to choose the Chinese medicinal herbs of different action directions correctly.

In terms of the attributions of yin and yang, ascending and floating pertain to yang, while descending and sinking pertain to yin. Generally, the Chinese medicinal herbs of ascending and floating natures act to elevate yang, relieve the exterior pattern, eliminate wind, remove cold, induce vomiting, open aperture, etc., while the Chinese medicinal herbs of descending and sinking natures act to reduce-purge, clear heat, promote urination, remove damp, calm and tranquilize mind, subdue yang, eliminate wind, digest food, dissolve food accumulation, subdue up-reverse flowing qi, stop nausea, restrain and astringe, stop cough, soothe asthma, etc.

升降浮沉的阴阳属性为升浮属阳，沉降属阴。升浮性的药物大多具有升阳发表、祛风散寒、涌吐、开窍等功效。沉降性的药物大多具有泻下、清热、利水渗湿、重镇安神、潜阳息风、消导积滞、降逆止呕、收敛固涩、止咳平喘等功效。

Ascending, descending, floating and sinking, as one of the theories of herb natures, are closely related to the property, flavor and quality of the Chinese medicinal herbs. Generally, the Chinese medicinal herbs of ascending and floating are mostly pungent or sweet in flavor and warm or hot in property, while the Chinese medicinal herbs of descending and sinking are mostly sour, bitter, salty or astringent flavor and cold or cool in property. The

升降浮沉是药性理论之一，与性味、药物质地轻重关系密切。一般来说，升浮性药大多具有辛甘之味和温热之性。沉降性药大多具有酸苦咸涩之味和寒凉之性。药物质地的轻重是药物作用趋势形成的重要因素，一般认为质轻的花、叶、皮、枝等药

Chinese medicinal herbs vary in quality, which is an important factor of the action direction of the Chinese medicinal herbs. Generally, the Chinese medicinal herbs in light quality, as the flower, leaf, bark and twig, are mostly ascending and floating, while the Chinese medicinal herbs in heavy quality, as the semen, fruit, mineral and shell, are mostly descending and sinking. But it is not absolute, there are some exceptions. For example, *Inulae Flos* (xuan fu hua) is a kind of flower, but acts to subdue the lung and stomach qi, as the Chinese medicinal herb of descending and sinking.

物，大多数是升浮性的，而质重的种子、果实、矿物、贝壳等药物，大多是沉降性的。当然，此非绝对如此，亦有例外，如旋覆花虽用花，但却能降肺胃之气，属沉降性药。

Processing and compatibility may influence the action directions of the Chinese medicinal herbs to change the original action directions. The Chinese medicinal herbs processed with different medicinal adjuvant may be different in their action directions. Generally, the frying method with alcohol causes ascending, the frying method with ginger juice causes dispersing, the frying method with vinegar causes restraining, while the frying method with salty solution causes descending. The compatibility of Chinese medicinal herbs in the compound prescriptions may also change the action directions of the Chinese medicinal herbs. For example, if the Chinese medicinal herbs of ascending and floating are combined with more Chinese medicinal herbs of descending and sinking, their ascending and floating nature is somewhat inhibited. On the contrary, if the Chinese medicinal herbs of descending and sinking are combined with more Chinese medicinal herbs of ascending and floating, their descending and sinking nature is somewhat inhibited.

炮制和配伍对药物的作用趋势会产生改变趋势的影响。如药物与不同的辅料炮制，会改变作用趋势，一般认为酒炒则升，姜汁炒则散，醋炒则收敛，盐水炒则下行。复方配伍亦会改变药物原有的作用趋势，如性属升浮的药物在同较多沉降药配伍时，其升浮之性可受到一定的制约。反之，性属沉降的药物同较多的升浮药同用，其沉降之性亦能受到一定程度制约。

Section 4 Meridian tropism

第 4 节 归经

Tropism refers to the action location of the Chinese medicinal herbs, while meridian refers to the zang-fu organs and meridians of human body. Meridian tropism implies the concrete areas where the Chinese medicinal herbs works, indicating that the Chinese medicinal herbs possess the selective actions on certain parts of human body.

归，指药物作用的归属；经，指人体的脏腑经络。归经是表示药物作用部位，可以说明药物对机体某部分的选择性作用。

Originating from the long-term clinical practice, the theory of meridian tropism is based upon the theories of visceral manifestations and meridians, and also on the diseases and patterns in the treatment as well. The disease may affect the internal organs through the meridians, while the disease of zang-fu organs may be reflected on the body surface through the meridians. Due to this reason, the location of disease can be determined in the process of disease. Meridian tropism is a location concept of the actions of Chinese medicinal herbs, closely related to the location of disease. For example, if the heart is abnormal and fails to dominate the spirit, there can be the symptoms of poor sleep, dream-disturbed sleep, even coma, mental disorders, dementia, poor memory, etc. In such a condition, it is advisable to apply *Ziziphi Spinosae Semen* (suan zao ren) which acts to nourish the heart and calm the mind, *Moschus* (she xiang) which acts to wake up the spirit, *Cinnabaris* (zhu sha) which acts to tranquilize the spirit and calm the mind, and *Ginseng Radix et Raizoma* (ren shen) which acts to reinforce qi and benefit the intelligence, because all the Chinese medicinal herbs are

归经理论来源于长期的临床实践，是以脏腑经络理论为基础，以所治病证为依据的。疾病可以通过经络影响内脏，脏腑病变亦可反映到体表，在疾病过程中可以确定病位。归经是药物作用的定位概念，与疾病定位关系密切。如心主神明的功能异常，可出现失眠、多梦，甚则昏迷、癫狂、呆痴、健忘等，可分别选择养心安神的酸枣仁、开窍醒神的麝香、镇惊安神的朱砂、补气益智的人参，这些药物皆入心经。

attributed to the Heart Meridian.

Based upon the theories of visceral manifestations and meridians, the theory of meridian tropism is originally based upon the meridian system. For example, *Notopterygii Rhizoma et Radix* (qiang huo) attributed to the Bladder Meridian is applied to treat headache and general aching caused by the attack of the exogenous wind, cold and damp, so it is based upon the pattern identification according to meridians. It is said that the Bladder Meridian of Foot-Taiyang dominates the exterior, so qiang huo is attributed to the Bladder Meridian. For another example, *Alismatis Rhizoma* (ze xie) attributed to the Bladder Meridian acts to promote urination and remove the damp, so it is based upon the pattern identification according to zang-fu organs. Pattern identification according to no matter the meridians or the zang-fu organs, is the theoretical basis for the establishment of the meridian tropism of the Chinese medicinal herbs.

归经理论虽以脏腑经络为基础,但早期曾有以经络体系为依据确立药物归经的记载。如归膀胱经的羌活,为疗外感风寒湿邪所致的头痛身痛证所用,其归膀胱经即依据经络辨证,有足太阳膀胱经主表之说,故羌活归膀胱经。同样归膀胱经的泽泻,具有利水渗湿之功,其归经是依据了脏腑辨证。无论是脏腑还是经络辨证,都为药物归经的确定提供了理论依据。

Combined with the natures of the Chinese medicinal herbs, the selection of the Chinese medicinal herbs with the confirmed location attribution may increase the precision in the prescribing of the Chinese medicinal herbs. For example, the interior heat pattern of excess can be further divided into the lung heat pattern, the heart fire patter, the liver fire pattern and the stomach heat pattern due to the different affected areas, so it is advisable to choose the cold-cool property Chinese medicinal herbs with heat-clearing action, and to confirm the action locations of the Chinese medicinal herbs as well, such as *Scutellariae Radix* (huang qin) attributed to the Lung Meridian is applied to clear the

结合药物的药性,选择定位归属明确的药物,可更好地提高用药的准确性。如里实热证因其发病部位不同,有肺热、心火、肝火、胃热之不同,在选用寒凉性的清热药的同时,还应确定药物的作用部位,如用归肺经的黄芩清肺热,归心经的淡竹叶清心火,归肝经的夏枯草清肝火,归胃经的黄连清胃热。这样具有针对性的用药能更好地发挥药效,使用药更趋合理。

lung heat, *Lophatheri Herba* (dan zhu ye) attributed to the Heart Meridian is applied to clear the heart fire, *Prunellae Spica* (xia ku cao) attributed to the Liver Meridian is applied to clear the liver fire, and *Coptidis Rhizoma* (huang lian) attributed to the Stomach Meridian is applied to clear the stomach heat. Such a directional application of the Chinese medicinal herbs makes full use of herb efficiency and makes the prescription of Chinese medicinal herbs more reasonable.

In guidance of the clinical application of Chinese medicinal herbs with the theory of meridian tropism, it is necessary to notice that the disease of the zang-fu organs or meridians may transfer to and influence the other organs or meridians. Therefore, it is not advisable to only apply the Chinese medicinal herbs attributed to the meridian which is affected, but advisable to apply the Chinese medicinal herbs attributed to several meridians according to the physiological relations and transferring regulations of the zang-fu organs and meridians. For example, the liver yang hyperactivity pattern is often caused by the insufficiency of the kidney yin, so it is advisable to apply the Chinese medicinal herbs attributed to the Liver Meridian with the action to subdue the liver yang, and also the Chinese medicinal herbs attributed to the Kidney Meridian with the action to moisturize and nourish the kidney yin. In the treatment of cough with bloody sputum caused by the liver fire attacking the lung, it is advisable to apply the Chinese medicinal herbs attributed to the Lung Meridian with the action to purify the lung and dissolve the phlegm, and also the Chinese medicinal herbs attributed to the Liver Meridian with

在掌握归经理论指导临床用药的同时,应明白脏腑经络的病变可以相互传变、影响,临床用药选择不只是某经病单纯使用某经药,而是应根据脏腑经络之间的生理关系、传变规律,选择多经药配伍合用。肝阳上亢常因肾阴不足,可选用归肝经的平肝阳药和归肾经的滋养肾阴药同用。肝火犯肺的咳嗽痰血,应该选择归肺经的清肺化痰药,与归肝经的清热凉肝药同用。若拘泥于见肺治肺,见肝治肝的单纯分经用药,疗效必受影响。

the action to clear the heat and cool the liver as well. If the simple treatment for the lung is applied for the lung disease, or if the simple treatment for the liver is applied for the liver disease, the therapeutic effect will be definitely decreased.

Section 5 Toxicity

第5节 有毒无毒

The toxicity refers to the harmful effect of the Chinese medicinal herbs to the human body. It is necessary to understand the toxicity of the Chinese medicinal herbs and the causes of the toxicity, and to master the resolving methods and preventive measures for the Chinese medicinal herb poisoning in order to ensure the safety in the application of Chinese medicinal herbs.

毒性是指药物对人体产生的危害性。为了确保用药安全,必须认识中药的毒性,了解毒性反应产生的原因,掌握中药中毒的解救方法和预防措施。

"Toxicity" in Chinese Materia Medica has the implication in wide sense and narrow sense. In wide sense, "toxicity" firstly refers to all types of herbs. The Chinese medicinal herbs were called "the toxic herbs" before the Western Han Dynasty (206 BCE—23 CE). It secondly refers to the deviation of the Chinese medicinal herbs. It is believed that the reason why the Chinese medicinal herbs act to treat diseases, it is because of their deviation, which is applied to correct the deviation of yin or yang of human body. Such a deviation is so called "toxicity". In narrow sense, "toxicity" refers to the "toxicity" of the Chinese medicinal herbs which may cause the adverse herb reaction on human body, the so-called "untoward effect".

"毒"在中药学中的含义有广义、狭义之分。广义的"毒"有二层含义,一是泛指一切药物。在西汉之前,将药物称之为"毒药"。其二是指药物的偏性,认为药物之所以可以治病,就是用利用了它的偏性,来纠正人体的阴阳之偏,这种偏性,亦称之为"毒"。狭义的"毒",则是指药物对人体造成伤害的"毒性",或称之为不良反应。

In all types of monographs of Chinese Materia

在古代与现代本草专著

Medica in both the ancient and modern times, the Chinese medicinal herbs are marked with signs to tell the toxicity, and even the different degrees of toxicity, as mild toxicity, extreme toxicity, etc. are recorded, in order for the physicians to pay attention to the toxicity in the application of the toxic herbs. Besides, those Chinese medicinal herbs without marks of toxicity may also produce the toxicity in over-dose or improper application, because the deviation of the Chinese medicinal herbs is applied to correct the deviation of yin or yang of human body. Therefore, the mark of toxicity is only a prompt, but the most important thing is to pay attention to the toxicity of the Chinese medicinal herbs, and also to prevent the adverse herb reations produced by the nontoxic herbs as well in the practical application.

中，可以看到对药物的有毒无毒进行了标注，尤其对毒性的大小有较为细致的区分，如有小毒、大毒等记载，以告知医家在使用这些有毒药物时应加以注意。其实，即使未标注的无毒药，因其是利用药物的偏性来纠正人体的阴阳之偏的，若过量或使用不当，亦会产生毒性。所以说，有毒无毒的标注只是种提示，重要的是在实际应用药物时既要注意毒性药，也要防止无毒性药产生的不良反应。

It does not mean that those toxic herbs have no a single redeeming feature and can never be applied. The toxic herbs are also beneficial in a sense. The ancient physicians advanced a kind of therapeutic principle to fight the poison with the poison, i.e. to apply the toxicity of the toxic herbs to treat diseases. A great number of experiences have been accumulated in the clinical practice in both the ancient and modern times in the treatment of furuncles, abscess, psora, scabies, leprosy, scrofula, simple goiter, tumor, carcinoma, abdominal masses, etc., and the therapeutic effect is confirmed. The key to the application is to master the proper quantity of the toxic herbs.

当然，有毒药并非一无是处，不可应用。有毒性的药物也有可利用的一面。古代医家有以毒攻毒的治则，即利用有毒药的毒性来治疗疾病。古今利用某些有毒药物治疗恶疮肿毒、疥癣、麻风、瘰疬、瘿瘤、癌肿癥瘕等，积累了大量的经验，并获得了肯定疗效。把握适当的度和量是其关键所在。

There are various causes of the toxicity of Chinese medicinal herbs, as confused species, unclear sources, different parts of the Chinese medicinal

影响有毒无毒的因素很多，如品种的混乱，来源不清，入药部位的不同，产地、

herbs, different places of production, acquisition time, processing and manufacturing, herb forms, technological levels, compatibilities, dosages, administrative methods, etc. Therefore, it is necessary to make checks and control qualities in all the above-mentioned links, so as to decrease the probability of the toxic production, for the purpose to guarantee the safety in the application of Chinese medicinal herbs.

采集时间，炮制加工，剂型工艺，以及配伍、用量，给药途径等等。故应在以上各个环节加以把关控制，减少产生毒性的概率，以保证用药的安全。

In order to decrease the production of the adverse reactions of Chinese medicinal herbs, the following notes should be highly paid attention in the application of the toxic herbs: Firstly, it is necessary to control the dose which is started from the small dose and gradually increased. Secondly, it is necessary to strictly make checks in the links of collection and processing, to eradicate the fake and poor products or obscured products, and to standardize the processing, so as to ensure the effect of Chinese medicinal herbs. Thirdly, it is necessary to apply the appropriate herbs according to the different individuals without heavy or arbitrary application of herbs.

为减少药物不良反应的产生，使用有毒药时需注意：掌控用量，从小剂量开始投药，逐渐增量；其次，严格把关采集、炮制各环节，保证杜绝伪劣品、混淆品，规范炮制，保证药效；其三，做到根据不同对象合理用药，不滥用乱投。

In terms of the resolving methods of the poisoning of Chinese medicinal herbs, there are many records in the medical literatures at both ancient and modern times. At the same time when studying the ancient experiences, it is necessary to combine the modern medical knowledge, diagnosis, resolving measures and methods, so as to realize the better effect in resolving toxicity.

对于药物中毒的解救，古今文献均有不少记载。可在学习古代经验的同时，结合现代知识及诊断、解救措施和方法，以求取得更好的解救效果。

Chapter 2 Processing of Chinese Medicinal Herbs

第 2 章 中药的炮制

Processing refers to the necessary processes of preparing crude pharmaceutical materials before the application or preparations of forms. The reason why the processing is necessary is that it is necessary to treat the crude of part of crude pharmaceutical materials according to the different requirements of clinical treatment, prescription and preparing forms, so as to produce the satisfactory medicinal effects, to avoid or decrease the adverse herb reactions, and to match the clinical administration of medicinal herbs at the most extent.

炮制是指药物在应用或制成各种剂型以前所进行的必要的加工处理。炮制的理由是中医临床用药、配方、制剂对药物均有不同要求，故必须对原药材进行修治整理，对部分药材进行特殊处理，使药物充分发挥疗效，且避免或减轻不良反应，在最大程度上符合临床用药的目的。

Section 1 Processing purpose

第 1 节 炮制的目的

The purposes of processing Chinese medicinal herbs are as follows:

(1) Decrease or remove the toxicity and side effect of the medicinal herbs. The Chinese medicinal herbs, as *Aconiti Radix Praeparata* (fu zi), *Aconiti Radix* (chuan wu), *Pinelliae Rhizoma* (ban xia), *Arisaematis Rhizoma* (tian nan xing), etc., are toxic, and their toxicity can be decreased by processing. *Radix Dichroae* (chang shan) is used to

中药炮制的目的大致有以下方面：

（1）降低或消除药物的毒副作用。如附子、川乌、半夏、天南星等药物生用有毒，通过炮制能降低其毒性；常山能截疟，但易致呕吐，经酒炒炮制后，减轻了致呕吐的副作用，有利于药物作用的

treat malaria, but easily induces vomiting. After stir-baked processing with millet wine, its side effect to induce vomiting is reduced and its pharmacodynamic action can be fully realized.

发挥。

(2) Increase the pharmacodynamic action and promote the therapeutic effect. During processing Chinese medicinal herbs, it is advisable to add some medicinal adjuvant which possesses certain actions to increase the pharmacodynamic action and promote the therapeutic effect. For example, *Eriobotryae Folium* (pi pa ye) and *Stemonae Radix* (bai bu) prepared with honey act to moisturize the lung and stop cough. *Chuanxiong Rhizoma* (chuan xiong) and *Salviae Miltiorrhizae Radix et Rhizoma* (dan shen) stir-baked with millet wine can promote their blood-activating action. *Corydalis Rhizoma* (yan hu suo) and *Cyperi Rhizoma* (xiang fu) prepared with vinegar can promote their pain-relieving action. *Coptidis Rhizoma* (huang lian) and *Bambusae Caulis in Taenias* (zhu ru) prepared with ginger juice can promote their vomit-stopping action. *Atractylodis Rhizoma Macrocephalae* (bai zhu) fried with wheat bran can promote its spleen-strengthening action.

(2) 增强药物的作用，提高临床疗效。在中药的炮制过程中，加入一些本身具有一定功效的辅料共同加工，可增强药物的作用，提高临床疗效。如蜂蜜与枇杷叶、百部同制，可润肺止咳；酒炒川芎、丹参，活血作用得增；醋制延胡索、香附，能增强止痛之效；姜汁与黄连、竹茹同制，可增强止呕之功；麸皮炒白术，可加强健脾功效。

(3) Modify the properties or actions of Chinese medicinal herbs so as to make them more suitable for the therapeutic requirements. For example, *Radix Rehmanniae* (sheng di huang) is sweat and bitter in flavor and cold in property, acting to clear heat and cool blood to treat the blood heat pattern. After processing with the repeated steaming method, it becomes *Rehmanniae Radix Praeparata* (shu di huang), which is slightly warm in property, acting to reinforce blood to treat blood deficiency pattern. *Rhei Radix et Rhizoma* (da huang) in raw form acts

(3) 改变药物的性能或功效，使之更能适应病情的需要。如生地黄本为甘苦寒之品，长于清热凉血，适用于血分有热，经反复蒸制后为熟地黄，药性微温，以补血见长，适宜于血虚证；大黄生用攻积通便，为治热结便秘之要药，制后则泻下力减，功偏活血，炒炭后通便作用全失，长于止血。

to attack the accumulation and promote defecation, as an important medicinal herb to treat constipation due to heat. After processing, its purging action decreases, but it acts to activate blood. After stir-baked into charcoal, its purging action loses completely, but is acts to stanch bleeding.

(4) Facilitate application in easy storage and preparation. For convenient storage, it is necessary to dry and grind the Chinese medicinal herbs. For convenient form preparation, some medicinal herbs need to be cut into sections or slices. For convenient grinding preparation, some medicinal herbs need to be calcined.

（4）便于贮存和制剂。为了便于贮存，对药材必须进行干燥、粉碎等处理。为便于制剂和调剂，有些药需切段或切片，有的药需进行煅制，便于粉碎等。

(5) Remove non-pharmaceutical parts and impurities, to purify the medicinal herbs, so as to guarantee the high quality, precise dosage in application and convenient administration. For example, the rhizomes or roots of plants are often mixed with mud, which should be cleared away. *Thallus Sargassi Pallidi* (hai zao) and *Thallus Laminariae Japonicae* (kun bu) should be washed and rinsed repeatedly to eliminate their fishy odor.

（5）除去非药用部分和杂质，使药物纯净，保证药材品质和用量准确，并便于服用。如以植物根茎或根入药者，须去除须根和泥土；海藻、昆布等应反复漂洗，去除腥味等。

Section 2　Commonly-used processing methods

第 2 节　常用炮制方法

The commonly-used methods of processing medicinal herbs are as follows.

中药的常用炮制方法大致有以下几类。

1　Roughly processing methods

1　修治

1.1　Purifying

1.1　纯净处理

Take away the ashes, impurities and non-pharmaceutical parts, to make the medicinal herbs clean and pure.

去掉灰屑、杂质及非药用部分，使药物清洁纯净。

1.2 Grinding

Smash or grind the medicinal herbs into powder, so as to meet the requirements of preparation, processing and administration.

1.2 粉碎处理

将药物压碎或捣碎，以符合制剂、炮制和服用的要求。

1.3 Cutting

Cut the medicinal herbs into slices, segments, dices, shreds, etc., for further processing, drying, storing and weighing in preparation.

1.3 切制处理

将药物切成片、段、块、丝等不同规格，便于进一步炮制，也利于干燥、贮藏以及调剂时称量。

2 Processing with water

Processing with water is a kind of method to treat the pharmaceutical materials with water, for the purpose to clean and soften the medicinal herbs, or to conveniently prepare by cutting or modifying the natures, or to make the mineral herbs pure, fine and smooth. The commonly-used methods are as follows:

2 水制

水制是用水处理药物的方法。主要目的是清洁、软化药材，以便于切制和调整药性，或使矿石类药纯净细腻。常用的方法有：

2.1 Washing

Wash away the mud or impurities on the surface of the pharmaceutical materials.

2.1 洗

用水洗去药材表面的泥土杂质。

2.2 Moisturizing

According to the soft or hard texture of the pharmaceutical materials, water-spray the herbs to make them soft, so as to make them easy to cut.

2.2 润

根据药材质地的软硬，反复用水淋润药材，使其软化，便于切制。

2.3 Rinsing

Put the pharmaceutical materials into the clear water or flowing water, rinse them repeatedly to eliminate the fishy or salty odor, for convenient preparation and administration.

2.3 漂

将药物置清水或长流水中，反复漂去腥味、咸味等，便于制剂和服用。

2.4 Powder-refining with water

Refine and get the fine powder by grinding the insoluble mineral pharmaceutical materials in water. It is to crush the pharmaceutical materials into particles, and then to grind them in a mortar which

2.4 水飞

将不溶于水的矿物类药与水共研，制成极细粉末的一种方法。先将药物粉碎成粗粉，加入容器中与水同研，

contains a certain amount of clean water. During grinding, the supernatant suspension is decanted and then water is added again. The procedures above may be repeated until all the coarse particles are ground into fine powder. The sediment of coarse particles will be left when the supernatant fluid of suspension is decanted, from which fine powder is precipitated, separated and then dried for use.

反复研磨，倾出含细粉的混悬液，粗粒再研，直至无沉渣。将混悬液沉淀、分离，获取细粉，干燥即得。

3 Processing with fire

This is a processing method to heat the pharmaceutical materials with fire, including frying, stir-baking, calcining, roasting, etc.

3 火制

用火加热处理药物的方法。主要制法有炒、炙、煅、煨等。

3.1 Frying

Frying method is divided into simple frying and complex frying.

(1) Simple frying: It is a kind of frying method without adding any adjuvant. According to the degrees required, simple frying is further divided into frying to yellow color, frying to burnt color and frying to carbonized color. Frying to yellow color means that the medicinal herbs are fried by a slow fire into yellow surface. Frying to burnt color means that the medicinal herbs are fried with a high fire into burnt yellow or burnt brown surface, while the color of the interior becomes deeper, and a delicate fragrance occurs. Frying to yellow color and frying to burnt color can modify the properties of the medicinal herbs, beneficial for the effective constituents to dissolve out. Frying to carbonized color means that the medicinal herbs are fried with a high fire into burnt-black surface and partially carbonized surface, while the color of the interior becomes burnt yellow, and the inherent smell is

3.1 炒

有清炒、加固体辅料同炒两种。

(1) 清炒：属不加任何辅料的炒法，根据炒制程度有炒黄、炒焦、炒炭的不同区分。炒黄，即用文火炒至药物表面微黄。炒焦，用武火炒至药材表面焦黄或焦褐色，内部颜色加深，并有悠香之气。炒焦和炒黄能缓和药性，有利于有效成分溶出。炒炭，用武火炒至药材表面焦黑，部分炭化，内部焦黄，但仍保留有药材固有气味，即炒炭存性，大多能增强其收敛止血的功效。

kept. Frying to carbonized color can preserve the properties of the medicinal herbs, while most carbonized medicinal herbs act to astringe the blood and stanch bleeding.

(2) Complex frying: It is a kind of frying method with certain amount of solid adjuvant, such as soil, wheat bran, rice, sand, talc, shell powder, etc. Frying with adjuvant can decrease the irritation of the medicinal herbs and to promote the therapeutic effects.

（2）固体辅料同炒：固体辅料包括土、麸皮、米、砂、滑石粉、蛤粉等，与这些辅料同炒，可减少药物的刺激性，增强疗效。

3.2 Stir-baking

Stir-baking method is to stir-bake the medicinal herbs with liquid adjuvant, such as honey, millet wine, vinegar, ginger juice, salt solution, etc. Since the adjuvant is different in stir-baking, the effects of the prepared medicinal herbs are different. For example, stir-baking with honey acts to increase the functions to moisturize lung and stop coughing, to reinforce the middle energizer and benefit qi. Stir-baking with millet wine acts to increase the functions to activate blood and dissolve stasis, or acts to elevate the herb actions so as to change the acting tendency of medicinal herbs. Stir-baking with vinegar acts to relieve pain. Stir-baking with salt solution acts to subdue the herbs actions to enter the kidney. Stir-baking with ginger juice acts to restrain the cold property, and to increase the function to stop vomiting, or to decrease the toxicity of medicinal herbs.

3.2 炙

将药材与液体辅料拌炒。常用的液体辅料有蜜、酒、醋、姜汁、盐水等。因辅料不同，加工后的作用亦有区别。如蜜炙可增润肺止咳、补中益气之效；酒制增强活血祛瘀之力，或上行而改变药物作用趋势；醋制止痛；盐水炙下行入肾；姜汁炙能制约寒性，增强止呕作用，或降低药物毒性。

3.3 Calcining

It is a method to prepare the medicinal herbs by direct or indirect burning with a strong fire, so as to make the medicinal herbs crispy for easy powdering. The direct calcining method means that the medicinal

3.3 煅

将药材用猛火直接或间接煅烧，使质地松脆，易于粉碎。其中直接放炉火上加热者，称为明煅，多用于矿物药

herbs are burnt directly on stove fire, used in the preparation of medicinal herbs of minerals and shells. The indirect calcining method means that the medicinal herbs are burnt inside the sealed refractory container, used in the preparation of medicinal herbs of loosen texture, easy to be carbonized.

或动物甲壳类药的加工；将药材置于密闭容器内加热煅烧者，称为焖煅，适用于质地轻松，易炭化的药材。

3.4 Roasting

It is a method to prepare the medicinal herbs by wrapping them with dough or wet paper and being roasted in smouldering ashes, or by heating the medicinal herbs with the rough straw paper as the spacer.

3.4 煨

将药材包裹于湿面粉、湿纸中，放入热火灰中加热，或用草纸与饮片隔层分放加热的方法，称为煨法。

3.5 Heat-drying

It is a method to prepare the medicinal herbs by heating them in a slow fire to make them dry. Heat-drying method acts to decrease the toxicity and fishy or foul odor of medicinal herbs, and to make medicinal herbs easy to be powdered.

3.5 烘焙

将药材用微火加热，使之干燥的方法称烘焙。烘焙后可降低毒性和腥臭气味，且便于粉碎。

4 Processing with both water and fire

The common processing methods with both water and fire include boiling, steaming, scalding and quenching.

4 水火共制

常见的水火共制包括蒸、煮、燀、淬等。

4.1 Boiling

It is a method to prepare the medicinal herbs by heating them in clean water or liquid adjuvant.

4.1 煮

用清水或液体辅料与药物共同加热的方法。

4.2 Steaming

It is a method to prepare the medicinal herbs by putting them in a steaming pot or heating them with steam. Steaming without adding adjuvant is called simple steaming, while steaming with adding adjuvant is called adjuvant-steaming. The steaming time is determined according to the processing requirements. Long steaming method or repeated steaming and sun-drying method makes medicinal herbs more

4.2 蒸

利用水蒸气或隔水加热药物的方法，不加辅料者，称为清蒸；加辅料者，称为辅料蒸。加热的时间，视炮制的目的而定。有久蒸或反复蒸晒的，亦有为便于贮存，加热蒸制杀死虫卵的。

convenient in storage, while regular steaming method acts to kill the worm eggs.

4.3 Scalding

It is a method to prepare the medicinal herbs by putting them into boiling water and stirring them for a short while before taking them out. Scalding method acts to remove the peels of the medicinal herbs of semen, and to dry medicinal herbs of juicy texture.

4.3 燀

将药物快速放入沸水中短暂潦过，立即取出的方法。多用于种子类药物的去皮和肉质多汁药物的干燥处理。

4.4 Quenching

It is a method to prepare the medicinal herbs by burning them red and then rapidly putting them into cold water or liquid adjuvant, so as to make them crispy. The quenching method acts to make medicinal herbs easy to be powdered and make the adjuvant to be absorbed, so as to promote the therapeutic effects.

4.4 淬

将药物煅烧红后，迅速投入冷水或液体辅料中，使其酥脆的方法。淬后既易于粉碎，又可吸收辅料，从而提高药效。

5 Other processing methods

Besides the four above-mentioned processing methods, there are some other specific processing methods, as the method to make frostlike powder, fermentation, germination, etc. The first method to make frostlike powder is to make medicinal herbs into frostlike powder through pressing and degreasing. The second method to make frostlike powder is to make medicinal herbs into fine precipitated crystalline powder after certain preparation, such as *Watermelon Frost* (xi gua shuang). Fermentation means that the medicinal herbs and adjuvants are fermented at certain humidity and temperature with a series of procedures, by using fungus, so as to obtain a new type of medicinal herbs. Germination means that the medicinal herbs of seeds are soaked in water and kept certain humidity and temperature, so as to make them germinate to buds.

5 其他制法

除上述四类以外，尚有一些特殊的制法，常用的有制霜、发酵、发芽等。制霜，一是将种子类药材压榨去油成霜；二是药物经过物料析出细小结晶后的制品，亦称为霜，如西瓜霜。发酵，是将药材与辅料拌和，置一定的湿度和温度下，利用真菌发酵，获取新的药物的方法，称为发酵法。发芽是将具有发芽能力的种子药材用水浸泡后，保持一定的湿度和温度，使其发出幼芽的方法，称为发芽。

Chapter 3 Application of Chinese Medicinal Herbs

第3章 中药的应用

The application methods of Chinese medicinal herbs are very important, practically significant to guide the correct application of Chinese medicinal herbs in the clinic. The application methods of Chinese medicinal herbs include compatibility, contraindication, dosage and administration.

中药的应用方法十分重要，对指导临床正确使用中药具有现实意义。中药的应用方法包括中药的配伍、禁忌，以及剂量、用法。

Section 1 Compatibility

第1节 配伍

Compatibility of Chinese medicinal herbs refers to the combination of more than two herbs with purpose in the light of the clinical requirements and medicinal properties and actions.

The record of compatibility was mentioned as early as in *Shen Nong's Herbal Canon* (Shen Nong Ben Cao Jing). The ancients generalized the application of Chinese medicinal herbs and their compatibility into seven situations, called "seven compatible relations", as single application, mutual reinforcement, mutual assistance, mutual restraint, mutual detoxification, mutual inhibition and mutual incompatibility. Single application refers to the application of a single medicinal herb, used for the sim-

配伍是指有目的地按病情需要和药性特点，有选择地将两味以上药物配合使用。

关于配伍的记载最早见于《神农本草经》。前人把单味药的应用及药物之间的配伍关系概括为七种情况，称为"七情"，有单行、相须、相使、相畏、相杀、相恶、相反等。单行即指用单味药，大多用于病情较为单纯，选用一味针对性较强的药物即能获效。亦有单味用于病情危

ple and mild condition for which a single targeted medicinal herb obtains a good result. Clinically, single application is also used for some critical and serious condition for which a single medicinal herb acts for emergency usage. Since the most conditions and patterns in clinic are often complicated, a single medicinal herb is limit in property and action to achieve the required effect, or produces toxicity and side-effect. Therefore, several Chinese medicinal herbs must be used in combination according to their properties and actions. According to the ancients' summarization, the combining relations of mutual reinforcement, mutual assistance, mutual restraint, mutual detoxification, mutual inhibition and incompatibility are shown as follows:

急者,乃取其功专力宏,以应急用。由于临床上所见证型较为复杂,单味药力有限,且难以兼顾,或有些药物具有毒副作用,故需要多种药物同时配伍使用。根据前人总结,除单行外,相须、相使、相畏、相杀、相恶、相反都是配伍关系的归纳,分述如下。

1.1 Mutual reinforcement

It is to combine the medicinal herbs with similar properties and actions, so as to reinforce their original effects. For example, *Gypsum Fibrosum* (shi gao) and *Anemarrhenae Rhizoma* (zhi mu), acting to clear heat and reduce fire, are used together to obviously promote their actions to clear heat and reduce fire. *Carthami Flos* (hong hua) and *Persicae Semen* (tao ren), acting to activate blood and dissolve stasis, are used together to promote their actions to dissolve stasis and dredge meridians.

1.1 相须

把性能功效相类似的药物配合一起应用,以增强原有的疗效。如同为清热泻火的石膏与知母,合用后能明显增强清热泻火的功效;同能活血祛瘀的红花、桃仁,配伍同用可增强祛瘀通经之效。

1.2 Mutual assistance

It is to combine the medicinal herbs with similar properties and actions, or without similarities but with some relations. In the combination, one type of medicinal herbs is taken as the dominant, while the other type of medicinal herbs as the assistant, for the purpose to promote the effect of the dominant medicinal herbs. For example, *Radix*

1.2 相使

性能功效有某些共性,或性能不尽相同,却存在某种联系的药物同用,以一种药为主,另一种药为辅,以提高主药的疗效。如黄芪补气利水为主,茯苓利水健脾为辅,两者同用,能提高黄芪补

Astragali (huang qi) acts to reinforce qi and promote waterflow, as the dominant, while *Poria* (fu ling) acts to promote waterflow and strengthen spleen, as the assistant. The combination of both medicinal herbs may increase the therapeutic effect of huang qi to reinforce qi and promote waterflow.

气利水的疗效。

1.3 Mutual restraint

It implies that in combination of medicinal herbs, the toxicity or side-effect of one medicinal herb can be decreased or relieved by another medicinal herb. For example, the toxicity of *Pinelliae Rhizoma* (ban xia) and *Arisaematis Rhizoma* (tian nan xing) can be decreased or relieved by *Zingiberis Rhizoma Recens* (sheng jiang), the so-called ban xia and tian nan xing restrained by sheng jiang.

1.3 相畏

一种药物的毒性反应或副作用，能被另一种药物减轻或消除。如生半夏和生南星的毒性能被生姜减轻或消除，即生半夏和生南星畏生姜。

1.4 Mutual detoxification

It implies that in combination of medicinal herbs, one medicinal herb can decrease or relieve the toxicity or side-effect of another medicinal herb. For example, *Zingiberis Rhizoma Recens* (sheng jiang) can decrease or relieve the toxicity of *Pinelliae Rhizoma* (ban xia) and *Arisaematis Rhizoma* (tian nan xing), the so-called Sheng jiang detoxifying for ban xia and tian nan xing.

It can be seen that mutual restraint and mutual detoxification are two different formulations in a same compatibility relation.

1.4 相杀

即一种药物能减轻或消除另一种药物的毒性或副作用。如生姜能减轻或消除生半夏和生南星的毒性或副作用，即生姜杀生半夏和生南星的毒。

可见，相畏、相杀是同一配伍关系的两种提法。

1.5 Mutual inhibition

It implies that in combination of medicinal herbs, one medicinal herb decreases or removes the original action of another medicinal herb. For example, *Ginseng Radix et Raizoma* (ren shen) acts to reinforce qi, while *Raphani Semen* (lai fu zi) acts to relieve stagnant qi. The combination of the two medicinal herbs

1.5 相恶

即两药合用，一种药物能使另一种药物原有功效降低，甚至丧失。如人参补气，莱菔子破气，两者合用，会削弱人参的补气作用。

may weaken the qi-reinforcing action of ren shen.

1.6 Incompatibility

It implies that the combination of two medicinal herbs may produce or increase the toxicity or side-effect, as the medicinal herbs in "eighteen incompatibilities" and "nineteen restraints".

In summary, mutual reinforcement and mutual assistance are the compatibility relations to increase the therapeutic effect of medicinal herbs, so they should be utilized fully in clinic application. Mutual restraint and mutual detoxification are the compatibility relations to decrease or relieve the toxicity and side-effect of medicinal herbs, so they are considered to be utilized in application of the medicinal herbs with toxicity or side-effect. Mutual inhibition and incompatibility are the compatibility relations to weaken the effect of medicinal herbs or to produce the toxicity, so they should be avoided. But in some situation, it is advisable to apply some compatibility relation to relieve some symptoms. For example, *Raphani Semen* (lai fu zi) may weaken the qi-reinforcing function of *Ginseng Radix et Raizoma* (ren shen). In the condition of abdominal distension due to over-taking ren shen, it is advisable to apply lai fu zi which acts to relieve stagnant qi, so as to treat distension and fullness in abdomen. But in other situations, incompatibility should be avoided.

1.6 相反

即两种药物合用，能产生或增强毒性反应或副作用。如“十八反”“十九畏”中的若干药物。

将上述六个方面的配伍关系加以概括，可以看出，相须、相使为增强药效的配伍关系，临床应用时应充分利用。相畏、相杀是通过互相作用，能减轻或降低毒副作用的配伍关系，在使用有毒药物或副作用明显的药物时应加以考虑。相恶、相反是使药物药效削减或产生毒性的配伍关系，应加以注意。相恶虽能削弱药物作用，但又是可以利用的配伍方法，如莱菔子能削弱人参的补气作用，但当服食人参导致腹胀时，则可利用莱菔子破气之功，消除胀满。而相反，属于配伍禁忌，应避免使用。

Section 2 Contraindication

Contraindication of Chinese medicinal herbs

第2节 用药禁忌

用药禁忌，包括配伍禁

includes prescription incompatibility, dietetic restraint and contraindication of Chinese medicinal herbs in pregnancy. According to the different degrees of adverse reactions to the patients, the application of Chinese medicinal herbs is divided into prohibiting application and cautious application.

忌、妊娠用药禁忌、服药食忌等内容。根据对患者造成的不良影响程度的不同，又常分为忌用和慎用。

2.1 Prescription incompatibility

In the application of Chinese medicinal herbs, the combination of some medicinal herbs may weaken their original actions, and even produce toxicity or adverse reaction, against the original intention of curing diseases with medicinal herbs. According to the ancients' summarizations and records in ancient classics in successive dynasties, the prescription incompatibility is divided into "eighteen incompatibilities" and "nineteen antagonisms". Different from "mutual restraint" in "seven compatible relations", "nineteen antagonisms" here refer to the incompatibilities of these medicinal herbs, falling into the category of "mutual incompatibility".

2.1 配伍禁忌

中药在配伍应用中，有些配伍会使药物原有的作用削弱，甚至产生毒性，导致不良反应，与用药治病的初衷相违背。根据历代医家总结和古籍记载，配伍禁忌有“十八反”和“十九畏”。其中“十九畏”的“畏”，与七情中相畏的含义不同，是指这些药为配伍禁忌，属“相反”的配伍范畴。

2.1.1 Eighteen incompatibilities

Glycyrrhizae *Radix et Rhizoma* (gan cao) is incompatible with *Kansui Radix* (gan sui), *Euphorbiae Pekinensis Radix* (da ji), *Sargassum* (hai zao) and *Genkwa Flos* (yuan hua). *Aconiti Radix* (wu tou) is incompatible with *Fritillariae Bulbus* (bei mu), *Trichosanthis Fructus* (gua lou), *Pinelliae Rhizoma* (ban xia), *Ampelopsis Radix* (bai lian) and *Bletillae Rhizoma* (bai ji). *Veratri Nigri Radix et Rhizoma* (li lu) is incompatible with *Ginseng Radix et Raizoma* (ren shen), *Adenophorae Radix* (sha shen), *Salviae Miltiorrhizae Radix et Rhizoma* (dan shen), *Scrophulariae Radix* (xuan shen), *Sophorae*

2.1.1 十八反

甘草反甘遂、大戟、海藻、芫花；乌头反贝母、瓜蒌、半夏、白蔹、白及；藜芦反人参、沙参、丹参、玄参、苦参、细辛、芍药。

Flavescentis Radix (ku shen), *Asari Radix et Rhizoma* (xi xin) and *Paeoniae Radix* (shao yao).

2.1.2 Nineteen antagonisms

Sulfur (liu huang) is antagonistic to *Mirabilitum* (pu xiao). *Hydrargyrum* (shui yin) is antagonistic to *Arsenicum Album* (pi shuang). *Euphorbiae Ebracteolatae Radix* (lang du) is antagonistic to *Lithargyrum* (mi tuo seng). *Crotonis Fructus* (ba dou) is antagonistic to *Pharbitidis Semen* (qian niu zi). *Flos Caryophylli* (ding xiang) is antagonistic to *Curcumae Radix* (yu jin). *Aconiti Radix* (chuan wu) and *Aconiti Radix Kusenzoffii* (cao wu) are antagonistic to *Cornu Rhinoceri Asiatici* (xi jiao). *Crystallized Mirabilite* (ya xiao) is antagonistic to *Sparganii Rhizoma Stoloniferi* (san leng). *Cinnamomi Cortex* (guan gui) is antagonistic to *Halloysitum Rubrum* (chi shi zhi). *Ginseng Radix et Raizoma* (ren shen) is antagonistic to *Trogopterorum Faeces* (wu ling zhi).

In terms of contraindications of eighteen incompatibilities and nineteen antagonisms, there were the strict conformists, and also the dissidents as well in the successive dynasties. There were quite a few formulas composed of Chinese medicinal herbs in eighteen incompatibilities and nineteen antagonisms. Therefore, some people believe that eighteen incompatibilities and nineteen antagonisms are not absolute taboos, and consider that the combination of the contrary medicinal herbs may be opposite and supplementary each other, so as to produce a better result.

The modern researches on eighteen incompatibilities and nineteen antagonisms are in progress. Before the confirmed conclusion is made, it is necessary to be cautious to treat eighteen incompatibili-

2.1.2 十九畏

硫黄畏朴硝，水银畏砒霜，狼毒畏密陀僧，巴豆畏牵牛子，丁香畏郁金，川乌、草乌畏犀角，牙硝畏三棱，官桂畏赤石脂，人参畏五灵脂。

对于将十八反、十九畏作为配伍禁忌，历代医药学家有遵循者，亦有持不同见解者。历代用十八反、十九畏中药组成的方剂亦有不少，故有人认为十八反、十九畏并非绝对禁忌，甚至有认为相反药同用，能相反相成，产生较强的功效。

十八反、十九畏的现代研究正在深入进行中，在尚未有明确结论之时，还是应慎重对待十八反、十九畏。

ties and nineteen antagonisms.

2 Contraindication of Chinese medicinal herbs in pregnancy

During pregnancy, some Chinese medicinal herbs may influence the development of fetus, even induce miscarriage. Therefore, it is necessary to consider the selection of medicinal herbs for the women in pregnancy. According to the different harmful degrees of medicinal herbs, they are divided into two categories of cautious application and prohibiting application. The medicinal herbs of cautious application category are those acting to activate blood and dredge meridians, move qi flow and break stasis, and those of pungent-hot properties. The medicinal herbs of prohibiting application category are those of fierce property or toxic property.

The Chinese medicinal herbs of cautious application are: *Achyranthis Bidentatae Radix* (niu xi), *Rhizoma Ligustici Chuanxiong* (chuan xiong), *Carthami Flos* (hong hua), *Persicae Semen* (tao ren), *Curcumae Longae Rhizoma* (jiang huang), *Moutan Cortex* (mu dan pi), *Aurantii Fructus Immaturus* (zhi shi), *Rhei Radix et Rhizoma* (da huang), *Folium Cassiae* (fan xie ye), *Aloe* (lu hui), *Natrii Sulfas* (mang xiao), *Aconiti Radix Praeparata* (fu zi), *Cinnamomi Cortex* (rou gui), etc.

The Chinese medicinal herbs of prohibiting application are: *Hydrargyrum* (shui yin), *Arsenicum Sublimatum* (pi shuang), *Realgar* (xiong huang), *Calomelas* (qing fen), *Mylabris* (ban mao), *Semen Strychni* (ma qian zi), *Bufonis Venenum* (chan su), *Aconiti Radix* (chuan wu), *Aconiti Radix Kusenzoffii* (cao wu), *Radix et Rhizoma Veratri*

2 妊娠用药禁忌

妊娠期间有些药物的应用会影响胎儿发育，甚则导致堕胎，故妊娠期间，应注意药物的选择。根据药物损害程度的不同，有慎用和禁用两类。慎用类大多为活血通经、行气破滞，以及辛热的药物。禁用药大多为药性峻烈、毒性较强的药物。

慎用药有：牛膝、川芎、红花、桃仁、姜黄、牡丹皮、枳实、大黄、番泻叶、芦荟、芒硝、附子、肉桂等药。

禁用药有：水银、砒霜、雄黄、轻粉、斑蝥、马钱子、蟾酥、川乌、草乌、藜芦、胆矾、瓜蒂、巴豆、甘遂、大戟、芫花、牵牛子、商陆、麝香、干漆、水蛭、虻虫、三棱、莪术等。

Nigri (li lu), *Chalcanthium* (dan fan), *Pedicellus Melo Fructus* (gua di), *Fructus Crotonis* (ba dou), *Radix Eupyorbiae Kansui* (gan sui), *Euphorbiae Pekinensis Radix* (da ji), *Genkwa Flos* (yuan hua), *Pharbitidis Semen* (qian niu zi), *Radix Phytolaccae* (shang lu), *Moschus* (she xiang), *Resina Rhois Praeparata* (gan qi), *Hirudo* (shui zhi), *Tabanus* (meng chong), *Sparganii Rhizoma* (san leng), *Curcumae Rhizoma* (e zhu), etc.

If there is no special need, it is necessary to avoid the Chinese medicinal herbs of cautious application and prohibiting application, so as to prevent any possible accidents. If it is really necessary, it is advisable to identify patterns correctly, to master the dosage and therapeutic course, and to reduce the harm of medicinal herbs to pregnancy as much as possible with proper processing and compatibility, so as to guarantee the safety and effect in application of Chinese medicinal herbs.

妊娠期间如无特殊必要,应尽量避免使用慎用药和禁用药,以免发生事故。若非用不可,则应注意辨证准确,掌握好剂量与疗程,并通过恰当的炮制和配伍,尽量减轻药物对妊娠的危害,做到用药安全而有效。

3 Dietetic restraint

Dietetic restraint implies that some sorts of foods are prohibited or limited to be eaten during taking Chinese medicinal herbs. In traditional Chinese medicine, it is paid attention to the relation between the food and medicinal herbs. It is believed that the dietetic restraint may avoid the production of adverse reactions or herb action decrease. In ancient classics, there were records of dietetic restraint in taking Chinese medicinal herbs. For example, green onion is taboo in taking *Radix Dichroae* (chang shan). Green onion, garlic and radish are taboo in taking *Radix Rehmanniae* (sheng di huang), *Polygoni Multiflori Radix* (he shou wu).

3 服药食忌

服药食忌简称食忌、忌口。中医较重视食药之间的关系,认为服药期间的饮食禁忌能避免产生不良反应或降低药效,在古代本草、方书中可以看到有为数不少的服药时食忌的记载,如常山忌葱,生地黄、何首乌忌葱、蒜、萝卜,薄荷忌鳖肉,茯苓忌醋等。另外,一般认为患病期间应忌食生冷、辛热、油腻、腥膻、有刺激性的食物。根据病情的不同,饮食禁忌也

Turtle meat is taboo in taking *Menthae Haplocalycis Herba* (bo he). Vinegar is taboo in taking *Poria* (fu ling). Besides, it is generally believed that a patient should abstain from raw, cold, pungent, hot, greasy, fishy and irritated foods. According to different conditions, the dietetic restraint is different. For example, a patient suffering from heat pattern should abstain from pungent, spicy, greasy, deep-fried foods. A patient suffering from cold pattern should abstain from raw and cold foods. A patient suffering from phlegm blocking chest pattern should abstain from fatty and greasy foods. A patient suffering from liver yang hyperactivity with the symptoms of dizziness, blurring of vision, restlessness, anger, etc. should abstain from foods as chili, garlic, chives, etc. A patient suffering from spleen and stomach deficiency pattern should abstain from deep-fried foods and foods which are not easy to digest.

有区别。如热性病应忌食辛辣、油腻、煎炸类食物，寒性病应忌食生冷，痰阻胸阳之胸痹应忌食肥腻；肝阳上亢，头晕目眩、烦躁易怒等应忌食辣椒、蒜、韭等，脾胃虚弱者应忌食油炸黏腻、不易消化的食物等。

Section 3 Dosage

第3节 剂量

Dosage refers to the amount of medicinal herbs, signifying the daily amount of one medicinal herb for an adult. Or it refers to the proportional measurements of medicinal herbs in one prescription, i.e. the relevant dosage.

The unit of measurement in Chinese medicinal herbs is gram. The most medicinal herbs are measured by weight, and a few medicinal herbs are measured by quantity and capacity. Generally, the dosage of medicinal herbs refers to that of the dried products, and it is necessary to specify the dosage if

剂量，即用药量，一般是指单味药的成人内服的一日用量。或指在方剂中药与药之间的比例分量，即相对剂量。

现今中药的计量单位采用公制克。中药的用量大多以重量单位表示，亦有少数以数量、容量表示。一般各药中所示的剂量均为干燥品的用量，用鲜品则需另注明

the fresh products are applied.

The determination of dosage of Chinese medicinal herbs is influenced by following factors:

3.1 The quality of Chinese medicinal herbs

Firstly, it is related to the quality of medicinal herbs. For example, the dosage of the light medicinal herbs as flower and folium is lighter, while the dosage of the heavy medicinal herbs as metal, stone and shell is heavier. The dosage of dried products is lighter, while the dosage of fresh products is heavier. Secondly, it is related to the property of medicinal herbs. The dosage of medicinal herbs of bland flavor and moderate action is heavier, while the dosage of medicinal herbs of strong flavor and fierce action is lighter.

3.2 Compatibility and dosage

Generally, the dosage of a single medicinal herb is heavier, while the dosage of medicinal herbs in prescription is lighter. In a prescription, the dosage of dominant medicinal herbs is heavier, while the dosage of adjuvant medicinal herbs is lighter. The dosage of medicinal herbs used for decoction is heavier, while the dosage of medicinal herbs used for pills and powder is lighter.

3.3 Conditions of patient

The dosage of medicinal herbs is also related to the patient's body constitution, age, disease course, etc.

(1) The dosage of medicinal herbs for a patient with strong body constitution is heavier, while the dosage of medicinal herbs for a patient with weak body constitution is lighter. The dosage of medicinal herbs for a patient with strong spleen and stomach is heavier, while the dosage of medicinal herbs for a patient with weak spleen and stomach is lighter.

用量。

中药剂量的确定，还受到如下各种因素的影响。

3.1 药物性质

一是与药物质地轻重有关，如花叶类质轻之品用量宜轻，金石、贝壳质重之品用量宜重；干品用量宜轻，鲜品用量宜重。二是与药性有关，气味平淡作用缓和的药，用量宜重；气味浓厚作用峻猛的药，用量宜轻。

3.2 配伍剂型

一般单味药用量较大，入复方则用量相对减小；复方中的主药用量相对大些，辅助药用量可低于主药。入汤剂时用量宜大；入丸、散剂时用量宜小。

3.3 患者情况

用药剂量与患者体质、年龄、病程等有关。

（1）身体壮实者用量宜重，身体虚弱者用量宜轻。脾胃强健者，用量宜稍大；脾胃虚弱者，用量宜轻小。

(2) The dosage of medicinal herbs for an old patient is lighter, while the dosage of medicinal herbs for a young or middle-aged patient is heavier. The dosage of medicinal herbs for a child below five is of 1/4 dose for an adult, while the dosage of medicinal herbs for a child above five is of 1/2 dose for an adult.

(2) 老年人用量宜减小，青壮年用量可大些。五岁以下小儿用量为成人量的1/4，五岁以上用成人量的1/2。

(3) The dosage of medicinal herbs for a patient with a new disease is heavier, while the dosage of medicinal herbs for a patient with a chronic disease is lighter. The dosage of medicinal herbs for a patient with an acute or severe disease is heavier, while the dosage of medicinal herbs for a patient with a moderate or mild disease is lighter.

(3) 新病患者用量可稍重，久病患者用量宜轻些。病急病重者用量宜重，病缓病轻者用量宜轻。

Section 4 Administration

第4节 用法

The administration of Chinese medicinal herbs mainly refers to the methods to decoct and take the medicinal herbs.

中药的用法主要简述中药汤剂的煎煮方法和服药法。

1 Methods to decoct Chinese medicinal herbs

1 煎药法

The decoction is the major dose form of Chinese medicinal herbs. If the decocting method is correct or not may directly influence the therapeutic effect. It is necessary to master the following key points.

中药以汤剂为常见剂型。中药煎煮方法的正确与否，将会对疗效产生直接的影响。煎煮中药时必须掌握以下要点。

1.1 Select a proper appliance for decocting Chinese medicinal herbs

1.1 选择合适的煎药器具

It might be just well to apply the marmite, enamel pot or stainless steel pot, which is stable in chemical composition, not easy to react chemically, even in heat conduction and good in heat retention.

最好用化学性质稳定，不易与药物成分发生化学反应，并且导热均匀，保暖性能好的砂锅、搪瓷烧锅或不锈

The metal appliances made of iron, copper or aluminum should not be applied, to avoid the chemical reaction on medicinal herbs, because this type of appliances may reduce the therapeutic effect and even produce toxicity or side-effect.

钢锅。忌用铁、铜、铝等金属器具，以免与药液中的中药成分发生化学反应，既可能使疗效降低，甚则产生毒副作用。

1.2 Select proper water for decocting Chinese medicinal herbs

It is advisable to select the clean drinking water without peculiar smell for decoction of Chinese medicinal herbs. The volume of water should be proper, usually about 2 cm over the surface of medicinal herbs. For decoction of medicinal herbs which need to be decocted for shorter time, it is advisable to add water just over the surface of medicinal herbs.

1.2 选择煎药用水

宜选择无异味、洁净澄清，可作饮用的水，作为煎煮中药用水。加水量不宜过多，以水液面淹没过饮片约2厘米为宜。煎煮时间较短的药物，液面淹没药物即可。

1.3 Soak time

Before decoction, it is advisable to soak the medicinal herbs in water, to make a full dissolution of the effective constituents in medicinal herbs. It is advisable to soak regular medicinal herbs in cold water for about 30 minutes. Under high temperature in summer, it is not advisable to soak medicinal herbs for too long time, so as to prevent medicinal herbs from being perishable.

1.3 浸泡时间

煎煮前需将中药饮片加水浸泡，以利于有效成分的充分溶出。一般药物用冷水浸泡 30 分钟左右。夏日高温时，浸泡时间不宜过长，以免腐败变质。

1.4 Fire level and time of decoction

It is necessary to decoct the medicinal herbs on strong fire first, and then on slow fire. It implies to decoct the medicinal herbs on strong fire before boiling, and to decoct them on slow fire after boiling to keep slightly boiling. In the decoction of the medicinal herbs to relieve the exterior and fragrant medicinal herbs, it is necessary to decoct them on strong fire to boiling, then to decoct them on slow fire for 10 to 15 minutes. In the decoction of the medicinal herbs of minerals, shells and crustaceans

1.4 煎煮火候及时间

一般煎药宜先武火后文火。即未沸前用大火，沸后用小火保持微沸状态。解表药及其他芳香性药物，用武火迅速煮沸后，文火煎煮10～15 分钟即可。矿物类、贝壳类、甲壳类药及补益药，一般武火煮沸后，文火再煎30 分钟以上，使有效成分充分溶出。

and those with reinforcing action, it is necessary to decoct them on strong fire to boiling, then to decoct them on slow fire for over 30 minutes, so as to make a full dissolution of the effective constituents.

1.5 Number of decoction

One dose of medicinal herbs is often decocted twice or three times. After first decoction, it is necessary to take out the decocted fluid, add some more water to the medicinal herbs for the second decoction. In order to fully utilize the medicinal herbs and avoid wasting, it is advisable to make the third decoction according to the requirements of herb dosage and treatment.

1.5 煎煮次数

一剂药大多煎煮两次或三次。第一次煎煮完成后，取出煎液，再加适量水，煎煮第二次。为充分利用药物，避免浪费，亦可根据药物剂量或治疗需要，再煎第三次。

1.6 Methods of decoction

Most of the medicinal herbs can be decocted at the same time. But a small amount of medicinal herbs, according to different parts or textures, or specific requirements in clinic application, can be decocted for different periods of time in different ways.

1.6 入药方法

大多药物可同时入煎，少部分药物因其入药部位或材质的不同，或临床应用的特殊需要，可能有不同煎煮时间的要求，入药方法有所不同。

1.6.1 Decoction first

Some medicinal herbs, such as *Magnetitum* (ci shi) and *Ostreae Concha* (mu li) of minerals and shells, *Aconiti Radix Lateralis Praeparata* (fu zi) and *Aconiti Radix* (chuan wu) of toxic medicinal herbs which toxicity may be reduced after long-term decoction, should be decocted first for 20 to 30 minutes, then decocted with other medicinal herbs together.

1.6.1 先煎

较其他药物先行煎煮20～30分钟，再与其他药同煎。如矿石类、贝壳类药的磁石、牡蛎等。还有宜久煎去毒的药物，如附子、川乌等。

1.6.2 Decoction later

Some fragrant medicinal herbs, such as *Menthae Haplocalycis Herba* (bo he) and *Semen Amomi Fructus Rotundus* (bai dou kou) which should not be decocted for too long time for guarantee of their

1.6.2 后下

即在其他药物煎煮即将完成之前，投入药物。需后下的药物大多气味芳香，不可久煎，为了保证药效而后

effects, should be put in to decoct before completion of decoction of other medicinal herbs. Besides, the medicinal herbs with purging action, as *Rhei Radix et Rhizoma* (da huang) and *Folium Cassiae* (fan xie ye), should also be decocted later or put into the decoction after it is done, or made decoction with boiling water, so as to avoid weakening their effects after decoction for too long time.

下，如薄荷、白豆蔻等。生大黄、番泻叶若久煎则减弱了泻下通便之力，故宜后下或开水泡服。

1.6.3 Decoction by wrapping

The medicinal herbs of tiny seeds, pollens, fine powder and tomenta, such as *Typhae Pollen* (pu huang), *Plantaginis Semen* (che qian zi), *Talcum* (hua shi) powder, *Inulae Flos* (xuan fu hua), etc. should be put into a cloth bag before decoction, so as to avoid floating or sinking in decoction, or to avoid stimulation to throat.

1.6.3 包煎

对于细小种子、花粉、细粉、带绒毛类药物可用布袋薄后入煎，以免漂浮在上或沉于锅底，或刺激咽喉，如蒲黄、车前子、滑石粉、旋覆花等。

1.6.4 Decoction singly

A very few of expensive medicinal herbs, such as *Radix Ginseng* (ren shen) and *Panacis Quinquefolii Radix* (xi yang shen), should be decocted separately. The decocted juice is taken and then added to the decoction made of other medicinal herbs.

1.6.4 另煎

少数价格昂贵的药物可另煎取汁，与其他药汁兑服，如人参、西洋参等。

1.6.5 Melt with heat

The medicinal herbs of gelatins, such as *Asini Corii Colla* (e jiao) and *Colla Cornus Cervi* (lu jiao jiao), should be melted and added to the decoction made of other medicinal herbs, so as to prevent them from adhering to other medicinal herbs or the pot bottom.

1.6.5 烊化

胶类药容易粘附于其他药渣及锅底，应先行烊化，再与其他药汁兑服，如阿胶、鹿角胶等。

1.6.6 Infusion for oral administration

The medicinal herbs which are dissolved easily in water or the medicinal herbs in juice form, such as *Natrii Sulfas* (mang xiao), *Succus Bambosae* (zhu li) and *Mel* (feng mi), should be infused into

1.6.6 冲服

有些入水即化的药或原为汁液性的药，宜取煎液或开水冲服，如芒硝、竹沥、蜂蜜等。

the decocted juice or water for oral administration.

2 Methods to take Chinese medicinal herbs

In terms of decoction, it is need to be taken warmly, one dose and two serves a day. For the patient with severe or emergent disease, it is need to be taken 2 doses and three serves a day. For the patient with chronic disease, it is need to be taken 1 dose every 2 days.

Generally speaking, it is advisable to take the sweat-making medicinal herbs hot, so as to make sweating, to take the vomit-stopping or toxin-relieving medicinal herbs frequently in small dosage, and to take the purging and defecation-promoting medicinal herbs until inducing defecation, not to take for long time.

In terms of time of taking Chinese medicinal herbs, it is important to take medicinal herbs timely, so as to guarantee their effects. Usually, the decoction is taken between two meals. But some medicinal herbs should be taken at certain time according to the requirements of conditions and herb properties. For example, the purging, defecation-promoting and parasite-expelling medicinal herbs should be taken on an empty stomach, the reinforcing medicinal herbs should be taken before meals, the stomach-strengthening medicinal herbs or the medicinal herbs which stimulates the stomach and intestines should be taken after meals, while the mind-calming and sleep-assisting medicinal herbs should be taken before going to bed.

Furthermore, the patent medicinal herbs, such as pills and powders, should be taken by warm water according to the required dosage.

2 服药法

中药汤剂一般温服，每日1剂，煎2次服。若病重或病急者，可每日2剂，煎3次服。慢性病患者可1剂分2日服。

一般而言，发汗药宜热服，以汗出为度。止吐或解毒药可多次小量频服。若为泻下通便药，亦以便通为度，不可久服。

适时服药是保证药效的重要方面。一般中药的服用时间以两餐之间服用为宜。有些药物的服药时间需根据病情需要及药物特性来确定，如泻下通便、驱虫药多在空腹时服，滋补药在饭前服用，健胃药和对胃肠有刺激的药大多在饭后服，有安神助眠作用的药应在临睡前服。

此外，丸药、散剂等成药制剂，一般按照规定服用剂量用温开水送服。

Specific Introduction

各论

Chapter 1 Exterior-Relieving Herbs

第1章 解表药

The Chinese medicinal herbs, acting to dissipate the exterior pathogens and to relieve the exterior pattern, are called the exterior-relieving herbs.

以发散表邪,解除表证为主要作用的药物,称解表药,亦称发表药。

Since the exterior pattern varies from the wind-cold pattern to the wind-heat pattern, the medicinal herbs of this category are divided into the wind-cold-dissipating herbs and wind-heat-dissipating herbs according to the actions and properties of the medicinal herbs.

由于表证有风寒和风热的区别,故本类药物根据其性能特点,分为发散风寒药和发散风热药两类。

The wind-cold-dissipating herbs are mostly pungent in flavor and warm in property, acting to relieve the exterior and to dissipate wind and cold, also called the exterior-relieving herbs with pungent-warm property. This type of medicinal herbs are used to treat the exterior wind-cold pattern, manifested by aversion to cold, fever, absence of sweating or slight sweating, headache, general aching, absence of thirst, thin-white tongue coating, superficial pulse, etc.

发散风寒药大多味辛性温,功能发表、散风寒,又称辛温解表药,主要用于风寒表证,症见恶寒发热,无汗或有汗,头痛身痛,口不渴,舌苔薄白,脉浮等。

The wind-heat-dissipating herbs are mostly pungent in flavor and cool in property, acting to relieve the exterior and to dissipate wind and heat, also called the exterior-relieving herbs with pungent-cool property. This type of medicinal herbs are used to treat the exterior wind-heat pattern or early stage of febrile disease in which the pathogens locate in the

发散风热药大多味辛性凉,功能散风热、除表证,又称辛凉解表药,主要用于外感风热或温病初起、邪在卫分,症见发热重、恶寒轻、头痛、咽干口渴、舌苔薄黄而干、脉浮数者。

Wei (Defensive) Phase, manifested by high fever, slight aversion to cold, headache, dry throat, thirst, thin-yellow-dry tongue coating, superficial-rapid pulse, etc.

Several notes should be paid attention in the application of the exterior-relieving herbs. First, it is not advisable to apply the exterior relieving herbs with strong action to make sweating in high-dose, so as to avoid profuse sweating, which may damage yang, consume qi and injure the body fluid. Second, it is necessary to cautiously apply this type of medicinal herbs for the cases of the exterior pattern, with spontaneous sweating due to qi deficiency or nocturnal sweats due to yin deficiency, with chronic carbuncles and ulcers, urinary infection, or hemorrhage. Third, it is advisable to increase or decrease the dosage of this type of medicinal herbs according to the seasonal changes and different geographic conditions. Fourth, it is not advisable to decoct this type of medicinal herbs for too long time, since most medicinal herbs are pungent in flavor with dissipating action.

使用解表药时尚应注意，对发汗力较强的解表药，用量不宜过大，以免发汗太过，伤阳耗气，损及津液。气虚自汗、阴虚盗汗以及疮疡日久、淋病、失血者，虽有表证，也应慎用。并要注意因时(季节变化)、因地(南北不同地区)增减用量。本类药多为辛散之品，入汤剂不宜久煎。

Section 1 Wind-cold-dissipating herbs

第1节 发散风寒药

Ephedrae Herba (ma huang)

It is the dried product from the herbaceous stem of *Ephedra sinica* stapf, *Ephedra intermedia schrenk* et C. A. Mey, and *Ephedra equisetina* Bunge, family Ephedraceae. The medicinal herb is collected in autumn, applied in crude form or in honey-prepared form.

麻黄

为麻黄科植物草麻黄、中麻黄及木贼麻黄的干燥草质茎。秋末采收。生用或蜜炙。

Features Flavor: pungent and slightly bitter. Property: warm. Meridian tropism: the Lung Meridian and the Bladder Meridian.

性味归经 辛、微苦，温。归肺、膀胱经。

Actions Make sweating, relieve the exterior, disperse lung, soothe panting, promote waterflow and subside swell.

功效 发汗解表，宣肺平喘，利水消肿。

Application

应用

(1) Exterior wind-cold pattern of excess. The medicinal herb makes sweating so as to dissipate wind and cold, as the fierce herb of pungent-warm property to relieve the exterior. It is applied to treat the exterior wind-cold pattern of excess, manifested by fever, aversion to cold, absence of sweating, headache, superficial-taut pulse, in combination with *Cinnamomi Ramulus* (gui zhi), as in Ephedra Decoction (Ma Huang Tang).

(1) 风寒表实证。本品善发汗以散风寒，为辛温解表之峻品。治发热恶寒，无汗，头痛，脉浮紧的风寒表实证，常与桂枝相须为用，如麻黄汤。

(2) Coughing and panting of excess pattern. The medicinal herb acts to disperse lung, relieve coughing and soothe panting, used to treat coughing and panting of excess pattern. In the treatment of coughing and panting due to wind-cold, it is often combined with *Armeniacae Amarum Semen* (ku xing ren) and *Glycyrrhizae Radix et Rhizoma* (gan cao), to form up Three Disobediences Decoction (San Ao Tang). In the treatment of cold-rheum in lung, it is combined with *Asari Radix et Rhizoma* (xi xin) and *Zingiberis Rhizoma* (gan jiang), to form up Minor Green Dragon Decoction (Xiao Qing Long Tang). In the treatment of pathogenic heat blocking lung with panting, coughing and yellow sputum, it is combined with *Gypsum Fibrosum* (shi gao) and ku xing ren, to form up Ephedra, Apricot, Gypsum and Liquorice Decoction (Ma Xing Shi Gan Tang).

(2) 咳喘实证。本品善散邪宣肺以止咳平喘，主要用于肺实咳喘。治风寒咳喘，常与杏仁、甘草配伍，即三拗汤。治肺有寒饮，咳痰清稀，可配伍细辛、干姜等同用，如小青龙汤。治邪热壅肺，痰黄喘咳，可与石膏、杏仁配伍，如麻杏石甘汤。

(3) Edema due to wind-water. The medicinal

(3) 风水水肿。本品既

herb acts to relieve the exterior and dissipate wind, and also to regulate the water passage, promote urination and subside swell as well. In the treatment of edema due to wind-water, it is combined with *Glycyrrhizae Radix et Rhizoma* (gan cao), to form up Liquorice and Ephedra Decoction (Gan Cao Ma Huang Tang), or combined with *Zingiberis Rhizoma Recens* (sheng jiang) and *Atractylodis Rhizoma Macrocephalae* (bai zhu), to form up Edema-Relieving and Atractylodes Decoction (Yue Bi Jia Zhu Tang).

辛散发表，又下调水道，利尿消肿。治风水水肿，小便不利，可与甘草同用，即甘草麻黄汤，或与生姜、白术同用，如越婢加术汤。

Furthermore, the medicinal herb acts to warm and dissipate the pathogenic cold, often used to treat the Bi (Obturation) Pattern due to wind, cold and damp, dorsal furuncle, goiter, etc.

此外，麻黄能温散寒邪，常用于治风寒湿痹、阴疽、痰核等证。

Usage and dosage Apply 3～10 g in decoction. It is advisable to use its crude form to make sweating and relieve the exterior, and to use its honey-prepared form to relieve coughing and soothing panting. The medicinal herb can be pounded to tomentum so as to moderate its action to make sweating, often used for children, old persons, or those with weak body.

用法用量 煎服，3～10克。生用发汗解表，蜜炙止咳平喘。捣绒缓和发汗，小儿、年老体弱者宜用麻黄绒或炙用。

Precautions for use It is cautiously applied for the exterior deficiency pattern with spontaneous sweating, yin deficiency pattern with nocturnal sweats, or panting of deficiency type due to kidney failing to accept qi.

使用注意 表虚自汗及阴虚盗汗、肾不纳气的虚喘者慎用。

Cinnamomi Ramulus **(gui zhi)**

桂枝

It is the dried product from the tender branch of *Cinnamomum cassia* Presl, family Lauraceae. The medicinal herb is collected in spring and summer, applied in crude form.

为樟科植物肉桂的干燥嫩枝。春、夏季采收。生用。

Features Flavor: pungent and sweet. Property: warm. Meridian tropism: the Lung Meridian, the Heart Meridian and the Bladder Meridian.

性味归经 辛、甘，温。归肺、心、膀胱经。

Actions Make sweating, relieve the exterior, warm meridians, dredge vessels, assist yang and transform qi.

功效 发汗解肌，温经通脉，助阳化气。

Application

(1) Wind-cold pattern due to exogenous factors. The medicinal herb is applied to treat the exterior excess pattern due to exogenous wind-cold without sweating, and also the exterior deficiency pattern with sweating as well. In the treatment of exterior excess pattern due to exogenous wind-cold, it is often combined with *Ephedrae Herba* (ma huang). In the treatment of exterior deficiency pattern with sweating, it is often combined with *Paeoniae Radix Alba* (bai shao), to form up Cinnamon-Twig Decoction (Gui Zhi Tang).

(2) Bi (Obturation) Pattern due to wind-damp, irregular menstruation or dysmenorrhea. The medicinal herb acts to warm and dredge meridians and vessels, dispel cold and relieve pain. In the treatment of Bi (Obturation) Pattern due to wind-damp, it is often combined with *Aconiti Radix Lateralis Praeparata* (fu zi) and *Glycyrrhizae Radix et Rhizoma* (gan cao). In the treatment of Bi (Obturation) Pattern due to blood deficiency, it is often combined with *Astragali Radix* (huang qi) and *Radix Paeoniae* (shao yao), to form up Astraglalus, Cinnamon and Five Ingredients Decoction (Huang Qi Gui Zhi Wu Wu Tang). In the treatment of irregular menstruation or dysmenorrhea due to cold coagulation and blood stasis, it is often combined with *Angelicae Sinensis Radix* (dang gui), *Rhizoma*

应用

(1) 外感风寒证。本品治外感风寒表实无汗或表虚有汗皆可应用。治风寒表实无汗，常与麻黄配伍。治风寒表虚有汗，常与白芍配伍，如桂枝汤。

(2) 风湿痹痛，月经不调或痛经。本品温通经脉，散寒止痛。治风湿痹证，常配伍附子、甘草同用；血虚痹痛，可与黄芪、芍药等同用，如黄芪桂枝五物汤。治寒凝血滞之月经不调或痛经，可与当归、川芎、芍药等同用，如温经汤。

Chuanxiong (chuan xiong) and shao yao, to form up Meridian-Warming Decoction (Wen Jing Tang).

(3) Cold pain at epigastria and abdomen. The medicinal herb acts to dispel cold and relieve pain. In the treatment of cold pain at epigastria and abdomen, it is often combined with bai shao and *Mattose* (yi tang), to form up Minor Center-Fortifying Decoction (Xiao Jian Zhong Tang).

（3）脘腹冷痛。本品散寒止痛，治脘腹冷痛，常配白芍、饴糖等同用，如小建中汤。

(4) Bi (Obturation) Pattern at chest, palpitation, irregular pulse, phlegm-rheum and edema. The medicinal herb acts to support heart yang, assist yang and transform qi. In the treatment of Bi (Obturation) Pattern at chest due to heart yang insufficiency or blood stasis blocking heart vessels, it is often combined with *Bulbus Allii Macrostemi* (xie bai) and *Trichosanthis Fructus* (gua lou), to form up Snakegourd, Longstaner Onion Bulb and Cinnamon Decoction (Gua Lou Xie Bai Gui Zhi Tang). In the treatment of palpitation and irregular pulse, it is often combined with *Glycyrrhizae Radix et Rhizoma Praeparatae* (zhi gan cao) and *Ginseng Radix et Raizoma* (ren shen), to form up Honeyed Liquorice Decoction (Zhi Gan Cao Tang). In the treatment of phlegm-rheum manifested by distension and fullness at chest and hypochondria, dizziness, blurring of vision, palpitation, or shortness of breath and cough, it is often combined with *Atractylodis Rhizoma Macrocephalae* (bai zhu) and *Poria* (fu ling), to form up Poria, Cinnamon, Atractylodes and Liquorice Decoction (Ling Gui Zhu Gan Tang). In the treatment of edema and difficult urination due to deficiency of kidney qi which fails to act transformation, it is often combined with fu ling and *Alismatis Rhizoma* (ze xie), to form up Poria

（4）胸痹，心动悸、脉结代，痰饮，水肿。本品能通心阳，助阳化气。治心阳不振、瘀血痹阻的胸痹，常与薤白、瓜蒌配伍，即瓜蒌薤白桂枝汤。治心动悸、脉结代，可与炙甘草、人参等同用，如炙甘草汤。治痰饮，症见胸胁胀满，眩晕心悸，或短气而咳，常与白术、茯苓等同用，如苓桂术甘汤。治肾虚气化失司的水肿、小便不利，常与茯苓、泽泻等配伍，如五苓散。

Five Powder (Wu Ling San).

Usage and dosage Apply 3～10 g in decoction.

Precautions for use It is prohibited to apply in the febrile disease, yin deficiency and yang excess pattern and bleeding due to heat in blood. It is cautiously applied for pregnant women and those with heavy flow of blood in menstruation.

用法用量 煎服，3～10克。

使用注意 温热病、阴虚阳盛、血热出血忌用。孕妇及月经过多者慎用。

Perillae Folium (zi su ye)

紫苏叶

It is the dried product from the leaf of *Perilla frutescens* (L.) Britt. Var. *acuta* (Thunb.) Kudo., family Labiatae. The medicinal herb is collected in summer when it is fruitful and lefty, applied in crude form.

为唇形科植物紫苏的干燥叶。又名苏叶。夏季枝叶茂盛时采收。生用。

Features Flavor: pungent. Property: warm. Meridian tropism: the Lung Meridian and the Spleen Meridian.

性味归经 辛，温。归肺、脾经。

Actions Make sweating, relieve the exterior, promote qi flow, dilate middle energizer, and relieve toxin from fish and crab.

功效 发汗解表，行气宽中，解鱼蟹毒。

Application

(1) Wind-cold pattern due to exogenous factors. The medicinal herb acts to dispel wind and cold, and disperse the lung qi. In the treatment of wind-cold pattern due to exogenous factors manifested by auersion to cold, fever, absence of sweat and cough with sputum, it is combined with *Peucedani Radix* (qian hu), *Platycodonis Radix* (jie geng) and *Armeniacae Amarum Semen* (ku xing ren), to form up Almond and Perilla Powder (Xing Su San). In the treatment of the condition accompanied by qi stagnation and stuffy chest, it is combined with *Cyperi Rhizoma* (xiang fu) and *Citri Reticulatae*

应用

（1）外感风寒证。本品能散风寒、宣肺气。治外感风寒证，症见恶寒发热无汗，兼见咳嗽咳痰，可与前胡、桔梗、杏仁等同用，如杏苏散。若兼胸闷气滞者，与香附、陈皮等同用，如香苏散。

Pericarpium (chen pi), to form up Cyperus Tuber and Perilla Powder (Xiang Su San).

(2) Qi stagnation pattern of spleen and stomach. The medicinal herb acts to promote qi flow, dilate middle energizer, harmonize stomach and stop vomiting. In the treatment of qi stagnation pattern of spleen and stomach accompanied by cold, it is combined with *Pogostmonis Herba* (huo xiang), to form up Agastache Vital Force Powder (Huo Xiang Zheng Qi San). In the treatment of qi stagnation pattern of spleen and stomach accompanied by heat, it is combined with *Coptidis Rhizoma* (huang lian). In the treatment of qi stagnation pattern of spleen and stomach accompanied with qi-phlegm accumulation, it is combined with *Pinelliae Rhizoma* (ban xia) and *Magnoliae Officinalis Cortex* (hou po). In the treatment of morning sickness, it is combined with chen pi and *Amomi Fructus* (sha ren).

(2) 脾胃气滞证。本品能行气宽中、和胃止呕。治脾胃气滞偏寒者，与藿香等同用，如藿香正气散。偏热者，与黄连等同用。偏痰气互结者，与半夏、厚朴等同用。治妊娠呕吐，常与陈皮、砂仁同用。

(3) Vomiting and diarrhea due to toxin from fish and crab. The medicinal herb acts to relieve toxin from fish and crab. It can be decocted singly, or with *Zingiberis Rhizoma Recens* (sheng jiang), huo xiang and chen pi.

(3) 鱼蟹中毒之吐泻。本品能解鱼蟹毒。可水煎单用，或与生姜、藿香、陈皮同用。

Usage and dosage Apply 3～10 g in decoction. Apply 30～60 g to relieve toxin from fish and crab. It is not advisable to decoct it for long time.

用法用量 煎服，3～10克。治鱼蟹中毒，30～60克。不宜久煎。

Appendix *Perillae Caulis* (zi su geng)

It is the dried product from the stem of *Perilla frutescens.* The medicinal herb is warm in property, pungent in flavor and attributive to the Lung Meridian and the Spleen Meridian. It acts to promote qi flow, dilate middle energizer, relieve pain and pre-

附药 紫苏梗

为紫苏的干燥茎。性味辛，温。归肺、脾经。功能理气宽中，止痛，安胎。适用于胸膈痞满，胃脘疼痛，嗳气呕吐，胎动不安。煎服，5～10

vent miscarriage, to treat masses and fullness at chest and hypochondria, pain at epigastria, belching, vomiting and fetal irritability. Apply 5～10 g in decoction. It is not advisable to decoct it for long time.

克。不宜久煎。

Zingiberis Rhizoma Recens (sheng jiang)

It is the dried product from the fresh rhizome of Common Ginger, *Zingiber officinale* (Willd.) Rosc., family Zingiberaceae. It is collected in autumn, applied in crude form or reservedly applied by embedding in sand.

Features Flavor: pungent. Property: slightly warm. Meridian tropism: the Lung Meridian and the Spleen Meridian.

Actions Make sweating, relieve the exterior, warm middle energizer, stop vomiting, warm lung and stop coughing.

Application

(1) Wind-cold pattern due to exogenous factors. The medicinal herb is weak in making sweating and relieving the exterior, so it is added to other exterior-relieving herbs of pungent-warm property, so as to promote the action to make sweating. In the treatment of mild condition of wind-cold pattern, it is used to decoct singly by adding brown sugar.

(2) Vomiting. The medicinal herb acts to warm stomach, dispel cold, harmonize middle energizer and stop vomiting, a good medicine to stop vomiting. It is warm in property, so it is often used to treat vomiting due to cold attacking stomach, combined with *Pinelliae Rhizoma* (ban xia), to form up Minor Pinellia Decoction (Xiao Ban Xia Tang). In the treatment of vomiting in heat pat-

生姜

为姜科植物姜的新鲜根茎。秋末采挖。鲜用或埋入砂中备用。

性味归经 辛，微温。归肺、脾经。

功效 发汗解表，温中止呕，温肺止咳。

应用

（1）外感风寒证。本品发汗解表力弱，可入辛温解表剂，以增发汗之力。若治风寒轻症，可单煎加红糖热服。

（2）呕吐证。本品能温胃散寒、和中止呕，为止呕良药。性温而善治胃寒呕吐，常与半夏同用，如小半夏汤。治热证呕吐，可与竹茹、黄连等同用。

tern, it is combined with *Bambusae Caulis in Taenias* (zhu ru) and *Coptidis Rhizoma* (huang lian).

(3) Coughing due to wind-cold. The medicinal herb acts to warm lung, dispel cold, dissolve phlegm and stop coughing, often combined with other medicinal herbs of warming lung, dissolving phlegm and stopping cough.

(3) 风寒咳嗽。本品能温肺散寒、化痰止咳，常与其他温肺化痰止咳药同用。

Furthermore, the medicinal herb acts to relieve toxin from fish and crab, and to relieve toxin from *Pinelliae Rhizoma* (ban xia) and *Arisaematis Rhizoma* (tian nan xing).

此外，本品能解鱼蟹毒，解半夏、天南星毒。

Usage and dosage Apply 3～10 g in decoction, or take its juice orally.

用法用量 煎服，3～10克，或捣汁服。

Precautions for use It is prohibited to apply in yin deficiency and internal heat pattern and heat pattern of excess.

使用注意 阴虚内热及热盛之证忌用。

Moslae Herba (xiang ru)

香薷

It is the dried product from the aerial parts of the perennial herbaceous plants, herb of *Mosla-Chinensis Maxim*, family Labiatae. The medicinal herb is collected in summer and autumn when it is fruitful and lefty, applied in crude form.

为唇形科植物石香薷的干燥地上部分。夏、秋季茎叶茂盛、果实成熟时割取地上部分。生用。

Features Flavor: pungent. Property: slightly warm. Meridian tropism: the Lung Meridian, the Stomach Meridian and the Spleen Meridian.

性味归经 辛，微温。归肺、胃、脾经。

Actions Make sweating, relieve the exterior, dissolve damp, harmonize middle energizer, promote urination and subside swell.

功效 发汗解表，化湿和中，利水消肿。

Application

(1) Wind-cold pattern due to exogenous factors in summer. The medicinal herb acts to make sweating, relieve the exterior, dissolve damp and harmonize middle energizer. In the treatment of wind-

应用

(1) 夏季外感风寒证。本品能发汗解表，化湿和中。治夏季乘凉饮冷，或外感风寒、暑湿，症见发热恶寒、头

cold pattern in summer due to greed to cold in drinking and eating or due to exogenous wind-cold or summer-heat-damp, manifested by fever, aversion to cold, headache, absence of sweating, stuffy chest, nausea, or abdominal pain, vomiting, diarrhea, etc., it is combined with *Semen Dolichoris* (bian dou) and *Magnoliae Officinalis Cortex* (hou po), to form up Elsholtzia Powder (Xiang Ru San).

痛无汗、胸闷泛恶，或腹痛吐泻等，配扁豆、厚朴等同用，如香薷散。

(2) Edema and difficult urination. The medicinal herb acts to inspire yang qi, to promote urination and to subside swell. In the treatment of edema and difficult urination, it is applied singly or combined with *Atractylodis Rhizoma Macrocephalae* (bai zhu), to form up Elsholtzia and Atractylodes Pills (Ru Zhu Wan).

（2）水肿、小便不利。本品能发越阳气，利水消肿。治水肿、小便不利，可单用或配白术同用，即薷术丸。

Usage and dosage Apply 3～10 g in decoction. It is advisable to decoct it into a strong liquid to promote urination and to subside swell.

用法用量 煎服，3～10克。利水退肿须浓煎。

Precautions for use It is prohibited to apply for exterior deficiency pattern with sweating.

使用注意 表虚有汗者忌用。

Schizonepetae Herba (jing jie)

荆芥

It is the dried product from the aerial parts of the herbaceous plant, *Schizonepeta tenuifolia* Brig., family Labiatae. The medicinal herb is collected in summer and autumn when it is flowering, applied in crude form or carbonized form.

为唇形科植物荆芥的干燥地上部分。夏、秋开花时割取地上部分。生用或炒炭用。

Features Flavor: pungent. Property: slightly warm. Meridian tropism: the Lung Meridian and the Liver Meridian.

性味归经 辛，微温。归肺、肝经。

Actions Dispel wind, relieve the exterior, promote eruption, relieve itching and stanch bleeding.

功效 祛风解表，透疹止痒，止血。

Application

应用

(1) Exterior pattern due to exogenous factors.

（1）外感表证。本品性

The medicinal herb is moderate, acting to dispel wind and relieve the exterior, so as to apply to treat exterior pattern of exogenous cold or heat. In the treatment of wind-cold pattern due to exogenous factors, it is combined with *Saposhnikoviae Radix* (fang feng) and *Notopterygii Rhizoma et Radix* (qiang huo), to form up Schizonepeta and Ledebouriella Detoxifying Powder (Jing Fang Bai Du San). In the treatment of wind-heat pattern due to exogenous factors, it is combined with *Lonicerae Japonicae Flos* (jin yin hua), *Forsythiae Fructus* (lian qiao) and *Menthae Haplocalycis Herba* (bo he), form up Lonicera and Forsythia Powder (Yin Qiao San).

较和缓,能祛风解表,外感表证不论寒热,皆可应用。治外感风寒者,常配伍防风、羌活等同用,如荆防败毒散;治外感风热者,常配金银花、连翘、薄荷等同用,如银翘散。

(2) Urticaria with itching. The medicinal herb acts to dispel wind, relieve itching and promote eruption. In the treatment of urticaria with itching, it is combined with fang feng, *Sophorae Flavescentis Radix* (ku shen) and *Radix Rehmanniae* (sheng di huang), to form up Wind-Dispelling Powder (Xiao Feng San). It is also applied to treat measles with unsmooth eruption.

(2) 风疹瘙痒。本品能祛风止痒、宣散透疹。治风疹瘙痒,常与防风、苦参、生地黄等同用,如消风散。亦治麻疹透发不畅。

(3) Early stage of carbuncle and ulcer with exterior pattern. The medicinal herb acts to dissolve carbuncle and relieve the exterior, combined with fang feng, *Lonicerae Japonicae Flos* (jin yin hua) and *Forsythiae Fructus* (lian qiao).

(3) 疮疡初起兼有表证。本品能消疮解表。常与防风、金银花、连翘等同用。

(4) Hemoptysis, epistaxis and heavy blood flow in menstruation. The carbonized form of the medicinal herb acts to stanch bleeding, so as to treat various bleeding diseases combined with other medicinal herbs.

(4) 吐衄下血。本品炒炭能止血,配合其他药物同用,治多种出血证。

Usage and dosage Apply 3～10 g in decoction. It is not advisable to decoct for too long time.

用法用量 煎服,3～10克,不宜久煎。生用发表、透

It is applied in crude form to relieve the exterior, promote eruption and relieve carbuncle, while in carbonized form to stanch bleeding.

疹、消疮,炒炭止血。

Saposhnikoviae Radix (fang feng)

防风

It is the dried product from the root of *Saposhnikoviae divaricata* (Turcz.) Schischk, family Umbelliferae. The medicinal herb is collected in spring and autumn before sprouting, applied in crude form or carbonized form.

为伞形科植物防风的干燥根。春、秋季采挖未抽花茎植株的根。生用或炒炭用。

Features Flavor: pungent and sweet. Property: slightly warm. Meridian tropism: the Bladder Meridian, the Liver Meridian and the Spleen Meridian.

性味归经 辛、甘,微温。归膀胱、肝、脾经。

Actions Dispel wind, relieve the exterior, dissolve damp, relieve pain and relieve convulsion.

功效 祛风解表,胜湿止痛,止痉。

Application

应用

(1) Exterior pattern due to exogenous factors. The medicinal herb is slightly warm, sweet and moderate, acting to treat exterior patterns due to exogenous cold, heat or excess. In the treatment of wind-cold pattern due to exogenous factors, it is combined with *Schizonepetae Herba* (jing jie). In the treatment of wind-heat pattern due to exogenous factors, it is combined with *Menthae Haplocalycis Herba* (bo he), *Forsythiae Fructus* (lian qiao) and *Scutellariae Radix* (huang qin). In the treatment of urticaria due to wind-heat or itching of skin, it is combined with jing jie and *Tribuli Fructus* (bai ji li).

(1) 外感表证。本品微温,甘缓不峻,治外感表证,不论寒热实均可应用。治外感风寒,常与荆芥等同用。治外感风热,可配薄荷、连翘、黄芩等同用。治风热发疹或皮疹瘙痒,可与荆芥、白蒺藜等同用。

(2) Bi (Obturation) Pattern due to wind, cold and damp. The medicinal herb acts to dispel wind, dissolve damp and relieve pain, often applied to treat Bi (Obturation) Pattern, combined with *Notopterygii Rhizoma et Radix* (qiang huo), *Angelicae Sinensis*

(2) 风寒湿痹证。本品祛风、胜湿、止痛,为治痹证常用。常与羌活、当归、独活等同用,如蠲痹汤。

Radix (dang gui) and *Angelicae Pubescentis Radix* (du huo), to form up Bi (Obturation) Pattern-Alleviating Decoction (Juan Bi Tang).

(3) Tetanus. The medicinal herb, attributive to the Liver Meridian, acts to dispel wind and relieve convulsion. In the treatment of tetanus manifested by opisthotonos, spasm and convulsion, it is combined with *Gastrodiae Rhizoma* (tian ma), *Arisaematis Rhizoma* (tian nan xing) and *Rhizoma Typhonii* Gigantei (bai fu zi), to form up Jade Genius Powder (Yu Zhen San).

（3）破伤风。本品入肝经，能祛风止痉。治破伤风，症见角弓反张、抽搐痉挛，常配天麻、天南星、白附子等药同用，如玉真散。

Furthermore, the medicinal herb is also applied to treat abdominal pain, diarrhea and relieved pain after diarrhea due to liver qi over-acting on spleen or due to disharmony between liver and stomach. The medicinal herb in carbonized form is applied to treat bloody feces due to enteritis, heavy blood flow in menstruation, etc.

此外，本品还可用于肝气乘脾，肝胃不和之腹痛泄泻，泻后痛减者。炒炭可治肠风下血、妇女血崩等。

Usage and dosage Apply 3～10 g in decoction. It is applied in crude form to dispel wind, dissolve damp and relieve pain, while in carbonized form to stanch bleeding.

用法用量 煎服，3～10克。生用祛风、胜湿、止痛，炒炭止血。

Precautions for use It is cautious or prohibited to apply for convulsion due to blood deficiency and yin deficiency and internal fire pattern.

使用注意 血虚发痉及阴虚火旺者慎用或忌用。

Notopterygii Rhizoma et Radix (qiang huo)

羌活

It is the dried product from the rhizomes and roots of the perennial herbaceous plant, Rhizome of *Notopterygium incisum* Ting ex H. T. Chang or the Rhizome and root of *Notopterygium forbesii* Boiss, family Umbelliferae. The medicinal herb is collected in spring and autumn, applied in crude form.

为伞形科植物羌活或宽叶羌活的干燥根茎及根。春、秋季采挖。生用。

Features Flavor: pungent and bitter. Proper-

性味归经 辛、苦，温。

ty: warm. Meridian tropism: the Bladder Meridian and the Kidney Meridian.

归膀胱、肾经。

Actions Dispel wind and cold, dissolve damp and relieve pain.

功效 发散风寒，胜湿止痛。

Application

应用

(1) Wind-cold pattern due to exogenous factors. The medicinal herb acts to dispel wind and cold and relieve pain. In the treatment of wind-cold pattern due to exogenous factors manifested by fever, aversion to cold, headache and general aching, it is combined with *Saposhnikoviae Radix* (fang feng), *Angelicae Dahuricae Radix* (bai zhi) and *Asari Radix et Rhizoma* (xi xin), to form up Nine Ingredients Notoptreygium Decoction (Jiu Wei Qiang Huo Tang).

(1) 外感风寒证。本品发散风寒、止痛力较强。治外感风寒，症见发热恶寒，头痛身痛，常配防风、白芷、细辛等同用，如九味羌活汤。

(2) Bi (Obturation) Pattern due to wind, cold and damp. The medicinal herb acts to dispel wind, dissolve damp, eliminate cold and relieve pain, applied to treat Bi (Obturation) Pattern with pain in upper part of body, combined with *Curcumae Longae Rhizoma* (jiang huang), *Gentianae Radix et Rhizoma Macrophyllae* (qin jiao) and *Ramulus Mori* (sang zhi).

(2) 风寒湿痹证。本品能祛风除湿，散寒止痛，善治上半身痹痛。可配伍姜黄、秦艽、桑枝等同用。

Usage and dosage Apply 3～10 g in decoction.

用法用量 煎服，3～10克。

Precautions for use It is prohibited to apply for yin deficiency pattern and dryness-heat pattern. Too large dose of the medicinal herb may cause vomiting.

使用注意 阴虚、燥热证忌用。用量过大，易致呕吐。

Angelicae Dahuricae Radix (bai zhi)

白芷

It is the dried product from the root of *Angelica dahurica* (Fisch. ex Hoffm.) Benth. et Hook. F., or *Angelica dahurica* (Fisch. ex Hoffm.) Benth. et Hook. F. var. t *aiwaniana* (Boiss.) Shan et Yuan,

为伞形科植物白芷或杭白芷的干燥根。夏、秋间采挖。生用。

family Umbelliferae. The medicinal herb is collected in summer and autumn, applied in crude form.

Features Flavor: pungent. Property: warm. Meridian tropism: the Lung Meridian and the Stomach Meridian.

性味归经 辛，温。归肺、胃经。

Actions Dispel wind, eliminate cold, relieve pain, open aperture, subside swell, drain pus, dry the damp and check vaginal discharge.

功效 祛风散寒，止痛通窍，消肿排脓，燥湿止带。

Application

(1) Wind-cold pattern due to exogenous factors, sinusitis. The medicinal herb acts to dispel wind, eliminate cold, relieve pain and open aperture. In the treatment of wind-cold pattern due to exogenous factors manifested by headache and nasal obstruction, it is combined with *Notopterygii Rhizoma et Radix* (qiang huo) and *Asari Radix et Rhizoma* (xi xin), to form up Nine Ingredients Notoptreygium Decoction (Jiu Wei Qiang Huo Tang). In the treatment of sinusitis, it is combined with *Xanthii Fructus* (cang er zi) which acts to open the nose aperture.

(2) Headache of Yangming Meridians and toothache. The medicinal herb acts to treat headache of Yangming Meridians, applied singly as in Even Beam Pills (Du Liang Wan). In the treatment of toothache, it is combined with different medicinal herbs according to cold pattern and heat pattern.

(3) Carbuncle, ulcer, swelling and pus. The medicinal herb acts to subside swell, drain pus and relieve pain. In the treatment of early stage of carbuncle without ulcer, it is applied to subside swell, combined with *Lonicerae Japonicae Flos* (jin yin hua), *Moutan Cortex* (mu dan pi) and *Taraxaci Herba* (pu gong ying). In the treatment of carbuncle with pus, it is applied to drain pus, combined with carbunde-relie-

应用

（1）外感风寒证，鼻渊。本品能祛风散寒、止痛通窍。外感风寒，症见头痛、鼻塞，常与羌活、细辛等同用，如九味羌活汤。治鼻渊，可与苍耳子等通鼻窍药同用。

（2）阳明经头痛，齿痛。善治阳明头痛，可单用，如都梁丸。治齿痛，辨寒热而随证配伍。

（3）疮疡肿毒。本品能消肿排脓止痛。对疮痈初起未溃者可消肿，配伍金银花、牡丹皮、蒲公英等同用。对疮疡脓成者可排脓，可配伍消痈排脓之品同用。

ving and pus-draining herbs.

(4) Excessive vaginal discharge. The medicinal herb acts to dry the damp and check vaginal discharge. In the treatment of excessive vaginal discharge due to cold and damp, it is combined with *Atractylodis Rhizoma Macrocephalae* (bai zhu) and *Poria* (fu ling). In the treatment of excessive vaginal discharge due to damp and heat, it is combined with *Phellodendri Cortex Chiensis* (huang bo) and *Plantaginis Semen* (che qian zi).

(4) 寒湿带下。本品能燥湿止带。治寒湿带下，配伍白术、茯苓等同用。治湿热带下，可配伍黄柏、车前子等同用。

Furthermore, the medicinal herb acts to dispel wind, dry the damp and relieve itching, applied to treat itching of skin.

此外，本品还能祛风燥湿止痒，治皮肤瘙痒等。

Usage and dosage Apply 3～10 g in decoction.

用法用量 煎服，3～10克。

Asari Radix et Rhizoma (xi xin)

细辛

It is the dried product from the roots and rhizomes of the perennial herbaceous plant, *Asarum heterotropoides* Fr. Schmidt var. *mandshuricum* (maxim) Kitag., and *Asarum sieboldii* Miq., family Aristolochiaceae. It is collected in summer or early autumn when it is fruitful, applied in crude form.

为马兜铃科植物北细辛、汉城细辛或华细辛的干燥根和根茎。夏季果熟期或初秋采挖。生用。

Features Flavor: pungent. Property: warm, slightly poisonous. Meridian tropism: the Lung Meridian, the Kidney Meridian and the Heart Meridian.

性味归经 辛，温；有小毒。归肺、肾、心经。

Actions Dispel wind, eliminate cold, dispel wind, relieve pain, warm lung, dissolve rheum and open aperture.

功效 祛风散寒，祛风止痛，温肺化饮，通窍。

Application

应用

(1) Wind-cold pattern due to exogenous factors. The medicinal herb acts to dispel wind, eliminate cold and relieve pain. In the treatment of exte-

(1) 外感风寒证。本品能祛风散寒止痛。治风寒表证，寒邪偏盛，症见头身疼痛

rior wind-cold pattern due to preponderance of pathogenic cold manifested by severe headache and general aching, it is combined with *Notopterygii Rhizoma et Radix* (qiang huo) and *Saposhnikoviae Radix* (fang feng). In the treatment of yang deficiency pattern with exogenous factors manifested by fever, aversion to cold and deep pulse, it is combined with *Aconiti Radix Praeparata* (fu zi) and *Ephedrae Herba* (ma huang), to form up Ephedra, Monkshood and Asarum Decoction (Ma Huang Fu Zi Xi Xin Tang).

甚者,可与羌活、防风等同用。亦治阳虚外感,症见发热恶寒,脉反沉者,配伍附子、麻黄等同用,即麻黄附子细辛汤。

(2) Headache, Bi (Obturation) Pattern and toothache. The medicinal herb acts to dispel wind, eliminate cold and relieve pain. In the treatment of headache due to wind and cold, it is combined with *Chuanxiong Rhizoma* (chuan xiong) and *Angelicae Dahuricae Radix* (bai zhi), to form up Tea-Blended Ligusticum Powder (Chuan Xiong Cha Tiao San). In the treatment of Bi (Obturation) Pattern due to wind and damp, it is combined with fang feng, *Angelicae Pubescentis Radix* (du huo) and *Gentianae Radix et Rhizoma Macrophyllae* (qin jiao). In the treatment of toothache, it is applied singly or combined with bai zhi to decoct into mouthwash.

(2) 头痛,痹痛,牙痛。本品祛风、散寒、止痛力强。治风寒头痛,常配伍川芎、白芷等同用,如川芎茶调散。治风湿痹痛,可配伍防风、独活、秦艽等同用。治牙痛,可单用,或与白芷煎汤漱口。

(3) Coughing and panting due to cold and rheum. The medicinal herb acts to eliminate cold exteriorly and warm lung to dissolve rheum interiorly. In the treatment of wind-cold pattern due to exogenous factors manifested by coughing, panting and white, clear and thin sputum caused by cold and rheum hidden in lung, it is combined with *Zingiberis Rhizoma* (gan jiang) and *Schisandrae Chinensis Fructus* (wu wei zi), to form up Minor Green Dragon Decoction (Xiao Qing Long Tang).

(3) 寒饮咳喘。本品外散表寒,内温肺饮。治外感风寒,寒饮伏肺,咳嗽气喘,痰白清稀,配伍干姜、五味子等,如小青龙汤。

(4) Sinusitis. The medicinal herb acts to open the nose aperture. In the treatment of sinusitis manifested by nasal obstruction, headache and running nose, it is combined with *Magnoliae Flos* (xin yi) and bai zhi.

（4）鼻渊。本品能通鼻窍。治鼻渊，症见鼻塞头痛流涕，可与辛夷、白芷等同用。

Usage and dosage Apply 3～5 g in decoction. Add 0.5～1 g to pills or powder. Apply it in proper volume for external use.

用法用量 煎服，3～5克。入丸散剂，0.5～1克。外用适量。

Precautions for use It is prohibited to apply for qi deficiency pattern with profuse sweating, yin deficiency and yang hyperactivity pattern or blood deficiency pattern with headache. The medicinal herb is incompatible with *Radix Veratri Nigri* (li lu). Large dose in application may cause poisoning.

使用注意 气虚多汗，阴虚阳亢或血虚头痛忌用。反藜芦。用量过大易引起中毒。

Xanthii Fructus **(cang er zi)**

苍耳子

Its source is from the dried fruit and involucre of *Xanthium sibiricum* Patr., family Compositae. The medicinal herb is collected in autumn, applied in crude form.

为菊科植物苍耳的干燥成熟带总苞的果实。秋季采收。生用。

Features Flavor: pungent and bitter. Property: warm, slightly poisonous. Meridian tropism: the Lung Meridian.

性味归经 辛、苦，温；有小毒。归肺经。

Actions Dispel wind and cold, open nose aperture and eliminate wind and damp.

功效 散风寒，通鼻窍，祛风湿。

Application

应用

(1) Headache, nasal obstruction, running nose and sinusitis due to wind-cold. The medicinal herb acts to dispel wind and cold and open nose aperture. In the treatment of headache and nasal obstruction due to exogenous wind-cold, it is combined with *Angelicae Dahuricae Radix* (bai zhi), *Saposhnikoviae Radix* (fang feng) and *Rhizoma Ligustici* (gao ben). In the treatment of sinusitis, thick and turbid

（1）风寒头痛，鼻塞流涕，鼻渊。本品能散风寒，通鼻窍。治外感风寒，头痛鼻塞，常与白芷、防风、藁本等同用。治鼻渊，流浊涕，不闻香臭者，常配辛夷、白芷等同用，如苍耳子散。

snivel and loss of smelling, it is combined with *Magnoliae Flos* (xin yi) and bai zhi, to form up Cocklebur Fruit Powder (Cang Er Zi San).

(2) Bi (Obturation) Pattern due to wind-damp. In the treatment of Bi (Obturation) Pattern, the medicinal herb is applied singly or combined with *Clematidis Radix et Rhizoma* (wei ling xian), fang feng and *Chuanxiong Rhizoma* (chuan xiong).

（2）风湿痹痛。治风湿痹痛，可单用，或与威灵仙、防风、川芎等同用。

Usage and dosage Apply 3～10 g in decoction or in pill form or powder form.

用法用量 煎服，3～10克。或入丸散剂。

Precautions for use It is not advisable to apply the medicinal herb for headache due to blood deficiency. Over dose of the medicinal herb causes poisoning.

使用注意 血虚头痛不宜用。过量服用易致中毒。

Magnoliae Flos (xin yi)

辛夷

It is the dried product from the flower bud of *Magnolia biondii* Pamp, *Magnolia denudate* Desr. and *Magnolia liliflore* Desr., family Magnoliaceae. The medicinal herb is collected in the early spring when the flower bud does not open, applied in crude form.

为木兰科植物望春花、玉兰或武当玉兰的干燥花蕾。早春花未开放时采收。生用。

Features Flavor: pungent. Property: warm. Meridian tropism: the Lung Meridian and the Stomach Meridian.

性味归经 辛，温。归肺、胃经。

Actions Dispel wind and cold, and open nose aperture.

功效 散风寒，通鼻窍。

Application

应用

(1) Headache and nasal obstruction due to wind-cold. The medicinal herb acts to dispel wind and cold and open nose aperture, combined with *Angelicae Dahuricae Radix* (bai zhi) and *Saposhnikoviae Radix* (fang feng).

（1）风寒头痛鼻塞。本品能散风寒、通鼻窍，常配白芷、防风等同用。

(2) Sinusitis and headache. The medicinal herb

（2）鼻渊头痛。本品为

is the major herb to treat sinusitis. In the treatment of sinusitis of cold pattern, it is combined with bai zhi and *Asari Radix et Rhizoma* (xi xin). In the treatment of sinusitis of heat pattern, it is combined with *Menthae Haplocalycis Herba* (bo he), *Scutellariae Radix* (huang qin) and *Anemarrhenae Rhizoma* (zhi mu).

治鼻渊之要药。治鼻渊属寒者，多与白芷、细辛等同用。属热者，多与薄荷、黄芩、知母等同用。

Usage and dosage Apply 3～10 g in decoction by wrapping. Apply proper dose for external use.

用法用量 煎服，3～10克。入煎剂宜包煎。外用适量。

Precautions for use It is prohibited to apply for yin deficiency and fire flaming pattern.

使用注意 阴虚火旺者忌服。

Section 2 Wind-heat-dissipating herbs

第2节 发散风热药

Menthae Haplocalycis Herba (bo he)

薄荷

It is the dried product from the branch and leaf of *Mentha haplocalyx* Briq., family Labiata. The medicinal herb is collected in summer and autumn when it is flowering and lefty, applied in crude form.

为唇形科植物薄荷的干燥地上部分。夏、秋季茎叶茂盛或花开至三轮时采割。生用。

Features Flavor: pungent. Property: cool. Meridian tropism: the Lung Meridian and the Liver Meridian.

性味归经 辛，凉。归肺、肝经。

Actions Dispel wind and heat, clear and benefit head and eyes, benefit throat, promote eruption, soothe liver and promote qi flow.

功效 发散风热，清利头目，利咽，透疹，疏肝行气。

Application

应用

(1) Wind-heat pattern due to exogenous factors and early stage of febrile disease. The medicinal herb, light, clear and cool, acts to dispel wind and heat and clear head and eyes, applied to treat wind-

（1）外感风热，温病初起。本品轻清凉散，善散风热、清头目，常用于外感风热、温病初起，症见头痛、发

heat pattern due to exogenous factors and early stage of febrile disease manifested by headache, fever and slight aversion to wind, combined with *Schizonepetae Herba* (jing jie), *Lonicerae Japonicae Flos* (jin yin hua) and *Forsythiae Fructus* (lian qiao), to form up Lonicera and Forsythia Powder (Yin Qiao San).

热、微恶风者,可与荆芥、金银花、连翘等配伍同用,如银翘散。

(2) Sore throat and unsmooth eruption. The medicinal herb acts to dispel wind and heat, clear and benefit throat, relieve the exterior and promote eruption. In the treatment of sore throat due to wind and heat, it is combined with *Chrysanthemi Flos* (ju hua) and *Platycodonis Radix* (jie geng). In the treatment of wind-heat restraining the body surface and unsmooth eruption, it is combined with *Cimicifugae Rhizoma* (sheng ma) and *Schizonepetae Herba* (jing jie).

(2) 咽痛肿痛,疹发不畅。本品能宣散风热,清利咽喉,疏表透疹。常与菊花、桔梗等同用,治风热咽痛。与升麻、荆芥等同用,治风热束于肌表,疹发不畅。

(3) Liver qi stagnation pattern. The medicinal herb, attributive to the Liver Meridian, acts to soothe liver and promote qi flow. In the treatment of liver qi stagnation pattern manifested by stuffy chest and distension at hypochondria, it is combined with *Bupleuri Radix* (chai hu) and *Paeoniae Radix Alba* (bai shao), to form up Free Wanderer Powder (Xiao Yao San).

(3) 肝气郁滞证。本品兼入肝经,有疏肝行气作用。治肝气郁滞,胸胁胀闷,常与柴胡、白芍等配伍同用,如逍遥散。

Usage and dosage Apply 3～6 g in decoction by decocting later.

用法用量 煎服,3～6克,后下。

Precautions for use It is not advisable to apply for exterior deficiency pattern with spontaneous sweating, while it is cautious to apply for yin deficiency pattern with dryness in blood.

使用注意 表虚自汗者不宜用,阴虚血燥者慎用。

Arctii Fructus (niu bang zi)

牛蒡子

It is the dried product from the ripening fruit of

为菊科植物牛蒡的干燥

Arctum lappa L., family Compositae. The medicinal herb is collected in autumn, applied in crude form or fried form.

成熟果实。秋季采收。生用或炒用。

Features Flavor: pungent and bitter. Property: cold. Meridian tropism: the Lung Meridian and the Stomach Meridian.

性味归经 辛、苦,寒。归肺、胃经。

Actions Dispel wind and heat, benefit throat, promote eruption, relieve toxin and subside swell.

功效 发散风热,利咽透疹,解毒消肿。

Application

应用

(1) Wind-heat pattern due to exogenous factors. The medicinal herb acts to dispel wind and heat and clear and disperse lung qi. In the treatment of wind-heat pattern due to exogenous factors manifested by cough and unsmooth spitting sputum, it is combined with *Lonicerae Japonicae Flos* (jin yin hua) and *Platycodonis Radix* (jie geng).

(1) 外感风热。本品既疏散风热,又清宣肺气。治外感风热,症见咳嗽、吐痰不利等,常与金银花、桔梗等配伍同用。

(2) Sore throat. The medicinal herb, pungent, bitter and cold, acts to dispel wind and heat. In the treatment sore throat caused by wind-heat or by heat-toxin, it is combined with *Menthae Haplocalycis Herba* (bo he), jin yin hua and jie geng.

(2) 咽喉肿痛。本品辛散风热、苦寒清利。风热或热毒所致的咽喉肿痛皆可应用。常与薄荷、金银花、桔梗等配伍同用。

(3) Urticaria due to wind-heat. The medicinal herb acts to dispel wind and heat and promote eruption. In the treatment of urticaria due to wind and heat, it is combined with bo he, *Periostracum Cicadae* (chan tui) and *Puerariae Lobatae Radix* (ge gen).

(3) 风热发疹。本品能散风热,透疹。治风热发疹,常与薄荷、蝉蜕、葛根等同用。

(4) Carbuncle due to heat-toxin and mumps. The medicinal herb acts to dispel and relieve heat and toxin. In the treatment of carbuncle and mumps, it is combined with *Forsythiae Fructus* (lian qiao), *Isatidis Radix* (ban lan gen) and *Chrysanthemi Flos Indici* (ye ju hua).

(4) 热毒疮肿,痄腮。本品能清解热毒。治疮肿或痄腮,常与连翘、板蓝根、野菊花等配伍同用。

Usage and dosage Apply 6～12 g in decoction after smashing it. Its bitter flavor and cold property slightly decrease in prepared form by stir-frying.

用法用量 煎服，6～12克；入汤剂宜捣碎。炒用苦寒性略减。

Precautions for use Due its intestine lubricating action, it is cautious to apply for spleen deficiency pattern with loose feces.

使用注意 有滑肠之弊，脾虚便溏者慎用。

Mori Folium (sang ye)

桑叶

It is the dried product from the leaf of *Morus alba* L., family Moraceae. The medicinal herb is collected after early frost, applied in crude form.

为桑科植物桑的干燥叶。初霜后采收。生用。

Features Flavor: sweet and bitter. Property: cold. Meridian tropism: the Lung Meridian and the Liver Meridian.

性味归经 甘、苦，寒。归肺、肝经。

Actions Dispel wind and heat, clear lung, moisturize the dry, clear liver and brighten eyes.

功效 发散风热，清肺润燥，清肝明目。

Application

应用

(1) Wind-heat pattern due to exogenous factors and early stage of febrile disease. The medicinal herb acts to dispel wind and heat, applied to treat wind-heat pattern due to exogenous factors and early stage of febrile disease, combined with *Chrysanthemi Flos* (ju hua), *Forsythiae Fructus* (lian qiao) and *Platycodonis Radix* (jie geng), form up Mulberry and Chrysanthemum Drink (Sang Ju Yin).

（1）外感风热，温病初起。本品能轻疏风热，治外感风热、温病初起，常与菊花、连翘、桔梗等同用，如桑菊饮。

(2) Cough due to dryness-heat. The medicinal herb acts to clear heat from lung and moisturize lung from being dry. In the treatment of cough, scanty sputum, dry nose and throat, etc. due to dryness-heat, it is combined with *Armeniacae Amarum Semen* (ku xing ren), *Fritillariae Cirrhosae Bulbus* (chuan bei mu) and *Adenophorae Radix Tetraphyllae* (nan sha shen), form up Mulberry and Almond Decoction (Sang Xing Tang).

（2）燥热咳嗽。本品能清肺热、润肺燥。治燥热咳嗽痰少，鼻咽干燥等，常与杏仁、贝母、沙参等同用，如桑杏汤。

(3) Redness of eyes and blurring of vision. The medicinal herb acts to clear liver and brighten eyes. In the treatment of redness of eyes, dryness and pain of eyes, lacrimation, etc., due to excessive heat in Liver Meridian or due to wind-heat, it is combined with ju hua, *Cassiae Semen* (jue ming zi) and *Plantaginis Semen* (che qian zi). In the treatment of blurring of vision due to liver yin insufficiency, it is combined with *Semen Sesami Nigrum* (hei zhi ma) and made into honey pills of Mulberry and Sesame Pills (Sang Ma Wan).

（3）目赤昏花。本品能清肝明目。治肝经实热或风热所致目赤、涩痛、多泪等症，可与菊花、决明子、车前子等同用。若属肝阴不足，目暗昏花，可与黑芝麻配伍，作蜜丸服，如桑麻丸。

Usage and dosage　Apply 5～10 g in decoction.

用法用量　煎服，5～10克。

Chrysanthemi Flos (ju hua)

菊花

It is the dried product from the capitulum of the perennial herbaceous plant, *Chrysanthemum morifolium* Ramat, family Compositae. The medicinal herb is collected in late autumn when it is flowering. Due to different origins, its Chinese name varies as "bo ju", "chu ju" or "gong ju" produced in Anhui Province, "hang ju" produced in Zhejiang Province, and "huai ju", one of four "huai" herbs in Henan Province, produced in Henan Province. It is applied in crude form.

为菊科植物菊的干燥头状花序。秋末花盛开时分批采收。主产于安徽者，称"亳菊""滁菊""贡菊"。主产于浙江者，称"杭菊"。主产于河南者，称"怀菊"，为河南四大怀药之一。生用。

Features　Flavor: sweet and bitter. Property: slightly cold. Meridian tropism: the Lung Meridian and the Liver Meridian.

性味归经　甘、苦，微寒。归肺、肝经。

Actions　Dispel wind and heat, soothe liver, brighten eyes, clear heat and relieve toxicin.

功效　发散风热，平肝明目，清热解毒。

Application

应用

(1) Wind-heat pattern due to exogenous factors and early stage of febrile disease. The medicinal herb acts to dispel wind and cold. In the treatment

（1）外感风热，温病初起。本品能疏散风热，治外感风热或温病初起的发热、

of wind-heat pattern due to exogenous factors and early stage of febrile disease manifested by fever and headache, it is combined with *Mori Folium* (sang ye) and *Menthae Haplocalycis Herba* (bo he), to form up Mulberry and Chrysanthemum Drink (Sang Ju Yin).

头痛，常与桑叶、薄荷等同用，如桑菊饮。

(2) Headache and vertigo. The medicinal herb acts to soothe liver and subdue yang. In the treatment of liver yang hyperactivity pattern manifested by headache and vertigo, it is combined with *Haliotidis Concha* (shi jue ming), *Paeoniae Radix Alba* (bai shao) and *Uncariae Ramulus cum Uncis* (gou teng).

（2）头痛眩晕。本品能平肝阳，治肝阳上亢的头痛眩晕，常与石决明、白芍、钩藤等同用。

(3) Redness of eyes due to heat in liver and blurring of vision due to liver deficiency. The medicinal herb acts to clear heat from liver. In the treatment of redness, swelling and pain of eyes due to wind-heat in the Liver Meridian or due to liver fire flaring-up, it is combined with sang ye and *Prunellae Spica* (xia ku cao) which acts to clear heat from liver. In the treatment of blurring of vision due to liver deficiency, it acts to brighten eyes, combined with *Lycii Fructus* (gou qi zi) and *Rehmanniae Radix Praeparata* (shu di huang), to form up Lycium, Chrysanthemun and Rehmannia Pills (Qi Ju Di Huang Wan).

（3）肝热目赤，肝虚目昏。本品治肝经风热或肝火上攻的目赤肿痛，能清肝热，常与桑叶、夏枯草等清肝热药同用。治肝虚目昏，视物不清，能明目，可与枸杞子、熟地黄等同用，如杞菊地黄丸。

(4) Carbuncles and ulcers due to toxin. The medicinal herb acts to treat carbuncles and ulcers, combined with *Lonicerae Japonicae Flos* (jin yin hua) and *Glycyrrhizae Radix et Rhizoma* (gan cao).

（4）疔疮肿毒。本品尤善治疔毒，常与金银花、生甘草等同用。

Usage and dosage Apply 5～10 g in decoction. The medicinal herb in yellow is applied to dispel wind and heat, while that in white is applied to soothe liver and brighten eyes.

用法用量 煎服，5～10克。疏散风热多用黄菊花；平肝明目多用白菊花。

Bupleuri Radix (chai hu)

It is the dried product from the root of the Perennial herbaceous plant, *Bulpleurum chinense* Dc. or *Bulpleurum scorzonerifolium* Willd., family Umbelliferae. The medicinal herb is collected in spring and autumn, applied in crude form or vinegar-baked form.

Features　Flavor: bitter and pungent. Property: slightly cold. Meridian tropism: the Liver Meridian and the Gallbladder Meridian.

Actions　Dispel wind, eliminate heat, soothe liver, relieve depression and elevate yang qi.

Application

(1) Fever due to exogenous factors and alternate chills and fever. The medicinal herb acts to relieve the exterior and eliminate heat. In the treatment of fever due to exogenous factors, it is combined with *Puerariae Lobatae Radix* (ge gen), *Scutellariae Radix* (huang qin) and *Gypsum Fibrosum* (shi gao), to form up Bupleurum and Pueraria Muscle-Relaxing Decoction (Chai Ge Jie Ji Tang). The medicinal herb acts to dispel the pathogens locating in Shaoyang or the semi-exterior and semi-interior part. In the treatment of alternate chills and fever in Shaoyang pattern, it is combined with huang qin and *Pinelliae Rhizoma* (ban xia), to form up Minor Bupleurum Decoction (Xiao Chai Hu Tang).

(2) Liver qi stagnation pattern. The medicinal herb acts to soothe liver and relieve depression. In the treatment of irregular menstruation or dysmenorrheal due to liver qi stagnation, it is combined with *Angelicae Sinensis Radix* (dang gui) and *Paeoniae Radix Alba* (bai

柴胡

为伞形科植物柴胡和狭叶柴胡的干燥根。前者称“北柴胡”,后者称“南柴胡”。春、秋季采挖。生用,或醋炙。

性味归经　苦、辛,微寒。归肝、胆经。

功效　疏散退热,疏肝解郁,升举阳气。

应用

(1) 外感发热,寒热往来。本品能透表泄热,治外感发热,常与葛根、黄芩、石膏等同用,如柴葛解肌汤。本品尤善疏散少阳半表半里之邪,治少阳证寒热往来,可与黄芩、半夏等同用,如小柴胡汤。

(2) 肝郁气滞证。本品功善疏肝解郁。治肝郁月经不调或痛经,常与当归、白芍等配伍同用,如逍遥散。治肝郁胁痛,常与香附、川芎等

shao) to form up Free Wanderer Powder (Xiao Yao San). In the treatment of hypochondriac pain due to liver qi stagnation, it is combined with *Cyperi Rhizoma* (xiang fu) and *Chuanxiong Rhizoma* (chuan xiong), to form up Bupleurum Liver-Soothing Powder (Chai Hu Shu Gan San).

同用，如柴胡疏肝散。

(3) Qi deficiency and sinking pattern. The medicinal herb acts to elevate yang qi. In the treatment of qi deficiency and sinking pattern manifested by chronic diarrhea and prolapse of rectum, it is combined with *Cimicifugae Rhizoma* (sheng ma) and *Astragali Radix* (huang qi), to form up Center-Supplementing Qi-Boosting Decoction (Bu Zhong Yi Qi Tang).

(3) 气虚下陷证。本品能升举阳气。治气虚下陷的久泻脱肛诸证，常与升麻、黄芪等同用，如补中益气汤。

Usage and dosage Apply 3～10 g in decoction. The medicinal herb in crude form is applied to relieve the exterior and dispel heat, while that in prepared form with vinegar is applied to soothe liver and relieve depression.

用法用量 煎服，3～10克。生用疏散退热，醋炙疏肝解郁。

Precautions for use It is prohibited to apply for liver yang inducing wind pattern and yin deficiency and fire flaring-up pattern.

使用注意 阳亢风动，阴虚火旺者忌用。

Cimicifugae Rhizoma (sheng ma)

升麻

It is the dried product from the rhizome of *Cimicifuga heracleifolia* kom., *Cimicifuga dahurica* (Turcz.) Maxim. and *Cimicifuga foetida* L., family Ranunculaceae. The medicinal herb is collected in autumn, applied in crude form.

为毛茛科植物大三叶升麻、兴安升麻或升麻的干燥根茎。秋季采挖。生用。

Features Flavor: pungent and slightly sweet. Property: slightly cold. Meridian tropism: the Lung Meridian, the Spleen Meridian, the Stomach Meridian and the Large Intestine Meridian.

性味归经 辛、微甘，微寒。归肺、脾、胃、大肠经。

Actions Relieve the exterior, promote

功效 发表透疹，清热

eruption, clear heat, relieve toxin and elevate yang qi.

解毒,升举阳气。

Application

(1) Headache due to wind-heat and unsmooth eruption. The medicinal herb acts to relieve the exterior, dispel heat and promote eruption. In the treatment of headache due to wind-heat or unsmooth eruption, it is combined with *Puerariae Lobatae Radix* (ge gen) and *Glycyrrhizae Radix et Rhizoma* (gan cao), to form up Cimicifuga and Pueraria Decoction (Sheng Ma Ge Gen Tang).

(2) All of heat-toxin patterns. The medicinal herb acts to clear heat and relieve toxin, especially to remove heat-toxin in the Yangming Meridians. In the treatment of excessive heat in the Yangming Meridians pattern manifested by headache, toothache, ulcers on tongue and in mouth, it is combined with *Coptidis Rhizoma* (huang lian) and *Gypsum Fibrosum* (shi gao), to form up Stomach-Clearing Powder (Qing Wei San). In the treatment of sore throat due to wind-heat, it is combined with *Platycodonis Radix* (jie geng) and *Scrophulariae Radix* (xuan shen). In the treatment of carbuncles and ulcers due to heat-toxin, it is combined with *Taraxaci Herba* (pu gong ying), *Lonicerae Japonicae Flos* (jin yin hua) and *Forsythiae Fructus* (lian qiao).

(3) Qi deficiency and sinking pattern. The medicinal herb acts to elevate yang qi. In the treatment of qi deficiency and sinking pattern manifested by chronic diarrhea and prolapse of rectum, it is combined with *Bupleuri Radix* (chai hu) and *Astragali Radix* (huang qi), to form up Center-Supplementing Qi-Boosting Decoction (Bu Zhong Yi Qi Tang). In the treatment of heavy uterine bleeding

应用

(1) 风热头痛,疹发不畅。本品能升散发表,解热透疹。治风热头痛,或疹发不畅,可配伍葛根、甘草等同用,如升麻葛根汤。

(2) 热毒诸证。本品善清热解毒,尤善清阳明热毒。治阳明热盛的头痛、牙龈肿痛、口舌生疮等证,常与黄连、石膏等配伍同用,如清胃散。治风热咽痛,常配伍桔梗、玄参等同用。治热毒疮痈,常与蒲公英、金银花、连翘等同用。

(3) 气虚下陷证。本品能升气举陷。治气虚下陷的久泻脱肛等证,常与柴胡、黄芪等同用,如补中益气汤;治气不摄血的崩漏不止,可与人参、黄芪等同用。

due to qi failing to check blood, it is combined with *Ginseng Radix et Raizoma* (ren shen) and huang qi.

Usage and dosage Apply 3～10 g in decoction.

用法用量 煎服，3～10克。

Precautions for use It is prohibited to apply for yin deficiency and yang floating pattern, panting due to up-reverse flow of qi and erupted measles.

使用注意 阴虚阳浮，喘满气逆，麻疹已透者忌用。

Puerariae Lobatae Radix (ge gen)

葛根

It is the dried product from the roots of *Pueraria lobata* (Willd.) Ohwi, family Leguminosae. The medicinal herb is collected in autumn and winter, applied in crude form.

为豆科植物野葛的干燥根。秋、冬季采挖。生用。

Features Flavor: sweet and pungent. Property: cool. Meridian tropism: the Spleen Meridian and the Stomach Meridian.

性味归经 甘、辛，凉。归脾、胃经。

Actions Relieve the exterior, reduce heat, promote eruption, produce fluid, stop thirst, elevate yang and stop diarrhea.

功效 解肌退热，透疹，生津止渴，升阳止泻。

Application

应用

(1) Exterior pattern due to exogenous factors. The medicinal herb acts to relieve the exterior and reduce heat. In the treatment of exterior pattern due to exogenous wind-cold manifested by aversion to cold, absence of sweating, stiffness and pain at nape and upper back, it is combined with *Ephedrae Herba* (ma huang) and *Cinnamomi Ramulus* (gui zhi). In the treatment of exterior pattern due to exogenous wind-heat, it is combined with *Bupleuri Radix* (chai hu), *Gypsum Fibrosum* (shi gao) and *Scutellariae Radix* (huang qin), to form up Bupleurum and Pueraria Muscle-Relaxing Decoction (Chai Ge Jie Ji Tang).

(1) 外感表证。本品能发表解肌退热。治外感风寒表证，恶寒无汗、项背强痛者，可配麻黄、桂枝等同用。外感表证郁而化热者，常与柴胡、石膏、黄芩等同用，如柴葛解肌汤。

(2) Unsmooth eruption. The medicinal herb

(2) 疹发不畅。本品能

acts to promote eruption. In the treatment of early stage of measles with unsmooth eruption, it is combined with *Cimicifugae Rhizoma* (sheng ma) and *Radix Paeoniae* (shao yao).

发散透疹。治麻疹初起，疹出不畅，常与升麻、芍药等同用。

(3) Restlessness and thirst in febrile disease and diabetes due to internal heat. The medicinal herb acts to produce fluid and stop thirst. In the treatment of restlessness and thirst due to febrile disease which consumes body fluid, it is combined with *Phragmitis Rhizoma* (lu gen) and *Trichosanthis Radix* (tian hua fen). In the treatment of diabetes due to internal heat, it is combined with tian hua fen and *Ophiopogonis Radix* (mai men dong), to form up Jade Spring Pills (Yu Quan Wan).

（3）热病烦渴，内热消渴。本品能生津止渴。治热病伤津烦渴，常与芦根、天花粉等同用；治内热消渴，常与天花粉、麦冬等配伍，如玉泉丸。

(4) Diarrhea and dysentery due to damp-heat, diarrhea due to spleen deficiency. The medicinal herb acts to elevate yang so as to stop diarrhea. In the treatment of diarrhea and dysentery due to damp-heat, it is combined with *Coptidis Rhizoma* (huang lian) and huang qin, to form up Pueraria, Scutellaria and Copitis Decoction (Ge Gen Qin Lian Tang). In the treatment of diarrhea due to spleen deficiency, it is combined with *Codonopsis Radix Pilosulae* (dang shen), *Atractylodis Rhizoma Macrocephalae* (bai zhu) and *Poria* (fu ling), to form up Atractylodes Powder with Seven Ingredients (Qi Wei Bai Zhu San).

（4）湿热泻痢，脾虚泄泻。本品能升发清阳而止泻。治湿热泻痢，可与黄连、黄芩等配伍同用，如葛根芩连汤。治脾虚泄泻，常配伍党参、白术、茯苓等同用，如七味白术散。

Usage and dosage　Apply 10～15 g in decoction.

用法用量　煎服，10～15克。

Sojae Semen Praeparatum (dan dou chi)

淡豆豉

It is the product prepared by fermenting the seed of *Glycine max* (L.) Merr., family Leguminosae, applied in crude form.

为豆科植物大豆的成熟种子的发酵加工品。生用。

Features Flavor: bitter and pungent. Property: cool. Meridian tropism: the Lung Meridian and the Stomach Meridian.

性味归经 苦、辛，凉。归肺、胃经。

Actions Relieve the exterior, reduce restlessness, disperse and dispel heat.

功效 解表，除烦，宣发郁热。

Application

应用

(1) Exterior pattern due to exogenous factors. The medicinal herb acts to relieve the exterior with a slight effect. In the treatment of exterior pattern due to exogenous wind-heat and early stage of febrile disease, it is combined with *Lonicerae Japonicae Flos* (jin yin hua), *Forsythiae Fructus* (lian qiao) and *Menthae Haplocalycis Herba* (bo he). In the treatment of exterior pattern due to exogenous wind-cold, it is combined with *Bulbus Allii Fistulosi* (cong bai) and *Platycodonis Radix* (jie geng).

(1) 外感表证。本品能解表，单用力薄。治外感风热，温病初起，常与金银花、连翘、薄荷等同用。治风寒表证，常与葱白、桔梗等同用。

(2) Restlessness and boredom in febrile disease. The medicinal herb acts to dispel exogenous factors and disperse heat. In the treatment of restlessness, boredom and poor sleep in febrile disease, it is combined with *Gardeniae Fructus* (zhi zi), to form up Capejasmine and Fermented Soy Bean Decoction (Zhi Zi Chi Tang).

(2) 热病烦闷。本品能透散外邪，宣发郁热。治热病胸中烦闷、不眠，每与栀子配伍同用，即栀子豉汤。

Usage and dosage Apply 6～12 g in decoction.

用法用量 煎服，6～12克。

Brief summary

小　结

1 Wind-cold-dissipating herbs

1 发散风寒药

Both *Ephedrae Herba* (ma huang) and *Cinnamomi Ramulus* (gui zhi) act to make sweating and relieve the exterior. Ma huang has a strong effect to make sweating, often applied to treat exterior ex-

麻黄、桂枝，均能发汗解表。其中麻黄发汗力强，多用于风寒表证表实无汗；桂枝发汗力弱，治风寒表证无

cess pattern due to wind-cold manifested by absence of sweating, while gui zhi has a slight effect to make sweating, it is advisable to treat exterior excess pattern with absence of sweating, and exterior deficiency pattern with sweating as well. Ma huang also acts to disperse lung, soothe panting, promote waterflow and subside swell, as the major herb to soothe panting, applied to treat coughing and panting due to lung qi failing to disperse. Gui zhi also acts to warm meridians and dredge vessels, assist yang and transform qi, applied to treat cold coagulation and blood stasis manifested by joint pain due to wind-damp, cold pain at epigastria and abdomen and dysmenorrhea, heart yang dispiritedness pattern manifested by chest pain, and edema, phlegm and rheum due to yang deficiency.

论表实无汗还是表虚有汗皆宜。麻黄又能宣肺平喘、利水消肿，尤为平喘要药，善治肺气不宣之喘咳。桂枝又温经通脉、助阳化气，治寒凝血滞之风湿痹痛、脘腹冷痛、痛经，以及心阳不振的胸痹，阳虚水肿、痰饮等。

Both *Perillae Folium* (zi su ye) and *Zingiberis Rhizoma Recens* (sheng jiang) act to make sweating, relieve the exterior and relieve toxin from fish and crab. Zi su ye has a strong effect to make sweating and acts to promote qi flow, applied to treat exterior pattern due to wind-cold without sweating or with qi stagnation. It also acts to promote qi flow and dilate middle energizer, applied to treat qi stagnation of spleen and stomach, or morning sickness. Sheng jiang has a slight effect to make sweating, applied to treat mild condition of exterior pattern due to wind-cold. It also acts to warm middle energizer, stop vomiting, warm lung and stop coughing, applied to stop vomiting and relieve toxin from herbs.

紫苏、生姜，均能发汗解表、解鱼蟹毒。其中紫苏发汗力强，兼能行气，常用于风寒表证无汗或兼气滞者；又能行气宽中，治脾胃气滞证或妊娠呕吐。生姜发汗力弱，常用于风寒表证治轻证；又能温中止呕、温肺止咳，尤善止呕，还能解药物毒。

Herba Elsholtziae (xiang ru) acts to make sweating and relieve the exterior, but it is pungent but not hot, and also acts to dissolve damp and harmonize middle energizer, so it is taken as the major herb to

香薷虽能发汗解表，但其辛而不热，兼能化湿和中，故为治暑天外感风寒证之要药，有“夏月麻黄”之称，又能

treat exterior pattern due to exogenous wind-cold in summer, known as "ma huang in summer". It also acts to promote waterflow and subside swell.

利水消肿。

Both *Schizonepetae Herba* (jing jie) and *Saposhnikoviae Radix* (fang feng) are pungent in flavor and lightly warm in property. Due to their moderate property, they are applied to treat exterior patterns due to exogenous wind-cold and due to exogenous wind-heat. Jing jie is good at dispelling wind, as the commonly-used herb to disperse wind. It also acts to relieve carbuncles, promote eruption and stop itching, applied to treat carbuncles and ulcers with exterior pattern, and itching due to urticaria as well. Its carbonized form is astringent in property and acts to stanch bleeding, applied to treat various types of bleeding. Fang feng has a strong effect to dispel wind, sweet and moderate in property, and good at dispelling wind, dissolving damp and relieving pain, applied to treat Bi (Obturation) Pattern due to wind and damp, and also acting to dispel wind and relieve convulsion, applied to treat tetanus.

荆芥、防风，均味辛性微温，药性和缓，无论风寒、风热表证皆可应用。其中荆芥长于散风，为发表散风的通用药；又能消疮、透疹止痒，治疮疡兼表证以及风疹瘙痒；炒炭性涩止血，治多种出血。防风祛风力佳，甘缓不峻，且善祛风胜湿止痛，常用于风湿痹痛；还能祛风止痉，治破伤风。

All Rhizoma seu *Radix Notopterygii* (qiang huo), *Angelicae Dahuricae Radix* (bai zhi) and *Asari Radix et Rhizoma* (xi xin) act to relieve the exterior and dispel cold. Rhizoma seu qiang huo is pungent, bitter, warm and dry in property, has a strong effect to dispel cold and relieve pain, and acts to dissolve damp and relieve pain, applied to treat exterior pattern due to exogenous wind-cold manifested by obvious headache and general aching. Its action direction is ascending, so it is applied to treat Bi (Obturation) Pattern in upper part of body. Bai zhi acts to dispel wind and cold, open nose aperture and relieve pain with a slight effect in disper-

羌活、白芷、细辛，均能解表散寒。其中羌活辛苦温燥，散寒止痛力强，且能胜湿止痛，善治外感风寒头痛身痛明显者，其性善上行，可治上半身风湿痹痛。白芷功能祛风散寒，兼通鼻窍、止痛，发散力弱，善治阳明经头痛、齿痛；且能消肿排脓、燥湿止带，既为疮疡常用，又治妇女带下。细辛味辛性温，有小毒，功能祛风散寒，既治风寒表证，又疗阳虚外感；尤以散

sing, applied to treat headache and toothache of the Yangming Meridians. It acts to subside swell, drain apus, dry the damp and reduce vaginal discharge, applied to treat carbuncles and ulcers, and morbid leucorrhea as well. Xi xin is pungent in flavor and warm in property and slightly toxic. It acts to dispel wind and cold, applied to treat exterior pattern due to exogenous wind-cold, and also treat exterior pattern due to yang deficiency as well. It is good at dispelling cold and relieving pain, applied to treat various types of pain. It also acts to warm lung and dissolve rheum, applied to treat coughing and panting due to cold and rheum.

寒止痛力佳，善治多种疼痛；还能温肺化饮，治寒饮咳喘。

Both *Magnoliae Flos* (xin yi) and *Xanthii Fructus* (cang er zi) act to dispel wind and cold and open nose aperture. Xin yi is good at opening nose aperture, applied to treat nasal obstruction in exterior pattern due to exogenous wind-cold, and sinusitis as well. Cang er zi also acts to dispel wind and damp, applied to treat Bi (Obturation) Pattern due to wind and damp.

辛夷、苍耳子，均能散风寒、通鼻窍。其中辛夷功善通鼻窍，专治风寒表证兼鼻塞或鼻渊等证。苍耳子还能祛风湿，治风湿痹痛。

2 Wind-heat-dissipating herbs

2 发散风热药

Both *Menthae Haplocalycis Herba* (bo he) and *Arctii Fructus* (niu bang zi) act to dispel wind and heat, benefit throat and promote eruption, applied to treat exterior pattern due to exogenous wind-heat, early stage of febrile disease and itching due to urticaria. Bo he, pungent in flavor and cool in property, has a strong effect to make sweating with its action direction of ascending, and acts to clear and benefit head and eyes, mostly applied to treat exterior pattern due to exogenous wind-heat manifested by headache and absence of sweating. Besides, it acts to soothe

薄荷、牛蒡子，均能疏散风热、利咽透疹，治风热外感或温病初起，风疹瘙痒等证。其中薄荷辛凉，发汗力较强，性善上行，能清利头目，多用于风热表证头痛、无汗之证；且能疏肝解郁，治肝气郁滞，胸胁闷痛等证。牛蒡子辛苦性寒，发汗力虽较弱，兼能清宣肺气，多用于风热表证兼咳嗽痰多；且苦寒清泄，兼能

liver and relieve depression, applied to treat liver qi stagnation pattern manifested by stuffiness and pain at chest and hypochondria. Niu bang zi, pungent in flavor and cold in property, with slight effect to make sweating, acts to clear and disperse lung qi, applied to treat exterior pattern due to exogenous wind-heat manifested by cough with excessive sputum. Besides, the medicinal herb, bitter and cold, acts to lubricate intestines, applied to treat carbuncles and mumps due to heat-toxicity.

滑肠，多用于热毒疮肿痄腮等证。

Both *Mori Folium* (sang ye) and *Chrysanthemi Flos* (ju hua) acts to dispel wind and heat, soothe liver and brighten eyes, applied to treat exterior pattern due to exogenous wind-heat, early stage of febrile disease, dizziness due to liver yang, redness, swelling and pain of eyes due to the Liver Meridian wind-heat or liver fire, and blurred vision due to liver deficiency. Sang ye acts to clear heat from lung and moisturize lung, applied to treat cough due to heat or dryness in lung. Ju hua acts to soothe liver yang and clear heat from liver, applied to treat dizziness due to liver yang hyperactivity and redness of eyes due to liver fire. It also acts to clear heat and relieve toxicity, applied to treat carbuncles, ulcers and swelling due to toxicity.

桑叶、菊花，均能疏散风热、平肝明目，治风热外感或温病初起，肝阳眩晕，肝经风热或肝火之目赤肿痛，以及肝虚视物不清。其中桑叶功善清肺热、润肺燥，善治肺热或肺燥咳嗽。菊花功善平肝阳、清肝热，善治肝阳上亢之眩晕，以及肝火目赤等证；且能清热解毒，治疗疮肿毒。

All *Bupleuri Radix* (chai hu), *Cimicifugae Rhizoma* (sheng ma) and *Puerariae Lobatae Radix* (ge gen) act to relieve the exterior and elevate yang, applied to treat exterior pattern and qi deficiency and sinking pattern. Chai hu, bitter, pungent in flavor and slightly cold in property, acts to dispel heat, and attributive to the Liver Meridian, acts to dispel pathogens in Shaoyang and semi-exterior-semi-interior part, applied to treat alternate chills

柴胡、升麻、葛根，均能发表、升阳，均治表证及气虚下陷证。其中，柴胡苦辛微寒，能疏散退热，入肝胆经，尤善疏散少阳半表半里之邪，治少阳寒热往来及外感发热；且能疏肝解郁。升麻辛微甘微寒，能发表透疹，为治疹发不畅所常用；且能清

and fever due to Shaoyang disease and fever due to exogenous factors. It also acts to soothe liver and relieve depression. Sheng ma, pungent and slightly sweet in flavor and slightly cold in property, acts to relieve the exterior and promote eruption, applied to treat unsmooth eruption in measles. It also acts to relieve heat-toxicity in the Yangming part, applied to treat headache, toothache and ulcers in mouth due to excessive heat in the Yangming Meridians. Ge gen, sweet and pungent in flavor and cool in property, acts to relieve the exterior and dispel heat, applied to treat exterior pattern manifested by stiffness and pain at nape and upper back. It acts to produce fluid and stop thirst, applied to treat thirst due to febrile disease and diabetes due to yin deficiency. It also acts to stop diarrhea and promote eruption, applied to treat diarrhea, dysentery and unsmooth eruption. In terms of action to elevate yang, chai hu and sheng ma act to elevate the clear yang, applied to treat qi deficiency and sinking pattern, and prolapse of internal organs, while ge gen acts to inspire ascent of clear yang of spleen and stomach so as to stop diarrhea and dysentery, applied to treat diarrhea and dysentery due to damp-heat, and diarrhea due to spleen deficiency as well.

解阳明热毒，治阳明热盛的头痛、牙龈肿痛、口疮等证。葛根甘辛性凉，能发表解肌退热，善治表证兼项背强痛者；且能生津止渴，治热病口渴及阴虚消渴；还能止泻、透疹，治泻痢及疹发不畅。就升阳功效而言，柴胡、升麻为升清阳以举陷，多治气虚下陷、脏器脱垂诸证；葛根则以鼓舞脾胃清阳上升而止泻痢，无论湿热泻痢还是脾虚泄泻，皆可应用。

Semen Sojae Praeparatum (dan dou chi), bitter and pungent in flavor and cool in property, acts to relieve the exterior, reduce restlessness, and disperse and dispel depressed heat, applied to treat exterior pattern due to exogenous factors, and to treat restlessness and boredom in febrile disease as well. It is weak in action, so the medicinal herb is often applied with combination of other medicinal herbs.

淡豆豉苦辛性凉，功能解表除烦，宣发郁热，既治外感表证，又治热病烦闷，单用力薄，多配伍应用。

Chapter 2 Heat-Clearing Herbs

第2章 清热药

The Chinese medicinal herbs acting to reduce the interior heat, applied to treat the interior heat patterns are called the heat-clearing herbs.

Since the interior heat patterns possess different pathogenic factors, different diseases stages, different locations of disease and different patterns, it is advisable to select targeted heat-clearing herbs. The heat clearing herbs act to clear the interior heat, but some act to reduce fire, some act to cool blood, some act to relieve toxicity, some act to remove damp-heat, and some act to treat false heat, so they have their own strengthens. According to their major actions, the heat-clearing herbs are divided into heat-clearing and fire-reducing herbs, heat-clearing and damp-desiccating herbs, heat-clearing and toxin-relieving herbs, heat-clearing and blood-cooling herbs and false heat-clearing herbs.

The heat-clearing and fire-reducing herbs, mostly bitter in flavor and cold in property or sweet in flavor and cold in property, act to clear heat and reduce fire, applied to treat excessive heat pattern in Qi (Energy) Phase manifested by high fever, restlessness and thirst, or to treat heat of various zang-fu organs. The heat-clearing and damp-desiccating herbs, mostly bitter in flavor and dry and cold in property, act to clear heat and desiccate damp, applied to treat damp-heat patterns manifested by diarrhea, dysentery and jaun-

以清解里热为主要作用,用治里热证的药物,称为清热药。

由于里热证有不同的致病因素和疾病阶段,以及发病部位的不同,证型多种,宜选择针对性强的清热药进行治疗。清热药虽均能清里热,然或功偏泻火、或能凉血、或善解毒、或祛湿热、或疗虚热,各有所长。根据清热药的主要性能,清热药可分为清热泻火药、清热燥湿药、清热解毒药、清热凉血药、清虚热药。

清热泻火药性味多属苦寒或甘寒,功能清热泻火,主要用于气分实热的高热烦渴,或诸脏腑之热。清热燥湿药性味多苦燥性寒,功能清热燥湿,主要用于湿温、湿热泻痢、湿热黄疸等湿热病证。清热解毒药性味多苦寒,功能清解热毒或火毒,主要用于热毒炽盛的疮痈、泻

dice. The heat-clearing and toxin-relieving herbs, mostly bitter in flavor and cold in property, act to clear and relieve heat-toxin or fire-toxin, applied to treat heat-toxin flaming pattern manifested by sores, carbuncle, diarrhea, dysentery and sore throat. The heat-clearing and blood-cooling herbs, mostly sweet, bitter and salty in flavor and cold in property, act to clear heat from Ying (Nutrient) Phase and to nourish yin, applied to treat heat entering Ying (Nutrient) Phase and Xue (Blood) Phase pattern, manifested by high fever, loss of consciousness, hemoptysis and skin plaques. The false heat-clearing herbs, mostly cool in property, act to clear false heat and reduce fever, applied to treat heat pattern due to deficiency manifested by tidal fever, or feverish sensation at night and cool sensation during day.

痢、咽喉肿痛等证。清热凉血药性味大多甘苦咸寒，功能清解营血之热，兼能养阴，主要用于热入营血，高热神昏、吐衄发斑等证。清虚热药性凉，功能清虚热、退骨蒸，用于骨蒸潮热、或夜热朝凉等虚热证。

Notes for attention in application of heat-clearing herbs: The heat-clearing herbs are cool or cold in property and easy to injure spleen and stomach, so it is cautious to apply them for those with spleen and stomach deficiency, poor appetite and loose feces. The bitter and dry herbs are easy to consume yin, so it is cautious to apply them or advisable to apply them with yin-nourishing and fluid-producing herbs for those with yin deficiency. It is remarkable to stop applying the medicinal herbs when the disease is cured, for the purpose to prevent damage of the Zheng (Anti-Pathogenic) Qi.

使用清热药应注意：清热药药性寒凉，易伤脾胃，故脾胃虚弱、食少便溏者慎用。苦燥容易伤阴，阴虚者慎用，或与养阴生津药同用。注意中病即止，避免损伤正气。

Section 1 Heat-clearing and fire-reducing herbs

第1节 清热泻火药

Gypsum Fibrosum (shi gao)

It is the product from the monoclinic system of

石膏

为硫酸盐类矿物硬石膏

gypsum ore, containing hydrous calcium surfate ($CaSO_4 \cdot 2H_2O$). The medicinal is collected in winter, applied in crude form or in baked form.

族石膏，主要成分为含水硫酸钙($CaSO_4 \cdot 2H_2O$)。冬季采挖。生用或煅用。

Features Property: greatly cold. Property: pungent and sweet. Meridian tropism: the Lung Meridian and the Stomach Meridian.

性味归经 辛、甘，大寒。归肺、胃经。

Actions Clear heat, reduce fire, relieve boredom and stop thirst. Astringe damp and restrain ulcers in external use.

功效 清热泻火，除烦止渴，外用收湿敛疮。

Application

应用

(1) Febrile disease due to exogenous factors, high fever, restlessness and thirst. The medicinal herb, greatly cold, acts to clear heat and reduce fire, and pungent and sweet, acts to reduce heat and stop thirst. In the treatment of febrile disease due to exogenous factors manifested by high fever, restlessness, thirst and surging pulse, it is combined with *Anemarrhenae Rhizoma* (zhi mu), to form up White Tiger Decoction (Bai Hu Tang).

（1）外感热病，高热烦渴。本品大寒清热泻火，辛甘除热止渴，善治外感热病，高热烦渴，脉洪大，常与知母配伍同用，如白虎汤。

(2) Coughing and panting due to heat in lung. The medicinal herb acts to clear heat from lung. In the treatment of cough, thick sputum and shortness of breath due to heat in lung, it is combined with *Ephedrae Herba* (ma huang), *Armeniacae Amarum Semen* (ku xing ren) and *Glycyrrhizae Radix et Rhizoma* (gan cao), to form up Ephedra, Apricot, Gypsum and Liquorice Decoction (Ma Xing Shi Gan Tang).

（2）肺热喘咳。本品善清肺热。治肺热咳嗽、痰稠气急，常配伍麻黄、杏仁、甘草同用，即麻杏石甘汤。

(3) Toothache due to heat in stomach. The medicinal herb acts to clear fire from stomach. In the treatment of stomach heat pattern or yin deficiency pattern manifested by swollen and painful gum, headache, restlessness and thirst, it is combined with zhi mu, *Achyranthis Bidentatae Radix* (niu xi) and *Ophiopogonis Radix* (mai men dong), to form

（3）胃火牙痛。本品又能清胃火。治胃热阴虚所致的牙龈肿痛、头痛烦渴，常与知母、牛膝、麦冬等同用，如玉女煎。

up Jade Lady Decoction (Yu Nü Jian).

(4) Incurred carbuncle and ulcer, itch due to eczema, scalded wound and burnt wound. The baked herb is smashed into powder and applied on the surface of wound, for the purpose to astringe damp and restrain ulcers, promote tissue regeneration and stanch bleeding, applied to treat incurred carbuncle and ulcer, eczema, scalded wound and burnt wound.

（4）疮疡不敛，湿疹瘙痒，水火烫伤。煅石膏外用研末撒敷能收湿敛疮、生肌止血，治疮疡溃烂不敛，湿疹、水火烫伤等。

Usage and dosage Apply 15～60 g in decoction, decocted first after smashing it. It is applied in crude form in oral administration for the purpose to clear heat, reduce fire, relieve restlessness and stop thirst. It is applied in baked form in external use for the purpose to astringe damp and restrain ulcer with its astringent property. A proper amount of the medicinal herb is smashed into powder and applied on the surface of wound.

用法用量 煎服，15～60 克。打碎先煎。内服生用，清热泻火，除烦止渴。煅后外用，性涩收湿敛疮，取适量，研末撒敷患处。

Precautions for use It is cautious to apply for those with deficiency and cold of spleen and stomach.

使用注意 脾胃虚寒者慎用。

Anemarrhenae Rhizoma (zhi mu)

知母

It is the dried product from the rhizome of a perennial herbaceous plant, *Anemarrhena asphodeloides* Bunge, family Liliaceae. The medicinal herb is collected in spring and autumn, applied in crude form or stir-baked form with salt solution.

为百合科植物知母的干燥根茎。春、秋季采挖。生用或盐水炙用。

Features Flavor: bitter and sweet. Property: cold. Meridian tropism: the Lung Meridian, the Stomach Meridian and the Kidney Meridian.

性味归经 苦、甘，寒。归肺、胃、肾经。

Actions Clear heat, reduce fire, nourish yin and moisturize dryness.

功效 清热泻火，滋阴润燥。

Application

应用

(1) Febrile disease due to exogenous factors,

（1）外感热病，高热烦

high fever, restlessness and thirst. The medicinal herb is bitter and cold and acts to clear heat and reduce fire, and sweet and cold and acts to relieve restlessness and stop thirst. In the treatment of febrile disease manifested by high fever, restlessness and thirst, it is combined with *Gypsum Fibrosum* (shi gao), to form up White Tiger Decoction (Bai Hu Tang).

渴。本品苦寒清泄泻火，甘寒除烦止渴。常与石膏同用，治热病高热烦渴，如白虎汤。

(2) Cough due to heat in lung and dry cough due to yin deficiency. The medicinal herb acts to clear heat from lung and moisturize lung to eliminate dryness. In the treatment of cough due to heat in lung with yellow-thick sputum, it is combined with *Bulbus Fritillariae Thunbergii* (zhe bei mu), *Scutellariae Radix* (huang qin) and *Cortex Mori Albae Radicis* (sang bai pi). In the treatment of cough due to yin deficiency with scanty sputum, it is combined with *Fritillariae Cirrhosae Bulbus* (chuan bei mu), to form up Anemarrhena and Fritillary Powder (Er Mu San).

（2）肺热咳嗽，阴虚燥咳。本品能清肺热、润肺燥。治肺热咳嗽，痰黄稠厚，常与贝母、黄芩、桑白皮等同用。治阴虚燥咳少痰，常配伍贝母同用，即二母散。

(3) Diabetes due to yin deficiency. The medicinal herb is sweet and cold and acts to nourish yin, moisturize dryness and produce fluid. In the treatment of diabetes due to yin deficiency, it is combined with *Trichosanthis Radix* (tian hua fen), *Puerariae Lobatae Radix* (ge gen) and *Dioscoreae Rhizoma* (shan yao), to form up Jade Fluid Decoction (Yu Ye Tang).

（3）阴虚消渴。本品甘寒滋阴，润燥生津。治阴虚消渴，可与天花粉、葛根、山药等同用，如玉液汤。

(4) Feverish sensation and tidal fever. The medicinal herb acts to nourish kidney, reduce fire, eliminate heat and relieve feverish sensation. In the treatment of kidney yin deficiency pattern manifested by feverish sensation, tidal fever, seminal emission and nocturnal sweats, it is combined with

（4）骨蒸潮热。本品能滋肾降火、除热退蒸。治肾阴亏虚所致骨蒸潮热，遗精盗汗，常与黄柏、山茱萸等同用，如知柏地黄丸，或配伍龟甲、黄柏、熟地黄等同用，如

Cortex Phellodendri (huang bo) and *Corni Fructus* (shan zhu yu), to form up Anemarrhena, Phellodendron, and Rehmannia Pills (Zhi Bai Di Huang Wan), or combined with *Testudinis Carapax et Plastrum* (gui ban), *Phellodendri Cortex Chiensis* (huang bo) and *Rehmanniae Radix Praeparata* (shu di huang), to form up Great Yin-Supplementation Pills (Da Bu Yin Wan).

大补阴丸。

Usage and dosage Apply 6～12 g in decoction. It is applied to clear heat and reduce fire in crude form, while to nourish yin and moisturize dryness in prepared form stir-baked with salt solution.

用法用量 煎服，6～12克。生用清热泻火，盐水炙滋阴润燥。

Precautions for use The medicinal herb is easy to lubricate intestines, so it is not advisable to apply for those with loose feces due to spleen deficiency.

使用注意 易滑肠，脾虚便溏者不宜用。

Gardeniae Fructus (zhi zi)

栀子

It is the dried product from the fruit of *Gardenia jasminoides* Ellis var. radicans (Thumb.) Makino, family Rubiaceae. The medicinal herb is collected in summer and autumn and applied in crude form, in stir-baked form or in carbonized form.

为茜草科植物栀子的干燥成熟果实。夏、秋季采收。生用、炒用或炒焦用。

Features Flavor: bitter. Property: cold. Meridian tropism: the Heart Meridian, the Lung Meridian and the Triple Energizer Meridian.

性味归经 苦，寒。归心、肺、三焦经。

Actions Reduce fire, relieve restlessness, clear heat, dissolve damp, cool blood and relieve toxin. Subside swell and relieve pain for external use.

功效 泻火除烦，清热利湿，凉血解毒，外用消肿止痛。

Application

应用

(1) Febrile disease with restlessness. The medicinal herb is bitter and cold and acts to reduce fire

(1) 热病烦闷。本品苦寒，能泻三焦之火、清心除

from triple energizer, applied to purify heart and relieve restlessness. In the treatment of febrile disease manifested by restlessness, uneasiness and agitation, it is combined with *Sojae Semen Praeparatum* (dan dou chi), to form up Capejasmine and Fermented Soy Bean Decoction (Zhi Zi Chi Tang). In the treatment of heat excess pattern manifested by high fever, restlessness, loss of consciousness and delirium, it is combined with *Scutellariae Radix* (huang qin), *Coptidis Rhizoma* (huang lian) and *Forsythiae Fructus* (lian qiao), to form up Scourge-Clearing Detoxifying Drink (Qing Wen Bai Du Yin).

烦。治热病心烦、躁扰不宁，常与淡豆豉配伍，即栀子豉汤。治热盛高热烦躁，神昏谵语，可与黄芩、黄连、连翘等同用，如清瘟败毒饮。

(2) Jaundice due to damp-heat. The medicinal herb acts to clear heat, dissolve damp, benefit gallbladder and reduce jaundice. In the treatment of jaundice due to damp-heat, it is combined with *Artemisiae Scopariae Herba* (yin chen hao) and *Rhei Radix et Rhizoma* (da huang), to form up Artemisia Decoction (Yin Chen Hao Tang), or combined with *Phellodendri Cortex Chiensis* (huang bo) and *Glycyrrhizae Radix et Rhizoma* (gan cao), to form up Capejasmine, Phellodendron and White Mulberry Bark Decoction (Zhi Zi Bai Pi Tang).

（2）湿热黄疸。本品能清利湿热、利胆退黄。治湿热黄疸，常与茵陈、大黄配伍，即茵陈蒿汤。或与黄柏、甘草配伍，即栀子柏皮汤。

(3) Bleeding due to heat in blood. The medicinal herb acts to reduce fire and cool blood. In the treatment of bleeding patterns due to heat in blood, it is combined with *Imperatae Rhizoma* (bai mao gen), *Radix Rehmanniae* (sheng di huang) and huang qin.

（3）血热出血。本品能泻火凉血。治血热妄行所致的出血证，可与白茅根、生地黄、黄芩等同用。

(4) Carbuncle and ulcer due to heat-toxin. The medicinal herb acts to clear heat, reduce fire, relieve toxin and subside swell. In the treatment of carbuncle and ulcer due to heat-toxin

（4）热毒疮疡。本品能清热泻火、解毒消肿。治热毒疮疡，红肿热痛，常与蒲公英、连翘等同用。

manifested by redness, swelling, hotness and pain, it is combined with *Taraxaci Herba* (pu gong ying) and lian qiao.

(5) Traumatic injuries. The medicinal herb acts to subside swell and relieve pain for external use. In the treatment of swelling and pain due to traumatic injuries, it is applied by grinding into powder and made into paste by combining with millet wine for external use.

（5）跌打伤痛。本品外用消肿止痛，以生品研末与黄酒调成糊状外敷，可治跌打损伤之肿痛。

Usage and dosage Apply 3～10 g in decoction. Apply a proper amount for external use. It is applied orally in crude form to reduce fire, relieve restlessness, clear heat and dissolve damp. It is applied externally to subside swell and relieve pain. Its bitter and cold property is decreased after stir-baked preparation. It is applied in carbonized form to stanch bleeding.

用法用量 煎服，3～10克。外用适量。生用内服泻火除烦、清热利湿，外用消肿止痛。炒用苦寒之性减弱。炒焦止血。

Phragmitis Rhizoma (lu gen)

芦根

It is the fresh or dried product from the underground rhizomes of perennial herbaceous plant, *Phragmites communis* Trin, family Gramineae. The medicinal herb is collected all through the year, applied in fresh form or in crude form by sun-drying.

为禾本科植物芦苇的新鲜或干燥根茎。全年可采挖。鲜用或晒干。生用。

Features Flavor: sweet. Property: Cold. Meridian tropism: the Lung Meridian and the Stomach Meridian.

性味归经 甘，寒。归肺、胃经。

Actions Clear heat, reduce fire, produce fluid, stop thirst, relieve restlessness, stop vomiting and promote urination.

功效 清热泻火，生津止渴，除烦，止呕，利尿。

Application

应用

(1) Febrile disease manifested by restlessness and thirst. The medicinal herb acts to clear heat, reduce fire, relieve restlessness and produce fluid.

（1）热病烦渴。本品能清热泻火、除烦生津。治热病伤津，烦热口渴，常配伍天

In the treatment of febrile disease manifested by restlessness, feverish sensation and thirst due to consumption of body fluid, it is combined with *Trichosanthis Radix* (tian hua fen), *Ophiopogonis Radix* (mai men dong) and *Gypsum Fibrosum* (shi gao).

花粉、麦冬、石膏等同用。

(2) Cough due to heat in lung and pulmonary abscess with thick-purulent sputum. The medicinal herb acts to purify lung, reduce heat, eliminate abscess and discharge purulence. In the treatment of cough with thick-yellow sputum due to heat in lung, it is combined with *Scutellariae Radix* (huang qin) and *Trichosanthis Fructus* (gua lou). In the treatment of pulmonary abscess with thick-purulent sputum, it is combined with *Coicis Semen* (yi yi ren) and *Persicae Semen* (tao ren).

（2）肺热咳嗽，肺痈吐脓。本品能清肺泄热、消痈排脓。治肺热咳嗽，痰稠色黄，常配伍黄芩、瓜蒌等同用。治肺痈吐脓，常与薏苡仁、桃仁等配伍。

(3) Vomiting due to heat in stomach. The medicinal herb acts to clear heat from stomach and stop vomiting. It is applied singly in decoction or combined with *Bambusae Caulis in Taenias* (zhu ru) and ginger juice.

（3）胃热呕吐。本品善清胃热、止呕。可单味煎汁饮服，或与竹茹、姜汁同用。

(4) Stranguria with difficult and painful urination. The medicinal herb acts to clear heat and promote urination. In the treatment of stranguria with difficult and painful urination, it is combined with *Imperatae Rhizoma* (bai mao gen) and *Plantaginis Herba* (che qian cao).

（4）热淋涩痛。本品能清热利尿。治热淋涩痛，常配伍白茅根、车前草等同用。

Usage and dosage Apply 15～30 g in decoction. It is applied in fresh form with doubled dose, or to smash to take out its juice.

用法用量 煎服，15～30 克。鲜品用量加倍，或捣汁服。

Trichosanthis Radix (tian hua fen)

天花粉

It is the dried product from the root of *Trichosanthes kirilowii* Maxim., family Cucurbitaceae.

为葫芦科植物栝楼或双边栝楼的干燥根。秋、冬季

The medicinal herb is collected in autumn and winter, applied in crude form.

采挖。生用。

Features Flavor: sweet and slightly bitter. Property: slightly cold. Meridian tropism: the Lung Meridian and the Stomach Meridian.

性味归经 甘、微苦，微寒。归肺、胃经。

Actions Clear heat, reduce fire, produce fluid, stop thirst, subside swell and drain pus.

功效 清热泻火，生津止渴，消肿排脓。

Application

应用

(1) Restlessness and thirst due to febrile disease and diabetes due to internal heat. The medicinal herb acts to clear heat, reduce fire, produce fluid and stop thirst. In the treatment of febrile disease manifested by restlessness, agitation and thirst due to consumption of body fluid, it is combined with *Phragmitis Rhizoma* (lu gen) and *Ophiopogonis Radix* (mai men dong). In the treatment of diabetes manifested by thirst due to internal heat, it is combined with *Puerariae Lobatae Radix* (ge gen), *Anemarrhenae Rhizoma* (zhi mu) and *Schisandrae Chinensis Fructus* (wu wei zi), to form up Jade Fluid Decoction (Yu Ye Tang).

（1）热病烦渴，内热消渴。本品能清热泻火、生津止渴。治热病伤津、烦躁口渴，常配伍芦根、麦冬等同用。治内热消渴多饮，常与葛根、知母、五味子等配伍，如玉液汤。

(2) Cough due to heat in lung or dry cough with scanty sputum. The medicinal herb acts to clear heat from lung and moisturize lung to eliminate dryness. In the treatment of cough with yellow-thick sputum due to heat in lung, it is combined with *Belamecandae Rhizoma* (she gan), *Cortex Mori Albae Radicis* (sang bai pi) and *Fructus Aristolochiae Debilis* (ma dou ling), to form up Belamecanda and Aristolochiae Decoction (She Gan Dou Ling Tang). In the treatment of pathogenic dryness damaging lung pattern manifested by dry cough with scanty sputum or bloody sputum, it is combined with *Adenophorae Radix Tetraphyllae*

（2）肺热咳嗽或燥咳少痰。本品既清肺热，又润肺燥。治肺热咳痰黄稠，常配伍射干、桑白皮、马兜铃等同用，如射干兜铃汤。燥邪伤肺，干咳少痰，或痰中带血，常与沙参、麦冬、生地黄等同用。

(nan sha shen), *Ophiopogonis Radix* (mai men dong) and *Radix Rehmanniae* (sheng di huang).

(3) Carbuncle and ulcer. The medicinal herb acts to clear heat, reduce fire, subside swell and drain pus. In the treatment of carbuncle and ulcer in early stage when pus is not formed or the formed pus is not ruptured, it is combined with *Lonicerae Japonicae Flos* (jin yin hua), *Angelicae Dahuricae Radix* (bai zhi), to form up Fairy Formula Life-Saving Drink (Xian Fang Huo Ming Yin).

（3）痈肿疮疡。本品能清热泻火、消肿排脓，疮痈初起肿痛或脓成未溃者皆宜。常配伍金银花、白芷等同用，如仙方活命饮。

Usage and dosage Apply 10～15 g in decoction.

用法用量 煎服，10～15克。

Precautions for use It is cautious to apply for pregnant women. It is not advisable to apply with *Aconiti Radix* (chuan wu), *Aconiti Radix Preparata* (zhi chuan wu), *Aconiti Radix Kusenzoffii* (cao wu), *Aconiti Radix Kusenzoffii Preparate* (zhi cao wu) and *Aconiti Radix Lateralis Praeparata* (fu zi).

使用注意 孕妇慎用。不宜与川乌、制川乌、草乌、制草乌、附子同用。

Lophatheri Herba (dan zhu ye)

淡竹叶

It is the dried product from the entire plant of a perennial herb, *Lophatherum gracile* Brongn, family Gramineae. The medicinal herb is collected in late summer before its heading stage, applied in crude form.

为禾本科植物淡竹叶的干燥茎叶。夏季末抽花穗前采收。生用。

Features Flavor: sweet and bland. Property: cold. Meridian tropism: the Heart Meridian, the Stomach Meridian and the Small Intestine Meridian.

性味归经 甘、淡，寒。归心、胃、小肠经。

Actions Clear heat, reduce fire, relieve restlessness, stop thirst and promote urination.

功效 清热泻火，除烦止渴，利尿。

Application

应用

(1) Febrile disease manifested by restlessness and thirst. The medicinal herb acts to purify heart,

（1）热病烦渴。本品甘寒清心泻火、除烦止渴。治

reduce fire, relieve restlessness and stop thirst. In the treatment of febrile disease manifested by restlessness and thirst, it is combined with *Ophiopogonis Radix* (mai men dong), *Phragmitis Rhizoma* (lu gen) and *Trichosanthis Radix* (tian hua fen).

热病心烦口渴，常配伍麦冬、芦根、天花粉等同用。

(2) Ulcers of mouth and tongue and difficult urination. The medicinal herb acts to clear fire from heart and small intestine, reduce fire and promote urination. In the treatment of heart fire flaming pattern manifested by ulcers of mouth and tongue, or heart fire transmitting to small intestine pattern manifested by difficult urination, dark urine and painful urination, it is combined with *Akebiae Caulis* (mu tong), *Plantaginis Semen* (che qian zi), *Radix Rehmanniae* (sheng di huang), and *Glycyrrhizae Radix et Rhizoma* (gan cao).

（2）口舌生疮，小便不利。本品善清心与小肠之火，能降火利尿。治心火炽盛之口舌生疮或热移小肠之小便不利、尿赤涩痛，常与木通、车前子、生地黄、甘草等配伍同用。

Usage and dosage　Apply 6～10 g in decoction.

用法用量　煎服，6～10克。

Prunellae Spica (xia ku cao)

夏枯草

It is the dried product from the spike of *Prunella vulgaris* L., family Labiatae. The medicinal herb is collected in summer when fruit cluster is becoming reddish, applied in crude form.

为唇形科植物夏枯草的干燥果穗。夏季果穗呈棕红色时采收。生用。

Features　Flavor: pungent and bitter. Property: cold. Meridian tropism: the Liver Meridian and the Gallbladder Meridian.

性味归经　辛、苦，寒。归肝、胆经。

Actions　Clear heat, reduce fire, brighten eyes, subside swell and dissipate stagnation.

功效　清热泻火、明目，消肿散结。

Application

应用

(1) Redness, swelling and pain of eyes, headache, dizziness and eye pain. The medicinal herb acts to clear fire from liver. In the treatment of liver fire pattern manifested by redness of eyes, head-

（1）目赤肿痛、头痛眩晕，目珠疼痛。本品善清肝火。治肝火目赤、头痛眩晕，可单用或与菊花、决明子等

ache and dizziness, it is applied singly or combined with *Chrysanthemi Flos* (ju hua) and *Cassiae Semen* (jue ming zi). The medicinal herb is the major herb to treat eye pain, combined with *Angelicae Sinensis Radix* (dang gui), *Radix Rehmanniae* (sheng di huang) and *Paeoniae Radix Alba* (bai shao).

同用。本品为治目珠疼痛之要药,可与当归、生地黄、白芍等同用。

(2) Scrofula and goiter. The medicinal herb acts to clear heat and dissipate stagnation. In the treatment of scrofula and goiter, it is applied singly or combined with *Fritillariae Cirrhosae Bulbus* (chuan bei mu) and *Scrophulariae Radix* (xuan shen) by making decoction or extract.

(2) 瘰疬、瘿瘤。本品善清热散结。治瘰疬瘿瘤,可单味煎服或熬膏,亦可与贝母、玄参等同用。

Usage and dosage Apply 9～15 g in decoction.

用法用量 煎服,9～15克。

Cassiae Semen (jue ming zi)

决明子

It is the dried product from the ripe seed of *Cassia obtusifolia* L. or *Cassia tora.*, family Leguminosae. The medicinal herb is collected in autumn, applied in crude form or stir-baked form.

为豆科植物决明或小决明的干燥成熟种子。秋季采收。生用或炒用。

Features Flavor: sweet, bitter and salty. Property: slightly cold. Meridian tropism: the Liver Meridian and the Large Intestine Meridian.

性味归经 甘、苦、咸,微寒。归肝、大肠经。

Actions Clear heat, brighten eyes, moisturize intestines and promote defecation.

功效 清热明目,润肠通便。

Application

应用

(1) Redness, swelling and pain of eyes, and dim and blurred vision. The medicinal herb acts to purify liver and brighten eyes. In the treatment of liver heat pattern manifested by redness of eyes, it is combined with *Prunellae Spica* (xia ku cao) and *Gardeniae Fructus* (zhi zi). In the treatment of the Liver Meridian wind-heat pattern manifested by photophobia and lacrimation, it is combined with

(1) 目赤肿痛,目暗不明。本品功善清肝明目。治肝热目赤,常配伍夏枯草、栀子等同用。若肝经风热、羞明多泪,可与菊花、桑叶等同用。治肝肾阴亏,目暗不明,可与山茱萸、沙苑子、枸杞子等同用。

Chrysanthemi Flos (ju hua) and *Mori Folium* (sang ye). In the treatment of liver and kidney yin deficiency pattern manifested by dim and blurred vision, it is combined with *Corni Fructus* (shan zhu yu), *Astragali Complanati Semen* (sha yuan zi) and *Lycii Fructus* (gou qi zi).

(2) Headache and dizziness. The medicinal herb acts to purify liver and reduce fire. In the treatment of liver fire flaming pattern manifested by headache and dizziness, it is applied singly or combined with ju hua, *Uncariae Ramulus cum Uncis* (gou teng) and *Ostreae Concha* (mu li).

（2）头痛眩晕。本品清肝泻火。治肝火所致的头痛眩晕，可单味水煎，或与菊花、钩藤、生牡蛎等配伍同用。

(3) Constipation due to dryness in intestines. The medicinal herb acts to clear heat, moisturize intestines and promote defecation. In the treatment of constipation due to dryness in intestines, it is applied singly or combined with *Cannabis Fructus* (huo ma ren) and *Pruni Semen* (yu li ren).

（3）肠燥便秘。本品能清热润肠通便。治肠燥便秘，可单用，或与火麻仁、郁李仁等同用。

Usage and dosage　Apply 9～15 g in decoction.

用法用量　煎服，9～15克。

Precautions for use　It is cautious to apply for those with loose feces due to spleen deficiency.

使用注意　脾虚便溏者慎用。

Section 2　Heat-clearing and damp-desiccating herbs

第2节 清热燥湿药

Scutellariae Radix (huang qin)

黄芩

It is the dried product from the root of *Scutellaria baicalensis* Georgi, family Labiatae. The medicinal herb is collected in spring and autumn, applied in crude form, in stir-baked form or in prepared form with millet wine.

为唇形科植物黄芩的干燥根。春、秋季采挖。生用、炒用或酒炙用。

Features Flavor: bitter. Property: cold. Meridian tropism: the Lung Meridian, the Spleen Meridian, the Gallbladder Meridian, the Large Intestine Meridian and the Small Intestine Meridian.

性味归经 苦，寒。归肺、脾、胆、大肠、小肠经。

Actions Clear heats, desiccate damp, reduce fire, relieve toxin, stanch bleeding and prevent miscarriage.

功效 清热燥湿，泻火解毒，止血，安胎。

Application

(1) Damp-heat pattern or summer-heat-damp pattern manifested by jaundice, diarrhea, dysentery, burning, painful and difficult urination. The medicinal herb is bitter and acts to desiccate damp, and is cold and acts to clear heat, applied to treat all types of damp-heat pattern. In the treatment of damp-heat pattern or summer-heat-damp pattern manifested by stuffy chest, distension in epigastria, nausea and vomiting, it is combined with *Talcum* (hua shi) and *Amomi Fructus Rotundus* (bai dou kou), to form up Scutellaria and *Talcum* Decoction (Huang Qin Hua Shi Tang). In the treatment of jaundice due to damp-heat, it is combined with *Artemisiae Scopariae Herba* (yin chen hao) and *Gardeniae Fructus* (zhi zi). In the treatment of damp-heat pattern manifested by diarrhea, dysentery, abdominal pain or tenesmus, it is combined with *Puerariae Lobatae Radix* (ge gen) and *Coptidis Rhizoma* (huang lian), to form up Pueraria, Scutellaria and Copitis Decoction (Ge Gen Qin Lian Tang). In the treatment of burning, painful and difficult urination, it is combined with *Radix Rehmanniae* (sheng di huang) and *Akebiae Caulis* (mu tong).

应用

（1）湿温暑湿，黄疸泻痢，热淋涩痛。本品味苦燥湿，性寒清热，善治湿热诸证。治湿温、暑湿所致的胸脘痞闷、恶心呕吐，常与滑石、白豆蔻等同用，如黄芩滑石汤。治湿热黄疸，常与茵陈、栀子等药同用。治湿热泻痢腹痛，或里急后重，与葛根、黄连等配伍，如葛根芩连汤。治热淋涩痛，与生地黄、木通等同用。

(2) Cough due to heat in lung. The medicinal herb acts to purify lung and reduce heat. In the

（2）肺热咳嗽。本品长于清肺泄热。治肺热咳嗽，

treatment of cough due to heat in lung, it is applied singly or combined with *Trichosanthis Fructus* (gua lou), *Aurantii Fructus Immaturus* (zhi shi) and *Arisaematis Rhizoma Cum Bile* (dan nan xing), to form up Qi-Purifying and Phlegm-Dissolving Pills (Qing Qi Hua Tan Wan).

可单味应用，或与瓜蒌、枳实、胆南星等配伍，如清气化痰丸。

(3) Febrile disease manifested by restlessness, thirst, alternate chills and fever. The medicinal herb acts to clear heat and reduce fire. In the treatment of febrile disease manifested by high fever, restlessness and thirst, it is combined with zhi zi, huang lian and *Gypsum Fibrosum* (shi gao). In the treatment of Shaoyang disease manifested by alternate chills and fever, it is combined with *Bupleuri Radix* (chai hu), to form up Minor Bupleurum Decoction (Xiao Chai Hu Tang).

（3）热病烦渴，寒热往来。本品能清热泻火。治热病高热烦渴，常与栀子、黄连、石膏等同用。治邪在少阳，寒热往来，可与柴胡同用，如小柴胡汤。

(4) Carbuncle and ulcer due to heat-toxin. The medicinal herb acts to clear heat and relieve toxin. In the treatment of carbuncle and ulcer due to heat-toxin, it is combined with *Lonicerae Japonicae Flos* (jin yin hua) and *Forsythiae Fructus* (lian qiao).

（4）痈肿疮毒。本品能清热解毒。治痈肿疮毒，可与金银花、连翘等同用。

(5) Bleeding due to heat in blood. The medicinal herb acts to reduce fire, clear heat, cool blood and stanch bleeding. In the treatment of blood heat pattern manifested by hemoptysis, epstaxis, blood feces and uterine bleeding, it is combined with the medicinal herbs acting to cool blood and stanch bleeding.

（5）血热出血。本品能泻火清热、凉血止血。治血热所致的吐血、衄血、便血、崩漏等，常与凉血止血药同用。

(6) Fatal irritability. The medicinal herb acts to clear heat and prevent miscarriage. In the treatment of fatal irritability due to heat, it is combined with *Atractylodis Macrocephalae Rhizoma* (bai zhu).

（6）胎动不安。本品能清热安胎。治胎动不安兼热者，常配伍白术等同用。

Usage and dosage　Apply 3～10 g in decoc-

用法用量　煎服，3～10

tion. It is applied in crude form to clear heat, desiccate damp, reduce fire and relieve toxin. It is applied in stir-baked form to prevent miscarriage. It is applied in prepared form with millet wine to clear heat from upper energizer. It is applied in carbonized form to stanch bleeding.

克。生用清热燥湿、泻火解毒,炒用安胎,酒炙清上焦热,炒炭止血。

Precautions for use It is cautious to apply for those with spleen and stomach deficiency.

使用注意 脾胃虚弱者慎用。

Coptidis Rhizoma (huang lian)

黄连

It is the dried product from the rhizome of *Coptis chinensis* Franch. And *Coptis deltoidea* C. Y. cheng et Hsiao or *Coptis teeta* Wall., family Ranunculaceae. The three types are respectively called "wei lian", "ya lian" and "yun lian" in Chinese, produced in Sichuan and Yunnan Provinces. The medicinal herb is collected in autumn, applied in crude form, in fried form, or in stir-baked form.

为毛茛科植物黄连、三角叶黄连或云连的干燥根茎。以上三种分别习称"味连""雅连""云连"。主产四川、云南。秋季采挖。生用或炒用、炙用。

Features Flavor: bitter. Property: cold. Meridian tropism: the Heart Meridian, the Spleen Meridian, the Stomach Meridian, the Liver Meridian, the Gallbladder Meridian and the Large Intestine Meridian.

性味归经 苦,寒。归心、脾、胃、肝、胆、大肠经。

Actions Clear heats, desiccate damp, reduce fire and relieve toxin.

功效 清热燥湿,泻火解毒。

Application

应用

(1) Damp-heat pattern manifested by distension in epigastria, diarrhea, dysentery and abdominal pain. The medicinal herb, bitter and cold, acts to clear heat and desiccate damp, especially acts to reduce damp-heat from middle energizer. In the treatment of damp-heat blocking middle energizer pattern manifested by distension in epigastria, nausea and vomiting, it is combined with *Pinelliae*

(1)湿热痞满,泻痢腹痛。本品苦寒而能清热燥湿,尤善清中焦湿热。治湿热阻于中焦所致的脘痞呕恶,常与半夏、干姜等配伍,如半夏泻心汤。治湿热泻痢,轻者单用;或与木香同用,即香连丸。治泻痢身热

Rhizoma (ban xia) and *Zingiberis Rhizoma* (gan jiang), to form up Pinellia Heart-Reducing Decoction (Ban Xia Xie Xin Tang). In the treatment of dysentery due to damp-heat, it is applied singly for mild condition, while combined with *Aucklandiae Radix* (mu xiang), to form up Aucklandia and Coptis Pills (Xiang Lian Wan). In the treatment of dysentery with fever, it is combined with *Scutellariae Radix* (huang qin), *Puerariae Lobatae Radix* (ge gen) and *Glycyrrhizae Radix et Rhizoma* (gan cao), to form up Pueraria, Scutellaria and Copitis Decoction (Ge Gen Qin Lian Tang). In the treatment of dysentery with purulent and bloody feces, it is combined with *Pulsatillae Radix* (bai tou weng) and *Fraxini Cortex* (qin pi), to form up Pulsatilla Decoction (Bai Tou Weng Tang).

者,可与黄芩、葛根、甘草等同用,即葛根芩连汤。若泻痢脓血,则与白头翁、秦皮等同用,如白头翁汤。

(2) Febrile disease manifested with high fever. The medicinal herb acts to clear heat, reduce fire and relieve toxin. In the treatment of febrile disease manifested by high fever and restlessness, it is combined with huang qin and *Gardeniae Fructus* (zhi zi), to form up Coptis Detoxifying Decoction (Huang Lian Jie Du Tang).

(2) 热病高热。本品能清热泻火解毒。治热病高热烦躁,常与黄芩、栀子等同用,如黄连解毒汤。

(3) Restlessness, insomnia, vomiting due to heat in stomach, and vomiting and acid regurgitation due to disharmony between liver and stomach. The medicinal herb acts to clear fire from heart and stomach and to clear heat from liver. In the treatment of fire flaming pattern manifested by restlessness and insomnia, it is combined with *Paeoniae Radix Alba* (bai shao) and *Asini Corii Colla* (e jiao), to form up Coptis and Ass-Hide Glue Decoction (Huang Lian E Jiao Tang). In the treatment of insomnia due to disharmony between heart and kidney, it is combined with

(3) 心烦失眠,胃热呕吐,肝胃失和的呕吐吞酸。本品善清心、胃之火,且清肝热。治火旺心烦失眠,常与白芍、阿胶等同用,如黄连阿胶汤。心肾不交而失眠者,可与肉桂同用,即交泰丸。治胃热呕吐,可与半夏、竹茹、橘皮等同用,如黄连橘皮竹茹汤。若治肝胃不和所致胁痛、呕吐、吞酸,常与吴茱

Cinnamomi Cortex (rou gui), to form up Coordination-Restoring Pills (Jiao Tai Wan). In the treatment of vomiting due to heat in stomach, it is combined with *Pinelliae Rhizoma* (ban xia), *Bambusae Caulis in Taenias* (zhu ru) and *Exocarpium Citri Leiocarpae* (ju pi), to form up Coptis, Tangerine Peel and Bamboo Shavings Decoction (Huang Lian Ju Pi Zhu Ru Tang). In the treatment of disharmony between liver and stomach manifested by hypochondriac pain, vomiting and acid regurgitation, it is combined with *Euodiae Fructus* (wu zhu yu), to form up Coptis and Evodia Pills (Zuo Jin Wan).

萸配伍,即左金丸。

(4) Carbuncle and ulcer due to heat-toxin, eczema and redness of eyes. The medicinal herb is especially good at relieving toxin to treat carbuncle and ulcer. In the treatment of carbuncle and ulcer due to heat-toxin, it is combined with huang qin, zhi zi, *Forsythiae Fructus* (lian qiao) and *Arctii Fructus* (niu bang zi). In the treatment of eczema and redness of eyes, it is applied in ointment form for external use or in diffusion juice for eye drops.

(4) 痈肿疮毒,湿疮,目赤。本品尤善解毒,以疗疔疮。治热毒疔疮,常与黄芩、栀子、连翘、牛蒡子等配伍。治湿疮、目赤,可制膏外用或浸汁滴眼。

(5) Bleeding due to heat in blood. The medicinal herb acts to reduce fire, cool blood and stanch bleeding. In the treatment of hemoptysis and epistaxis due to heat in blood, it is combined with *Rhei Radix et Rhizoma* (da huang) and huang qin, to form up Heart-Reducing Decoction (Xie Xin Tang).

(5) 血热出血。本品能泻火凉血止血。治血热所致的吐血、衄血等,常与大黄、黄芩配伍,即泻心汤。

Usage and dosage Apply 2～5 g in decoction. Apply a proper amount for external use. It is applied to clear heat, desiccate damp, reduce fire and relieve toxin in crude form. It is to reduce its bitter and cold property in fried form. It is applied to clear fire from upper energizer in fried form with millet wine. It is applied to soothe liver, harmonize

用法用量 煎服,2～5克。外用适量。生用清热燥湿、泻火解毒,炒用降低苦寒之性,酒炒可清上焦之火,吴茱萸汁拌炒疏肝和胃止呕,姜汁炙能清胃和胃止呕。

stomach and stop vomiting in fried form with *Euodiae Fructus* (wu zhu yu) juice. It is applied to purify stomach, harmonize stomach and stop vomiting in stir-baked form with ginger juice.

Precautions for use It is cautious to apply for those with spleen and stomach deficiency and those with yin deficiency and fluid consumption.

使用注意 脾胃虚弱及阴虚津伤者慎用。

Phellodendri Cortex Chiensis (huang bo)

黄柏

It is the dried product from the bark of a deciduous arbor, *Phellodendrou chinense* Schneid, or *Phellodendrou amurense* Rupr., family Rutaceae. The former is also called "chuan huang bo" produced in Sichuan Province, while the latter is also called "guan huang bo" produced in Liaoning and Jilin Provinces. After barking, remove the coarse part of the bark. The medicinal herb is applied in crude form or in stir-baked form.

为芸香科植物黄皮树或黄檗的干燥树皮。前者习称"川黄柏",主产于四川等地。后者习称"关黄柏",主产于辽宁、吉林等地。剥取树皮后,除去粗皮。生用或炙用。

Features Flavor: bitter. Property: cold. Meridian tropism: the Kidney Meridian and the Bladder Meridian.

性味归经 苦,寒。归肾、膀胱经。

Actions Clear heats, desiccate damp, reduce fire, eliminate false heat, relieve toxin and treat carbuncle.

功效 清热燥湿,泻火除蒸,解毒疗疮。

Application

(1) Damp-heat pattern manifested by diarrhea, dysentery, jaundice, dark urine, morbid leucorrhea, burning, difficult and painful urination, swelling and pain of foot and knee. The medicinal herb acts to eliminate damp-heat from lower energizer. In the treatment of damp-heat pattern manifested by diarrhea and dysentery, it is combined with *Pulsatillae Radix* (bai tou weng), *Coptidis Rhizoma* (huang lian) and *Fraxini Cortex* (qin pi), to form up Pulsatil-

应用

(1) 湿热泻痢,黄疸尿赤,带下阴痒,热淋涩痛,足膝肿痛。本品善清下焦湿热。治湿热泻痢,可与白头翁、黄连、秦皮等同用,即白头翁汤。治黄疸尿赤,与栀子、甘草配伍,即栀子柏皮汤。治带下腥臭,外阴瘙痒,常与车前子、白果等配伍。

la Decoction (Bai Tou Weng Tang). In the treatment of jaundice and dark urine, it is combined with *Gardeniae Fructus* (zhi zi) and *Glycyrrhizae Radix et Rhizoma* (gan cao), to form up Capejasmine, Phellodendron and White Mulberry Bark Decoction (Zhi Zi Bai Pi Tang). In the treatment of morbid leucorrhea with fishy or stinky odor, and vaginal itch, it is combined with *Plantaginis Semen* (che qian zi) and *Semen Ginkgo* (bai guo). In the treatment of burning, difficult and painful urination, it is combined with *Akebiae Caulis* (mu tong) and *Talcum* (hua shi). In the treatment of swelling and pain of foot and knee due to damp-heat, it is combined with *Achyranthis Bidentatae Radix* (niu xi) and *Atractylodis Rhizoma* (cang zhu), to form up Three Wonderful Herbs Pills (San Miao Wan).

治热淋涩痛，常配合木通、滑石等同用。治湿热所致足膝肿痛，多与牛膝、苍术配伍，即三妙丸。

(2) Feverish sensation, tidal fever, seminal emission and nocturnal sweats. The medicinal herb is attributive to the Kidney Meridian and acts to reduce the Xiang (Ministerial) Fire and decrease false heat. In the treatment of yin deficiency and fire flaming pattern manifested by feverish sensation, tidal fever, aching at low back, tinnitus, seminal emission and nocturnal sweats, it is combined with *Anemarrhenae Rhizoma* (zhi mu) and *Rehmanniae Radix* (sheng di huang), to form up Anemarrhena, Phellodendron, and Rehmannia Pills (Zhi Bai Di Huang Wan) and Great Yin Supplementation Pills (Da Bu Yin Wan).

（2）骨蒸劳热，遗精盗汗。本品入肾而泻相火、退虚热。治阴虚火旺，骨蒸劳热、腰酸耳鸣、骨蒸潮热、遗精盗汗等，常与知母、生地黄等配伍，如知柏地黄丸、大补阴丸。

(3) Carbuncle and ulcer due to heat-toxin, and eczema. The medicinal herb acts to reduce fire and relieve toxin, and also acts to clear heat and desiccate damp as well. In the treatment of carbuncle, ulcer and eczema, it is applied for oral administra-

（3）疮疡肿毒，湿疹湿疮。本品既泻火解毒，又清热燥湿。治疮痈或湿疹湿疮，内服外用皆可。治热毒疮疡，常与黄连、栀子等煎

tion or external use. In the treatment of carbuncle and ulcer due to heat-toxin, it is combined with huang lian and zhi zi in decoction, or is ground into fine powder and mixed with pig bile for external use. In the treatment of eczema, it is combined with *Sophorae Flavescentis Radix* (ku shen) and *Schizonepetae Herba* (jing jie) in decoction for oral administration or for external use.

Usage and dosage Apply 3～12 g in decoction. Apply a proper amount for external use. It is to clear heat, desiccate damp, reduce fire and relieve toxin in crude form. It is to reduce fire and eliminated feverish sensation in stir-baked form with salty solution.

Precautions for use It is cautious to apply for those with spleen and stomach deficiency.

Gentianae Radix et Rhizoma (long dan)

It is the dried product from the root and rhizome of a perennial plant, *Gentiana manshurica* Kitag., or *Gentiana scabra* Bge. or *Gentiana triflora* Pall., or *Gentiana rigescen Franch*, family Gentianaceae. The former three types are called "long dan", produced in northwest areas, while the latter is called "jian long dan", produced in Yunnan and Sichuan Provinces. The medicinal herb is collected in spring and autumn, applied in crude form.

Features Flavor: bitter. Property: cold. Meridian tropism: the Liver Meridian and the Gallbladder Meridian.

Actions Clear heats, desiccate damp, and reduce fire in liver and gallbladder.

Application

(1) Damp-heat pattern manifested by jaundice,

服,或研细末,加猪胆汁调敷外用。治湿疹湿疮,可与苦参、荆芥等配合煎服,或煎汁洗患处。

用法用量 煎服,3～12克。外用适量。生用清热燥湿、泻火解毒,盐水炙泻火除蒸。

使用注意 脾胃虚弱者慎用。

龙胆

为龙胆科植物条叶龙胆、龙胆、三花龙胆或滇龙胆的干燥根及根茎。前三种习称"龙胆",主产于东北地区。后一种习称"坚龙胆",主产于云南、四川等地。春、秋季采挖。生用。

性味归经 苦,寒。归肝、胆经。

功效 清热燥湿,泻肝胆火。

应用

(1) 湿热黄疸,阴肿阴

vaginal swelling and itch, morbid leucorrhea with fishy or stinky odor, eczema and skin itch. The medicinal herb acts to eliminate damp-heat from liver, gallbladder and lower energizer. In the treatment of damp-heat pattern manifested by jaundice and dark urine, it is combined with *Artemisiae Scopariae Herba* (yin chen hao) and *Gardeniae Fructus* (zhi zi). In the treatment of vaginal swelling and itch, morbid leucorrhea with fishy or stinky odor, or eczema and skin itch, it is combined with *Phellodendri Cortex Chiensis* (huang bo), *Sophorae Flavescentis Radix* (ku shen) and *Plantaginis Semen* (che qian zi).

痒,带下腥臭,湿疹瘙痒。本品善清肝胆及下焦湿热。治湿热黄疸,身黄尿赤,常与茵陈、栀子等配伍。治阴肿阴痒,带下腥臭,或湿疹瘙痒等,常与黄柏、苦参、车前子等配伍。

(2) Liver fire pattern manifested by headache, deafness, redness of eyes, convulsion and twitching. The medicinal herb acts to reduce fire of the Liver Meridian. In the treatment of liver fire pattern manifested by headache, bitter taste in mouth, deafness, redness, swelling and pain of eyes, it is combined with *Bupleuri Radix* (chai hu), zhi zi and *Scutellariae Radix* (huang qin), to form up Gentian Liver-Draining Decoction (Long Dan Xie Gan Tang). In the treatment of the Liver Meridian heat pattern or extreme heat producing wind pattern manifested by convulsion and twitching, it is combined with *Uncariae Ramulus cum Uncis* (gou teng), *Coptidis Rhizoma* (huang lian) and *Bovis Calculus* (niu huang).

(2)肝火头痛、耳聋目赤,惊风抽搐。本品善泻肝经之火。治肝火头痛、口苦耳聋,目赤肿痛,常与柴胡、栀子、黄芩等同用,如龙胆泻肝汤。治肝经热极生风所致的惊风抽搐,常与钩藤、黄连、牛黄等配伍。

Usage and dosage Apply 3～6 g in decoction.

用法用量 煎服,3～6克。

Precautions for use It is not advisable to apply for those with spleen and stomach deficienty and cold.

使用注意 脾胃虚寒者不宜用。

Sophorae Flavescentis Radix (ku shen)

苦参

It is the dried product from the *Sophora*

为豆科植物苦参的干燥

flavescens Ait., family Leguminosae. The medicinal herb is collected in spring and autumn, applied in crude form.

根。春、秋季采挖。生用。

Features Flavor: bitter. Property: cold. Meridian tropism: the Heart Meridian, the Liver Meridian, the Stomach Meridian, the Large Intestine Meridian and the Bladder Meridian.

性味归经 苦，寒。归心、肝、胃、大肠、膀胱经。

Actions Clear heat, desiccate damp, kill worms and promote urination.

功效 清热燥湿，杀虫，利尿。

Application

(1) Damp-heat pattern manifested by diarrhea, dysentery, jaundice, dark urine, morbid leucorrhea and vaginal itch. The medicinal herb is bitter and cold and acts to clear heat, desiccate damp and eliminate damp-heat in lower energizer. In the treatment of damp-heat pattern manifested by diarrhea, dysentery and abdominal pain, it is applied singly or combined with *Aucklandiae Radix* (mu xiang) and *Glycyrrhizae Radix et Rhizoma* (gan cao), to form up Aucklandia and Sophora Root Pills (Xiang Shen Wan). In the treatment of jaundice and dark urine, it is combined with *Artemisiae Scopariae Herba* (yin chen hao), *Gardeniae Fructus* (zhi zi) and *Gentianae Radix et Rhizoma* (long dan). In the treatment of damp-heat pattern manifested by morbid leucorrhea with fishy or stinky odor and vaginal itch, it is combined with *Phellodendri Cortex Chiensis* (huang bo), *Cortex Ailanthi* (chun pi) and *Cnidii Fructus* (she chuang zi), for oral administration or external wash.

应用

（1）湿热泻痢，黄疸尿赤，带下阴痒。本品苦寒，能清热燥湿，善清下焦湿热。治湿热泻痢腹痛，可单味煎服，或与木香、甘草同用，即香参丸。治黄疸尿赤，多与茵陈、栀子、龙胆草等同用。治湿热带下，腥臭阴痒，可与黄柏、椿皮、蛇床子等配伍，内服或外洗。

(2) Eczema, skin itch, scabies and leprosy. The medicinal herb acts to dispel wind, kill worms, desiccate damp and stop itching, for both oral administration and external use. In the treatment of

（2）湿疹湿疮，皮肤瘙痒，疥癣麻风。本品能祛风杀虫、燥湿止痒，内服外用皆宜。治湿疹湿疮，可与黄连、

eczema, it is combined with *Coptidis Rhizoma* (huang lian) and huang bo. In the treatment of skin itch, it is combined with *Schizonepetae Herba* (jing jie) and *Radix Ledebouriellae* (fang feng) in decoction used for oral administration, or with *Capsicum Annuum* (chuan jiao) and *Stemonae Radix* (bai bu) in decoction used for external wash. In the treatment of scabies, it is applied singly or combined with *Cnidii Fructus* (she chuang zi), *Spica Schizonepetae Tenuifolia* (jing jie sui) and *Alumen* (bai fan) in decoction for external wash. In the treatment of leprosy, it is combined with *Semen Hydnocarpi* (da feng zi) and *Xanthii Fructus* (cang er zi).

黄柏等同用。治皮肤瘙痒，可与荆芥、防风等煎服，或配伍川椒、百部煎汤外洗。治疥癣，可单用，或配伍蛇床子、荆芥穗、白矾等煎汤外洗。治麻风，常与大风子、苍耳子等配伍。

(3) Difficult and painful urination. The medicinal herb acts to clear heat and promote urination. In the treatment of damp-heat pattern manifested by dribbling urine, difficult and painful urination, it is combined with the medicinal herbs acting to promote urination and treat stranguria, as *Plantaginis Semen* (che qian zi) and *Talcum* (hua shi).

(3) 小便涩痛。本品有清热利尿之功。治湿热所致的小便淋沥涩痛，常配伍车前子、滑石等利尿通淋药同用。

Usage and dosage Apply 5～9 g in decoction. Apply a proper amount for external use.

用法用量 煎服，5～9克。外用适量。

Precautions for use It is cautious to apply for those with spleen and stomach deficiency or those with yin deficiency and fluid consumption. It is not advisable to apply with *Radix et Rhizoma Veratri Nigri* (li lu).

使用注意 脾胃虚弱及阴虚津伤者慎用。不宜与藜芦同用。

Section 3 Heat-clearing and toxin-relieving herbs

第3节 清热解毒药

Lonicerae Japonicae Flos (jin yin hua)

金银花

It is the dried product from the flower bud of

为忍冬科植物忍冬的干

Lonicera japonica thunb., *Lonicera japonica* Thunb., family Caprifoliaceae. The medicinal herb is collected in early summer before flowering, applied in crude form or in carbonized form.

燥花蕾或带初开的花。夏初花开放前采摘。生用。

Features Flavor: sweet. Property: cold. Meridian tropism: the Lung Meridian, the Heart Meridian and the Stomach Meridian.

性味归经 甘，寒。归肺、心、胃经。

Actions Clear heat, relieve toxin, dispel wind and reduce heat.

功效 清热解毒，疏散风热。

Application

应用

(1) Carbuncle and ulcer. The medicinal herb acts to clear heat, relieve toxin and subside swell. In the treatment carbuncle and ulcer in early stage manifested by redness, swelling, hotness and pain, it is combined with *Trichosanthis Radix* (tian hua fen), *Angelicae Dahuricae Radix* (bai zhi) and *Radix Ledebouriellae* (fang feng), to form up Fairy Formula Life-Saving Drink (Xian Fang Huo Ming Yin). In the treatment of carbuncle and ulcer which are hard and deep-seated, it is combined with *Violae Herba* (zi hua di ding), *Chrysanthemi Flos Indici* (ye ju hua) and Herba *Taraxaci Mongolici* (pu gong ying), to form up Five Ingredients Detoxifying Drink (Wu Wei Xiao Du Yin). In the treatment of carbuncle and ulcer which are ruptured, it is combined with *Scrophulariae Radix* (xuan shen), *Angelicae Sinensis Radix* (dang gui) and *Glycyrrhizae Radix et Rhizoma* (gan cao), to form up Four-Agents Brave and Peaceful Decoction (Si Miao Yong An Tang).

（1）疮痈疔肿。本品善清热解毒、消散痈肿。治疮痈初起，红肿热痛，常配伍天花粉、白芷、防风等同用，如仙方活命饮；治疗疮坚硬根深，常与紫花地丁、野菊花、蒲公英等配伍，如五味消毒饮；治疮痈溃烂，常配伍玄参、当归、甘草同用，即四妙勇安汤。

(2) Wind-heat pattern due to exogenous factors and febrile disease in early stage. The medicinal herb acts to dispel wind and reduce heat, and also to clear heat and relieve toxin as well, applied

（2）外感风热，温病初起。本品既能疏风透热，又能清解热毒，可用于温病卫气营血的各个阶段。治外感

to treat febrile disease in all phases of Wei (Defense), Qi (Energy), Ying (Nutrient) and Xue (Blood) Phases. In the treatment of wind-heat pattern due to exogenous factors or febrile disease in early stage, it is combined with *Forsythiae Fructus* (lian qiao), *Menthae Haplocalycis Herba* (bo he) and *Arctii Fructus* (niu bang zi), to form up Lonicera and Forsythia Powder (Yin Qiao San). In the treatment of heat entering Ying (Nutrient) and Xue (Blood) Phase pattern, it is combined with the medicinal herbs acting to reduce heat and cool blood.

风热或温病初起，常配伍连翘、薄荷、牛蒡子等同用，如银翘散。与泄热、凉血之品配伍，可用于热入营血等证。

(3) Dysentery with bloody feces due to heat-toxin. The medicinal herb acts to clear heat, relieve toxin, cool blood and stop dysentery. In the treatment of dysentery with bloody and purulent feces due to heat-toxin, it is applied singly or combined with *Pulsatillae Radix* (bai tou weng) and *Fraxini Cortex* (qin pi).

(3) 热毒血痢。本品能清热解毒、凉血止痢。治热毒血痢，大便脓血者，可单用或配伍白头翁、秦皮等同用。

Furthermore, the medicinal herb is prepared by distillation into Honeysucle Flower Distillate (Jin Yin Hua Lu), acting to clear summer-heat, applied to treat restlessness and thirst due to summer-heat, and infantile furuncle and miliaria.

此外，本品蒸馏制成的金银花露，能清解暑热，可用于暑热烦渴，以及小儿热疖、痱子等证。

Usage and dosage Apply 10～15 g in decoction.

用法用量 煎服，10～15 克。

Precautions for use It is cautious to apply for those with spleen and stomach deficiency and cold or those with carbuncle and ulcer in thin pus due to qi deficiency.

使用注意 脾胃虚寒或气虚疮疡脓稀者慎用。

Appendix *Lonicerae Japonicae Caulis* (ren dong teng)

附药 忍冬藤

It is the dried product from the stem and leaf of *Lonicera japonica* thunb., *L. hypoglauca* Miq. and

为忍冬的茎叶，又名银花藤。味甘性寒。归肺、胃

L. confuse DC., family Caprifoliaceae. The medicinal herb is sweet in flavor, cold in property, and attributive to the Lung Meridian and the Stomach Meridian. It acts to clear heat, relieve toxin, dispel wind and dredge collaterals, applied to treat febrile disease manifested by fever, heat-toxin pattern manifested by dysentery with bloody feces, furucles and carbuncles with swelling and pain, Bi (Obturation) Pattern due to wind, damp and heat, and redness, swelling and pain of joints. Apply 9～30 g in decoction.

经。功能清热解毒，疏风通络。适用于温病发热，热毒血痢，疮痈肿痛，风湿热痹，关节红肿疼痛等。煎服，9～30克。

Forsythiae Fructus (lian qiao)

It is the dried product from the fruit of *Forsythia Suspensa* (Thunb.) Vahl., family Oleaceae. The medicinal herb is collected in autumn, called "qing qiao" when the fruits are in initial ripe, and called "lao qiao" when the fruits are in full ripe. It is applied in crude after sifting out the seeds.

Features　Flavor: bitter. Property: slightly cold. Meridian tropism: the Lung Meridian, the Heart Meridian and the Small Intestine Meridian.

Actions　Clear heat, relieve toxin, dissolve carbuncle, dissipate stagnation, dispel wind and reduce heat.

Application

(1) Carbuncle and ulcer due to heat-toxin, scrofula. The medicinal herb acts to clear heat and relieve toxin, taken as the sacred herb to treat carbuncle and ulcer, and applied to treat carbuncle and ulcer both in early stage and when they are ruptured. In the treatment of early carbuncle and ulcer with redness and swelling, it is combined with *Taraxaci Herba* (pu gong ying) and *Andrographitis Herba* (chuan xin lian). In the treatment ruptured car-

连翘

为木犀科植物连翘的干燥果实。秋季果实初熟尚带绿色时采收，习称"青翘"；果实熟透时采收，习称"老翘"。筛去种子。生用。

性味归经　苦，微寒。归肺、心、小肠经。

功效　清热解毒，消痈散结，疏散风热。

应用

（1）疮痈肿毒，瘰疬结核。本品功善清热解毒，为疗疮痈圣药，疮痈初起或疮痈已溃均可应用。治疮痈初起红肿，常与蒲公英、穿心莲等同用；治疮疡溃烂，脓出不畅，可与天花粉、金银花等同用。本品散结，善治瘰疬，多配伍夏枯草、玄参、浙贝母等

buncle and ulcer with unsmooth eruption, it is combined with *Trichosanthis Radix* (tian hua fen) and *Lonicerae Japonicae Flos* (jin yin hua). The medicinal herb acts to dissipate stagnation, applied to treat scrofula, with combination of *Prunellae Spica* (xia ku cao), *Scrophulariae Radix* (xuan shen) and *Bulbus Fritillariae Thunbergii* (zhe bei mu).

同用。

(2) Wind-heat pattern due to exogenous factors and febrile disease in early stage. The medicinal herb is bitter and cool and acts to clear heat, relieve toxin, dispel wind and reduce heat. In the treatment of wind-heat pattern due to exogenous factors or febrile disease in early stage, it is combined with jin yin hua, *Menthae Haplocalycis Herba* (bo he) and *Arctii Fructus* (niu bang zi), to form up Lonicera and Forsythia Powder (Yin Qiao San). In the treatment of heat entering Ying (Nutrient) and Xue (Blood) Phase pattern or heat entering pericardium pattern, it is combined with the medicinal herb acting to cool blood and clear heat.

(2) 外感风热，温病初起。本品苦凉，能清热解毒、疏风透热。治外感风热、温病初起，常与金银花、薄荷、牛蒡子等配伍，如银翘散。亦可与凉血清热之品配伍，用于热入营血或热陷心包诸证。

(3) Burning, difficult and painful urination. The medicinal herb is attributive to the Heart Meridian and the Small Intestine Meridian, and acts to purify heart, promote urination and treat stranguria. In the treatment of burning, difficult and painful urination, it is combined with *Plantaginis Semen* (che qian zi), *Akebiae Caulis* (mu tong) and *Lophatheri Herba* (dan zhu ye).

(3) 热淋涩痛。本品入心与小肠经，能清心利尿通淋，治热淋涩痛，可与车前子、木通、淡竹叶等同用。

Usage and dosage Apply 6～15 g in decoction.

用法用量 煎服，6～15克。

Precautions for use It is cautious to apply for those with carbuncle and ulcer in thin pus due to qi deficiency.

使用注意 气虚疮疡脓稀者慎用。

Isatidis Radix (ban lan gen)

It is the dried product from the root of *Isatis indigotica* Fort, family Cruciferae. The medicinal herb is collected in autumn, applied in crude form.

Features Flavor: bitter. Property: cold. Meridian tropism: the Heart Meridian and the Stomach Meridian.

Actions Clear heat, relieve toxin, cool blood and benefit throat.

Application

(1) Febrile disease manifested by fever, sore throat and general macula. The medicinal herb acts to clear heat and relieve toxin, and to cool blood and benefit throat as well. In the treatment of febrile disease manifested by fever, headache, sore throat, or general macula, it is combined with *Flos Lonicerae* (jin yin hua), *Forsythiae Fructus* (lian qiao) and *Gypsum Fibrosum Cruda* (sheng shi gao).

(2) Encephalitis B, erysipelas and mumps. The medicinal herb is bitter and cold and acts to clear heat and relieve toxin. In the treatment of encephalitis B manifested by red and puffy face and sore throat, erysipelas and mumps, it is combined with lian qiao, *Arctii Fructus* (niu bang zi) and *Scrophulariae Radix* (xuan shen), to form up Universal Salvation Detoxifying Drink (Pu Ji Xiao Du Yin).

Usage and dosage Apply 9～15 g in decoction.

Precautions for use It is prohibited to apply for those with spleen and stomach deficiency and cold.

Appendix

(1) *Folium Isatidis* (da qing ye)

It is the dried product from the leaf of *Isatis*

板蓝根

为十字花科植物菘蓝的干燥根。秋季采挖。生用。

性味归经 苦，寒。归心、胃经。

功效 清热解毒，凉血利咽。

应用

(1) 温病发热咽痛，身发斑疹。本品苦寒，既清热解毒，又凉血利咽。治温病发热，头痛咽痛，或身发斑疹，常与金银花、连翘、生石膏等同用。

(2) 大头瘟疫，丹毒痄腮。本品苦寒清泄，善清热解毒。治大头瘟疫，头面红肿、咽喉不利，或丹毒痄腮，常与连翘、牛蒡子、玄参等配伍同用，如普济消毒饮。

用法用量 煎服，9～15克。

使用注意 脾胃虚寒者忌用。

附药

(1) 大青叶

为十字花科植物菘蓝的

indigotica Fort., family Cruciferae. The medicinal herb is bitter in flavor, cold in property, and attributive to the Heart Meridian and the Stomach Meridian. It acts to clear heat, relieve toxin, cool blood and dissipate macula, applied to treat febrile disease manifested by high fever, general macula, mumps, erysipelas and carbuncle. Apply 9～15 g in decoction. It is prohibited to apply for those with spleen and stomach deficiency and cold.

干燥叶。味苦性寒。归心、胃经。功能清热解毒，凉血消斑。适用于温病高热，身发斑疹，痄腮，丹毒，痈肿。煎服，9～15 克。脾胃虚寒者忌用。

(2) *Indigo Naturalis* (qing dai)

It is the dried product in powder or crumb prepared from the branch and leaf of *Baphicacanthus cusia* (Nees) Bremek, or *Polygonum tinctorium* Ait. or *Isatis indigotica Fort*., family Acanthaceae, Polygonaceae or Cruciferae. The medicinal herb is salty in flavor, cold in property, and attributive to the Liver Meridian. It acts to clear heat, relieve toxin, cool blood, dissipate macula, reduce fire and soothe convulsion, applied to treat febrile disease manifested by macula, hemoptysis and epistaxis due to heat in blood, cough with bloody sputum, mouth ulcer, mumps and infantile convulsion. It is prepared into pills or powder, applied 1.5～3 g. Apply a proper amount for external use.

(2) 青黛

为爵床科植物马蓝、蓼科植物蓼蓝或十字花科植物菘蓝的叶或茎叶经加工制得后的干燥粉末或团块。味咸性寒。归肝经。功能清热解毒，凉血消斑，泻火定惊。适用于温病发斑，血热吐衄，咳嗽痰血，口疮痄腮，小儿惊痫。入丸散，1.5～3 克。外用适量。

Dryopteris Crassirhizomatis Rhizoma (guan zhong)

It is the dried product from the rhizome with petiole base of *Dryopteris crassirhizoma* Nakai, family Dryopteridaceae and *Blechnum orientale* L., family Blechnaceae. The medicinal herb is collected in autumn, applied in crude form or in carbonized form.

Features Flavor: bitter. Property: slightly cold and slightly poisonous. Meridian tropism: the Liver Meridian and the Stomach Meridian.

贯众

为鳞毛蕨科植物粗茎鳞毛蕨的干燥根茎及叶柄残基。秋季采挖。生用或炒炭用。

性味归经 苦，微寒；有小毒。归肝、胃经。

Actions Clear heat, relieve toxin, stanch bleeding and kill worms.

Application

(1) Common cold, headache due to wind-heat, macula due to heat-toxin, carbuncle and ulcer with swelling and pain. The medicinal herb is bitter and cool and acts to clear heat, relieve toxin and cool blood. In the treatment of common cold, headache due to wind-heat, macula, carbuncle and ulcer, it is applied singly or combined with *Isatidis Radix* (ban lan gen), *Lonicerae Japonicae Flos* (jin yin hua) and *Forsythiae Fructus* (lian qiao).

(2) Hemoptysis, epistaxis and uterine bleeding. In the treatment of hemoptysis and epistaxis due to heat in blood, it is combined with *Caumen Biotae* (ce bai ye), *Imperatae Rhizoma* (bai mao gen). In the treatment of uterine bleeding and bloody feces, it is combined with *Halloysitum Rubrum* (chi shi zhi).

(3) Parasitic amassment with abdominal pain. The medicinal herb acts to kill worms, applied to treat various types of parasitic disease through combinations with other medicinal herbs. In the treatment of roundworms with abdominal pain, it is combined with *Fructus Meliae TooSendan* (chuan lian zi). In the treatment of hookworms, it is combined with *Arecae Semen* (bing lang). In the treatment of pinworms, it is applied singly in decoction or applied to wash perianal area before sleep.

Usage and dosage Apply 5～10 g in decoction. It is applied to clear heat, relieve toxin and kill worms in crude form, while to stanch bleeding in carbonized form.

Precautions for use It is not advisable to ap-

功效 清热解毒，止血，杀虫。

应用

（1）时疫感冒，风热头痛，热毒斑疹，疮疡肿痛。本品苦凉，能清热解毒、凉血。善治时疫感冒或风热头痛，斑疹、疮疡等证，可单用，或配伍板蓝根、金银花、连翘等同用。

（2）吐衄崩漏。治血热吐衄，常与侧柏叶、白茅根等同用。治崩漏下血，常与赤石脂等配伍。

（3）虫积腹痛。本品杀虫。通过配伍可用于多种肠寄生虫病。治蛔虫腹痛，配伍川楝子等；治钩虫，配伍槟榔等；治蛲虫，可单用煎汁，临睡前洗肛门周围。

用法用量 煎服，5～10克。生用清热解毒、杀虫，炒炭止血。

使用注意 不宜过量。

ply in overdose. It is cautious to apply for those with spleen and stomach deficiency and cold.

脾胃虚寒者慎用。

Taraxaci Herba (pu gong ying)

蒲公英

It is the dried product from the herb of Mongolian Dandelion, *Taraxacum mongolicum* Hand-Mazz., *Taraxacum sinicum* Kitag. or *Taraxacum heterolepis* Nakai et H. Koidz., family Compositae. The medicinal herb is collected in summer and autumn when it is initially flowering, applied in crude form.

为菊科植物蒲公英、碱地蒲公英或同属数种植物的干燥全草。夏至秋季花初开时采收。生用。

Features Flavor: bitter and sweet. Property: cold. Meridian tropism: the Liver Meridian and the Stomach Meridian.

性味归经 苦、甘,寒。归肝、胃经。

Actions Clear heat, relieve toxin, subside swell, dissipate stagnation, promote urination and treat stranguria.

功效 清热解毒,消肿散结,利尿通淋。

Application

(1) Carbuncle, acute mastitis, acute appendicitis and pulmonary abscess. The medicinal herb is bitter and cold and acts to clear heat, relieve toxin, dissolve abscess and dissipate stagnation. In the treatment of carbuncle and ulcer due to heat-toxin, it is combined with *Lonicerae Japonicae Flos* (jin yin hua), *Violae Herba* (zi hua di ding), to form up Five Ingredients Detoxifying Drink (Wu Wei Xiao Du Yin). In the treatment of acute mastitis, it is applied singly in fresh form by smashing to paste for external use, or combined with *Trichosanthis Fructus* (gua lou) and *Forsythiae Fructus* (lian qiao) for oral administration. In the treatment of acute appendicitis, it is combined with *Rhei Radix et Rhizoma* (da huang) and *Moutan Cortex* (mu dan pi). In the treatment of pulmonary abscess

应用

(1) 疮痈,乳痈,肠痈,肺痈。本品苦泄性寒,善清泄热毒、消痈散结。治热毒疮痈,常与金银花、紫花地丁等配伍,如五味消毒饮。治乳痈,可单用鲜品捣烂外敷,或配伍全瓜蒌、连翘等内服。治肠痈腹痛,与大黄、牡丹皮等同用。治肺痈吐脓,常配伍鱼腥草、芦根等同用。

with purulent sputum, it is combined with *Houttuyniae Herba* (yu xing cao), *Phragmitis Rhizoma* (lu gen).

(2) Stranguria due to heat and jaundice. The medicinal herb is bitter and cold and acts to dissolve damp, clear heat and treat stranguria. In the treatment of stranguria with difficult and painful urination due to heat, it is combined with *Lysimachiae Herba* (jin qian cao) and *Plantaginis Semen* (che qian zi). In the treatment of jaundice due to damp-heat, it is combined with *Artemisiae Scopariae Herba* (yin chen hao), *Gardeniae Fructus* (zhi zi) and da huang.

（2）热淋，黄疸。本品苦泄清利，能利湿热、通淋。治热淋涩痛，常与金钱草、车前子等同用。治湿热黄疸，常配伍茵陈、栀子、大黄等同用。

Usage and dosage Apply 10～30 g in decoction. Apply a proper amount for external use.

用法用量 煎服，10～30克。外用适量。

Precautions for use It is possible to cause moderate diarrhea in large dose.

使用注意 大量可致缓泻。

Violae Herba (zi hua di ding)

紫花地丁

It is the dried product from the herb of *Viola yedoensis* Makino, family Violaceae. The medicinal herb is collected in spring and autumn, applied in crude form.

为堇菜科多年生草本紫花地丁的干燥全草。春、秋季采收。生用。

Features Flavor: bitter and pungent. Property: cold. Meridian tropism: the Heart Meridian and the Liver Meridian.

性味归经 苦、辛，寒。归心、肝经。

Actions Clear heat, relieve toxin, cool blood and subside swell.

功效 清热解毒，凉血消肿。

Application

应用

(1) Furuncle, boil, carbuncle, ulcer and erysipelas. The medicinal herb acts to clear heat, relieve toxin, cool blood and subside swell, and it is the key herb to treat furuncles. In the treatment of early furuncle and boil with swelling and pain, it is

（1）疔疮，痈疽，丹毒。本品能清热解毒、凉血消肿，为治疔疮之要药。治疔疮初起肿痛，常与连翘、栀子等同用。治热毒痈疽，可与金银

combined with *Forsythiae Fructus* (lian qiao) and *Gardeniae Fructus* (zhi zi). In the treatment of carbuncle and ulcer due to heat-toxin, it is combined with *Lonicerae Japonicae Flos* (jin yin hua), *Taraxaci Herba* (pu gong ying). In the treatment of erysipelas, it is combined with *Rehmanniae Radix* (sheng di huang) and *Paeoniae Radix Rubra* (chi shao).

花、蒲公英花等配伍。治丹毒，可与生地黄、赤芍等配伍同用。

(2) Poisonous snake bite. The medicinal herb acts to relieve toxin from snake, subside swell and relieve pain. In the treatment of poisonous snake bite, it is applied singly in decoction or in fresh form, by taking its juice for oral administrating or by smashing to paste for external use.

（2）毒蛇咬伤。本品能解蛇毒、消肿痛。治毒蛇咬伤，可单用鲜品捣汁内服或捣烂外敷，亦可煎服。

Usage and dosage Apply 15～30 g in decoction. Apply a proper amount for external use.

用法用量 煎服，15～30 克。外用适量。

***Houttuyniae Herba* (yu xing cao)**

鱼腥草

It is the dried product from the herb of *Houttuynia cordata* Thunb, family Saururaceae. The medicinal herb is collected in summer when it is fully flourishing and flowering, applied in crude form.

为三白草科植物蕺菜的新鲜全草或干燥地上部分。夏季茎叶茂盛花穗多时采收。生用。

Features Flavor: pungent. Property: slight cold. Meridian tropism: the Lung Meridian.

性味归经 辛，微寒。归肺经。

Actions Clear heat, relieve toxin, dissolve carbuncle, drain pus, promote urination and treat stranguria.

功效 清热解毒，消痈排脓，利尿通淋。

Application

应用

(1) Pulmonary abscess with purulent sputum and cough due to phlegm-heat. The medicinal herb is cold and attributive to the Lung Meridian, and acts to clear heat from lung. In the treatment of pulmonary abscess with purulent sputum, it is combined with *Platycodonis Radix* (jie geng),

（1）肺痈吐脓，痰热咳嗽。本品药性寒凉，专入肺经而善清肺热。治肺痈吐脓，常与桔梗、芦根、薏苡仁等同用。治肺热咳嗽，痰黄黏稠，常与桑白皮、贝母、瓜

Phragmitis Rhizoma (lu gen) and *Coicis Semen* (yi yi ren). In the treatment of cough with yellow-thick sputum due to heat in lung, it is combined with *Cortex Mori Albae Radicis* (sang bai pi), *Bulbus Fritillariae Thunbergii* (zhe bei mu) and *Trichosanthis Fructus* (gua lou).

萎等同用。

(2) Carbuncle and ulcer. The medicinal herb acts to clear heat, relieve toxin, dissipate carbuncle and subside swell. In the treatment of carbuncle and ulcer with redness and swelling due to heat-toxin, it is combined with *Taraxaci Herba* (pu gong ying), *Forsythiae Fructus* (lian qiao), or applied singly in fresh form by smashing to paste for external use.

（2）热毒疮痈。本品能清热解毒、消散痈肿。治热毒疮痈红肿，常与蒲公英、连翘等配伍。亦可单用鲜品捣烂外敷。

(3) Stranguria due to heat. The medicinal herb is cold and acts to promote urination and treat stranguria. In the treatment of stranguria with difficult and painful urination due to heat, it is combined with *Plantaginis Semen* (che qian zi), *Lygodii Spora* (hai jin sha) and *Lysimachiae Herba* (jin qian cao).

（3）热淋。本品性寒且能利尿通淋。治热淋小便涩痛，常与车前子、海金沙、金钱草等同用。

Usage and dosage Apply 15～30 g in decoction. Apply its fresh product in double dose. Apply a proper amount for external use.

用法用量 煎服，15～30 克；鲜品用量加倍。外用适量。

Precautions for use It is not advisable to decoct for long time.

使用注意 不宜久煎。

Andrographitis Herba (chuan xin lian)

穿心莲

It is the dried product from the herb of *Andrographis paniculata* (Burm. f.) Nees., family Acanthaceae. The medicinal herb is collected in early autumn when it is flourishing, applied in crude form.

为爵床科植物穿心莲的干燥地上部分。秋初茎叶茂盛时采收。生用。

Features Flavor: bitter. Property: cold. Meridian tropism: the Lung Meridian, the Stomach

性味归经 苦，寒。归肺、胃、大肠、膀胱经。

Meridian, the Large Intestine Meridian and the Bladder Meridian.

Actions Clear heat, relieve toxin, cool blood and subside swell.

功效 清热解毒,凉血,消肿。

Application

应用

(1) Common cold manifested by fever and sore throat, and cough due to heat in lung. The medicinal herb is cold and acts to clear heat and relieve toxin, especially to clear heat from lung. In the treatment of febrile disease in early stage or wind-heat pattern due to exogenous factors manifested by fever, headache and sore throat, it is combined with *Lonicerae Japonicae Flos* (jin yin hua), *Forsythiae Fructus* (lian qiao) and *Menthae Haplocalycis Herba* (bo he). In the treatment of cough due to heat in lung, it is combined with *Scutellariae Radix* (huang qin) and *Trichosanthis Fructus* (gua lou). In the treatment of pulmonary abscess with purulent sputum, it is combined with *Houttuyniae Herba* (yu xing cao), *Phragmitis Rhizoma* (lu gen) and *Platycodonis Radix* (jie geng).

(1) 感冒发热,咽喉肿痛,肺热咳嗽。本品苦寒泄热,能清热解毒,尤善清肺热。治温病初起或外感风热,发热头痛,咽喉肿痛,常与金银花、连翘、薄荷等同用。治肺热咳嗽,常配伍黄芩、瓜蒌等同用。若肺痈吐脓,可与鱼腥草、芦根、桔梗等配伍。

(2) Carbuncle and ulcer, and poisonous snake bite. The medicinal herb acts to clear heat, relieve toxin, cool blood and dissolve carbuncle, and to relieve toxin from snake. In the treatment of carbuncle and ulcer due to heat-toxin, it is combined with *Taraxaci Herba* (pu gong ying), *Violae Herba* (zi hua di ding). In the treatment of poisonous snake bite, it is applied singly by smashing to paste for external use, or combined with eliminating heat and toxin in decoction for oral administration.

(2) 痈肿疮疡,毒蛇咬伤。本品能清热解毒、凉血散痈,且解蛇毒。治热毒疮痈肿痛,常配伍蒲公英、紫花地丁等。治毒蛇咬伤,可单用本品捣烂外敷,或配伍清热解毒药等水煎内服。

(3) Diarrhea and dysentery, and stranguria due to heat. The medicinal herb is bitter and acts to desiccate damp, and cold and acts to clear heat, ap-

(3) 泻痢,热淋。本品味苦燥湿,性寒清热,善治湿热诸证。治湿热泻痢,常与白

plied to treat various damp-heat patterns. In the treatment of diarrhea and dysentery due to damp-heat, it is combined with *Pulsatillae Radix* (bai tou weng) and *Coptidis Rhizoma* (huang lian). In the treatment of stranguria with difficult and painful urination due to heat, it is combined with *Plantaginis Semen* (che qian zi) and *Imperatae Rhizoma* (bai mao gen).

头翁、黄连等配伍。治热淋涩痛,可与车前子、白茅根等同用。

Usage and dosage Apply 6～9 g in decoction. Apply a proper amount for external use.

用法用量 煎服,6～9克。外用适量。

Precautions for use The medicinal herb is bitter in flavor, so it is not advisable to apply in too large dose.

使用注意 本品味苦,用量不宜过大。

Scutellariae Barbatae Herba (ban zhi lian)

半枝莲

It is the dried product from the herb of *Scutellaria barbata* D. Don, family Labiatae. The medicinal herb is collected in summer and autumn when it is fully flourishing, applied in crude form.

为唇形科植物半枝莲的干燥全草。夏、秋季茎叶茂盛时采收。生用。

Features Flavor: pungent and bitter. Property: cold. Meridian tropism: the Lung Meridian, the Liver Meridian and the Kidney Meridian.

性味归经 辛、苦,寒。归肺、肝、肾经。

Actions Clear heat, relieve toxin, dissolve stasis and promote urination.

功效 清热解毒,化瘀利尿。

Application

应用

(1) Carbuncle and ulcer due to heat-toxin, and poisonous snake bite. The medicinal herb is bitter and cold and acts to clear heat and relieve toxin from snake. In the treatment of carbuncle and ulcer due to heat-toxin or poisonous snake bite, it is applied singly by smashing to paste for external use, or combined with *Violae Herba* (zi hua di ding).

(1) 疮痈肿毒,毒蛇咬伤。本品性味苦寒,能清解热毒,且解蛇毒。治热毒疮痈肿痛,或毒蛇咬伤,可单用鲜品捣烂外敷,或配伍紫花地丁等同用。

(2) Traumatic injury. The medicinal herb is pungent and acts to dissolve stasis. In the treatment

(2) 跌打损伤。本品辛行祛瘀。治跌打损伤所致的

of bruise, swelling and pain due to traumatic injury, it is combined with *Olibanum* (ru xiang) and *Myrrha* (mo yao).

瘀肿疼痛，常与乳香、没药等配伍。

(3) Edema and jaundice. The medicinal herb acts to clear heat and promote urination. In the treatment of ascites, it is applied singly or combined with *Alismatis Rhizoma* (ze xie), *Plantaginis Semen* (che qian zi). In the treatment of jaundice due to damp-heat, it is combined with *Artemisiae Scopariae Herba* (yin chen hao) and *Gardeniae Fructus* (zhi zi).

（3）水肿，黄疸。本品能清热利水。治大腹水肿，可单用，或与泽泻、车前子等同用。治湿热黄疸，可与茵陈、栀子等同用。

Usage and dosage Apply 15～30 g in decoction. Apply its fresh product 30～60 g. Apply a proper amount for exernal use.

用法用量 煎服，15～30 克；鲜品 30～60 克；外用适量。

Precautions for use It is cautious to apply for pregnant women.

使用注意 孕妇慎用。

Sargentodoxae Caulis (da xue teng)

大血藤

It is the dried product from the stem of a deciduous woody vine, *Sargentodoxa cuneata* (Oliv.) Rehd. et Wits., family Lardizabalaceae, also called "hong teng". The medicinal herb is collected in autumn and winter, applied in crude form.

为木通科植物大血藤的干燥藤茎。又称红藤。秋、冬季采收。生用。

Features Flavor: bitter. Property: neutral. Meridian tropism: the Large Intestine Meridian and the Liver Meridian.

性味归经 苦，平。归大肠、肝经。

Actions Clear heat, relieve toxin, activate blood and stop pain.

功效 清热解毒，活血止痛。

Application

应用

(1) Acute appendicitis, carbuncle and ulcer. The medicinal herb acts to relieve toxin, activate blood and stop pain. In the treatment acute appendicitis manifested by abdominal pain, it is combined with *Lonicerae Japonicae Flos* (jin yin hua), *Forsythiae Fructus* (lian qiao) and *Moutan Cortex*

（1）肠痈，疮疡。本品长于解毒，且能活血止痛。治肠痈腹痛，常与金银花、连翘、牡丹皮等配伍。治热毒疮痈，多与蒲公英、紫花地丁等同用。

(mu dan pi). In the treatment of carbuncle and ulcer due to heat-toxin, it is combined with *Taraxaci Herba* (pu gong ying) and *Violae Herba* (zi hua di ding).

(2) Traumatic injury, dysmenorrheal, amenorrhea and Bi (Obturation) Pattern due to wind-damp. The medicinal herb acts to activate blood, dissolve stasis, dredge meridians and stop pain. In the treatment of bruise, swelling and pain due to traumatic injury, it is combined with *Paeoniae Radix Rubra* (chi shao) and *Olibanum* (ru xiang). In the treatment of dysmenorrheal and amenorrhea, it is combined with *Cyperi Rhizoma* (xiang fu), *Salviae Miltiorrhizae Radix et Rhizoma* (dan shen) and *Leonuri Herba* (yi mu cao). In the treatment of Bi (Obturation) Pattern due to wind-damp and impaired joints, it is combined with *Saposhnikoviae Radix* (fang feng) and *Angelicae Pubescentis Radix* (du huo).

（2）跌打损伤，痛经，经闭，风湿痹痛。本品能活血祛瘀、通络止痛。治跌打损伤所致的瘀肿疼痛，常与赤芍、乳香等同用。治痛经、经闭，常与香附、丹参、益母草等配伍。治风湿痹痛，关节不利，可与防风、独活等同用。

Usage and dosage　Apply 9～15 g in decoction.

Precautions for use　It is cautious to apply for pregnant women.

用法用量　煎服，9～15克。

使用注意　孕妇慎用。

Patriniae Herba (bai jiang cao)

It is the dried product from the root and stem of *Patrinias scabiosaefolia* Fisch. or *Patrinia villosa* Juss., family Valerianaceae. The medicinal herb is collected in summer and autumn, applied in crude form.

Features　Flavor: pungent and bitter. Property: slightly cold. Meridian tropism: the Liver Meridian, the Stomach Meridian and the Large Intestine Meridian.

败酱草

为败酱科植物黄花败酱、白花败酱的干燥带根全草。夏、秋季采收。生用。

性味归经　辛、苦，微寒。归肝、胃、大肠经。

Actions Clear heat, relieve toxin, dissolve carbuncle, drain pus, dissolve stasis and stop pain.

Application

(1) Acute appendicitis, pulmonary abscess, carbuncle and ulcer. The medicinal herb is bitter and acts to clear heat, dissolve carbuncle and drain pus. In the treatment of acute abscess in early stage, it is combined with *Sargentodoxae Caulis* (da xue teng) and *Moutan Cortex* (mu dan pi). In the treatment of acute appendicitis with purulence, it is combined with *Coicis Semen* (yi yi ren) and *Aconiti Radix Praeparata* (fu zi), to form up Jobstears Seed, Monkshood and Patrinia Powder (Yi Yi Fu Zi Bai Jiang San). In the treatment of pulmonary abscess with purulent sputum, it is combined with *Houttuyniae Herba* (yu xing cao), *Platycodonis Radix* (jie geng). In the treatment of carbuncle and ulcer with swelling and pain, it is applied singly in decoction for oral administration, or applied in fresh form by smashing to paste for external use.

(2) Abdominal pain after delivery. The medicinal herb acts to dissolve stasis and relieve pain. In the treatment of abdominal pain after delivery due to blood stasis, it is combined with *Carthami Flos* (hong hua) and *Typhae Pollen* (pu huang).

Usage and dosage Apply 6～15 g in decoction. Apply a proper amount for external use.

Precautions for use It is cautious to apply for those with spleen and stomach deficiency.

功效 清热解毒,消痈排脓,祛瘀止痛。

应用

(1)肠痈,肺痈,疮痈。本品苦泄清热、消痈排脓。治肠痈初起,常与红藤、牡丹皮等同用;肠痈脓成,则与薏苡仁、附子同用,即薏苡附子败酱散。治肺痈吐脓,可与鱼腥草、桔梗等同用。治疮痈肿痛,可单味煎汤顿服,或用鲜品捣烂外敷。

(2)产后腹痛。本品能祛瘀止痛。治产后瘀阻腹痛,可与红花、蒲黄等同用。

用法用量 煎服,6～15克。外用适量。

使用注意 脾胃虚弱者慎用。

Pulsatillae Radix (bai tou weng)

It is the dried product from the root of *Pulsatilla chinensis* (Bunge) Regel, family Ranunculaceae. The medicinal herb is collected in spring

白头翁

为毛茛科植物白头翁的干燥根。春、秋二季采挖。生用。

and autumn, applied in crude form.

Features Flavor: bitter. Property: cold. Meridian tropism: the Large Intestine Meridian.

Actions Clear heat, relieve toxin, cool blood and stop dysentery.

Application

(1) Dysentery with bloody feces due to heat-toxin. The medicinal herb acts to clear heat, cool blood and stop dysentery, as the major herb to treat dysentery. In the treatment of dysentery with blood feces due to heat-toxin, it is combined with *Coptidis Rhizoma* (huang lian), *Phellodendri Cortex Chiensis* (huang bo) and *Fraxini Cortex* (qin pi), to form up Pulsatilla Decoction (Bai Tou Weng Tang). In the treatment of diarrhea after delivery, it is combined with *Asini Corii Colla* (e jiao), huang bo and *Glycyrrhizae Radix et Rhizoma* (gan cao). In the treatment of chronic dysentery with bloody feces and cold pain at abdomen, it is combined with *Zingiberis Rhizoma* (gan jiang) and *Halloysitum Rubrum* (chi shi zhi).

(2) In the treatment of vaginal itch, the medicinal herb is decocted for external wash.

Usage and dosage Apply 9～15 g in decoction. Apply a proper amount for external use.

Precautions for use It is prohibited to apply for those with diarrhea or dysentery due to deficiency and cold.

性味归经 苦，寒。归大肠经。

功效 清热解毒，凉血止痢。

应用

（1）热毒血痢。本品功善清热凉血止痢，为治痢要药。治热毒血痢，常与黄连、黄柏、秦皮配伍，即白头翁汤。治产后下痢，常与阿胶、黄柏、甘草同用。若用于赤痢日久不愈，腹中冷痛，可与干姜、赤石脂等同用。

（2）此外，本品煎汤外洗，可治阴痒。

用法用量 煎服，9～15克。外用适量。

使用注意 虚寒泻痢者忌服。

Fraxini Cortex (qin pi)

It is the dried product from the bark of Korean Ash., *Fraxinus rhynchophylla* Hance or Chinese Ash., *Fraxinus chinensis* Roxb. or *Fraxinus stylosa* Lingelsh, family Oleaceae. The medicinal herb is col-

秦皮

为木犀科植物苦枥白蜡树、白蜡树或尖叶白蜡树、宿柱白蜡树等的干燥枝皮或干皮。春、秋季剥取。生用。

lected in spring and autumn, applied in crude form.

Features Flavor: bitter and astringent. Property: cold. Meridian tropism: the Liver Meridian, the Gallbladder Meridian and the Large Intestine Meridian.

性味归经 苦、涩,寒。归肝、胆、大肠经。

Actions Clear heat, relieve toxin, stop dysentery, treat morbid leucorrhea and brighten eyes.

功效 清热解毒,止痢,止带,明目。

Application

应用

(1) Dysentery due to heat-toxin and morbid leucorrhea due to damp-heat. The medicinal herb is cold and acts to reduce heat and desiccate damp, to stop dysentery and treat morbid leucorrhea. In the treatment of diarrhea or dysentery with tenesmus due to heat-toxin, it is combined with *Phellodendri Cortex Chiensis* (huang bo), *Coptidis Rhizoma* (huang lian) and *Pulsatillae Radix* (bai tou weng), to form up Pulsatilla Decoction (Bai Tou Weng Tang). In the treatment of morbid leucorrhea due to damp-heat, it is combined with huang bo.

(1) 热毒泻痢,湿热带下。本品苦寒泄热燥湿,能止痢、止带。治热毒泻痢,里急后重,常与黄柏、黄连、白头翁等配伍,如白头翁汤。治湿热带下,可配伍黄柏等同用。

(2) Redness, swelling and pain of eyes, and cataract. The medicinal herb acts to purify liver, reduce heat, brighten eyes and treat cataract. In the treatment of redness, swelling and pain of eyes due to liver fire or cataract, it is combined with *Cassiae Semen* (jue ming zi), *Chrysanthemi Flos* (ju hua) and *Prunellae Spica* (xia ku cao), or applied to decoct for external wash.

(2) 目赤肿痛,目生翳障。本品能清肝泄热、明目退翳。治肝火目赤肿痛或目生翳障,常与决明子、菊花、夏枯草等配伍同用,或煎汤外洗。

Usage and dosage Apply 6～12 g in decoction. Apply a proper amount for external use.

用法用量 煎服,6～12克。外用适量。

Belamecandae Rhizoma (she gan)

射干

It is the dried product from the rhizome of Blackberrylily, *Belamcanda chinensis* (L.) DC., family Iridaceae. The medicinal herb is collected in

为鸢尾科植物射干的干燥根茎。春初萌芽或秋末茎叶枯萎时采挖。生用。

early spring when it is sprouting or in late autumn when its leaves are withered, applied in crude form.

Features Flavor: bitter. Property: cold. Meridian tropism: the Lung Meridian.

Actions Clear heat, relieve toxin, dissolve phlegm and benefit throat.

Application

(1) Sore throat. The medicinal herb acts to clear heat, relieve toxin and benefit throat. In the treatment of sore throat, it is applied singly or combined with *Scutellariae Radix* (huang qin) and *Platycodonis Radix* (jie geng).

(2) Cough and panting due to phlegm accumulation. The medicinal herb is attributive to the Lung Meridian and acts to clear heat from lung and dissolve phlegm, applied to treat cough and panting due to phlegm accumulation. In the treatment of lung heat pattern with thick-yellow sputum, it is combined with *Cortex Mori Albae Radicis* (sang bai pi), jie geng, to form up Belamecanda. In the treatment of cough and panting with sputum due to cold, it is combined with *Asari Radix et Rhizoma* (xi xin) and *Ephedrae Herba* (ma huang), to form up Belamecanda and Ephedra Decoction (She Gan Ma Huang Tang).

Usage and dosage Apply 3～10 g in decoction.

性味归经 苦，寒。归肺经。

功效 清热解毒，消痰利咽。

应用

（1）咽喉肿痛。本品善清热毒、利咽喉。治咽喉肿痛，可单用，亦可配伍黄芩、桔梗等同用。

（2）痰壅咳喘。本品专入肺经，能清肺热、消痰涎，为咳喘痰多所常用。治肺热痰稠色黄，常与桑白皮、桔梗等配伍。治寒痰咳喘，可与细辛、麻黄等同用，如射干麻黄汤。

用法用量 煎服，3～10克。

Section 4 Heat-clearing and blood-cooling herbs

第4节 清热凉血药

Rehmanniae Radix (sheng di huang)

It is the dried product from the root of

生地黄

为玄参科植物地黄的干

Rehmannia glutinosa Libosch, family Scrophulariaceae. The medicinal herb is mainly produced in Henan Province, is also called "huai di huang". It is collected in autumn, applied in crude form.

燥块根。主产于河南，又称怀地黄。秋季采收，生用。

Features Flavor: sweet. Property: cold. Meridian tropism: the Heart Meridian, the Liver Meridian and the Kidney Meridian.

性味归经 甘，寒。归心、肝、肾经。

Actions Clear heat, cool blood, nourish yin and produce fluid.

功效 清热凉血，养阴生津。

Application

应用

(1) Heat entering Ying (Nutrient) and Xue (Blood) Phase pattern. The medicinal herb is attributive to the Xue (Blood) Phase, bitter and acts to clear heat and cool blood, and sweet and cold and acts to nourish yin and produce fluid. In the treatment of febrile disease of heat entering Ying (Nutrient) and Xue (Blood) Phase pattern manifested by feverish sensation, dry mouth, loss of consciousness and deep-red tongue, it is combined with *Scrophulariae Radix* (xuan shen) and *Coptidis Rhizoma* (huang lian), to form up Ying-Nutrient Phase-Purifying Decoction (Qing Ying Tang). In the treatment of febrile disease in late stage manifested by feverish sensation at night and cold sensation in morning due to vesidal heat, it is combined with *Herba Artemisiae Chinghao* (qing hao) and *Trionycis Carapax* (bie jia), to form up Sweet Wormwood and Turtle Shell Decoction (Qing Hao Bie Jia Tang).

（1）热入营血证。本品入血分，苦泄清热凉血，甘寒养阴生津。治温病热入营血，身热口干，神昏舌绛，常与玄参、黄连等配伍，如清营汤。治热病后期，余热未清，夜热早凉，常与青蒿、鳖甲等同用，如青蒿鳖甲汤。

(2) Hemoptysis, epistaxis and uterine bleeding, and macula due to heat-toxin. The medicinal herb acts to cool blood and stanch bleeding. In the treatment of hemoptysis, epistaxis and uterine bleeding due to heat, it is combined with fresh

（2）吐衄崩漏，热毒斑疹。本品能凉血止血。治血热吐衄崩漏，常与鲜荷叶、生艾叶、生侧柏叶同用，即四生丸。治热毒斑疹，色紫暗不

Folium Nelumbinis (he ye), *Folium Artemistae Argyi Cruda* (sheng ai ye) and *Caumen Biotae Cruda* (sheng ce bai ye), to form up Four Crude Ingredients Pills (Si Sheng Wan). In the treatment of macula with dark color due to heat-toxin, it is combined with *Paeoniae Radix Rubra* (chi shao), *Arnebiae Radix* (zi cao) and xuan shen.

红活，多与赤芍、紫草、玄参等配伍。

(3) Febrile disease manifested by thirst, diabetes, and constipation due to dryness in intestines. The medicinal herb is sweet and moist and acts to produce body fluid, and is cold and acts to clear heat. In the treatment of febrile disease damaging fluid manifested by red tongue and dry mouth, it is combined with *Adenophorae Radix* (nan sha shen) and *Ophiopogonis Radix* (mai men dong). In the treatment of diabetes due to yin deficiency, it is combined with *Puerariae Lobatae Radix* (ge gen) and *Trichosanthis Radix* (tian hua fen), to form up Jade Spring Powder (Yu Quan San). In the treatment of constipation due to fluid consumption, it is combined with xuan shen and mai men dong, to form up Humor-Increasing Decoction (Zeng Ye Tang).

（3）热病口渴，消渴，肠燥便秘。本品甘润生津，性寒清热。治热病伤津，舌红口干，常与沙参、麦冬等同用。治阴虚消渴，多与葛根、天花粉等同用，如玉泉散。若津伤便秘，常与玄参、麦冬配伍，即增液汤。

Usage and dosage Apply 10～30 g in decoction.

用法用量 煎服，10～30 克。

Precautions for use It is not advisable to apply for those with loose feces due to spleen deficiency.

使用注意 脾虚便溏者不宜用。

Scrophulariae Radix (xuan shen)

玄参

It is the dried product from the root of *Scrophalaria ningpoensis* Hemsl, family Scrophulariaceae. The medicinal herb is collected in winter when the twigs and leaves are withered, applied in crude form.

为玄参科植物玄参的干燥根。冬季茎叶枯萎时采挖。生用。

Features Flavor: sweet, bitter and salty. Property: cold. Meridian tropism: the Lung Meridian, the Stomach Meridian and the Kidney Meridian.

性味归经 甘、苦、咸，寒。归肺、胃、肾经。

Actions Clear heat, cool blood, nourish yin and relieve toxin.

功效 清热凉血，滋阴解毒。

Application

应用

(1) Heat entering Ying (Nutrient) and Xue (Blood) Phase pattern. The medicinal herb is salty to entering the blood, bitter to reduce heat and cold to clear heat, and acts to clear heat, cool blood, reduce heat and relieve toxin. In the treatment of febrile disease when heat entering Ying (Nutrient) and Xue (Blood) Phases manifested by feverish body, dry mouth, loss of consciousness and deep-red tongue, it is combined with *Rehmanniae Radix* (sheng di huang) and *Forsythiae Fructus* (lian qiao), to form up Ying-Nutrient Phase-Purifying Decoction (Qing Ying Tang). In the treatment of heat entering pericardium manifested by loss of consciousness and delirium, it is combined with *Forsythiae Fructus* (lian qiao) and *Lophatheri Herba* (dan zhu ye).

（1）热入营血证。本品咸入血，苦泄热，寒清热，善清热凉血、泻火解毒。治温病热入营血，身热口干，神昏舌绛，常与生地黄、连翘等同用，如清营汤。治热入心包，神昏谵语，常配连翘心、竹叶卷心等同用。

(2) Sore throat, carbuncle and ulcer due to heat-toxin, scrofula and goiter. The medicinal herb acts to reduce fire, relieve toxin, soften hardness and dissipate stagnation. In the treatment of sore throat due to heat-toxin, it is combined with lian qiao and *Isatidis Radix* (ban lan gen). In the treatment of carbuncle and ulcer due to heat-toxin, it is combined with *Taraxaci Herba* (pu gong ying) and *Violae Herba* (zi hua di ding). In the treatment of scrofula and goiter, it is combined with *Ostreae Concha* (mu li) and *Bulbus Fritillariae Thunbergii* (zhe bei mu).

（2）咽喉肿痛，痈肿疮毒，瘰疬痰核。本品善泻火解毒、软坚散结。治热毒咽痛，常与连翘、板蓝根等同用。治热毒疮痈，常与蒲公英、紫花地丁等配伍。治瘰疬痰核，常配牡蛎、贝母等同用。

Furthermore, the medicinal herb is also applied to treat tuberculosis with hemoptysis, fever due to yin deficiency, diabetes and constipation.

此外，本品还可用于劳嗽咳血，阴虚发热，消渴便秘等证。

Usage and dosage Apply 9～15 g in decoction.

用法用量 煎服，9～15克。

Precautions for use It is not advisable to apply for those with loose feces due to spleen deficiency. The medicinal herb is incompatible with *Radix et Rhizoma Veratri Nigri* (li lu).

使用注意 脾虚便溏者不宜用。反藜芦。

Moutan Cortex (mu dan pi)

牡丹皮

It is the dried product from the cortex of *Paeonia suffruticoas* Andr, family Ramunculaceae. The medicinal herb is collected in autumn, applied in crude form.

为毛茛科植物牡丹的干燥根皮。秋季采挖。生用。

Features Flavor: bitter and pungent. Property: slightly cold. Meridian tropism: the Heart Meridian, the Liver Meridian and the Kidney Meridian.

性味归经 苦、辛，微寒。归心、肝、肾经。

Actions Clear heats, cool blood, reduce false heat, activate blood and dissipate stagnation.

功效 清热凉血，退虚热，活血散瘀。

Application

应用

(1) Macula, hemoptysis and epistaxis due to heat in blood. The medicinal herb acts to clear heat and cool blood. In the treatment of heat entering Ying (Nutrient) and Xue (Blood) Phases manifested by macula, or bleeding due to heat in blood as hemoptysis and epistaxis, it is combined with *Rehmanniae Radix* (sheng di huang) and *Paeoniae Radix Rubra* (chi shao).

(1) 血热斑疹，吐衄。本品具有清热凉血之功。治热入营血，身发斑疹，或血热妄行，吐血衄血，常配生地黄、赤芍等同用。

(2) False heat pattern. The medicinal herb is pungent and bitter and acts to clear the false heat. In the treatment of febrile disease with residual heat manifested by feverish sensation at night and cool

(2) 虚热证。本品辛透苦泄，能清透阴分伏热，而具清虚热之功。治温病余热未清，夜热早凉，热退无汗，常

sensation in the morning, and absence of sweating without fever, it is combined with *Artemisiae Annuae Herba* (qing hao) and *Trionycis Carapax* (bie jia). The medicinal herb acts to treat fever, feverish sensation and tidal fever due to yin deficiency by combining with yin-nourishing herbs.

与青蒿、鳖甲等同用。与养阴药配伍，亦治阴虚发热，骨蒸潮热等证。

(3) Amenorrhea, dysmenorrhea and abdominal masses, traumatic injuries. The medicinal herb is pungent to move blood and acts to activate blood and dissipate stagnation. In the treatment of amenorrhea and dysmenorrhea due to blood stasis, it is combined with *Salviae Miltiorrhizae Radix et Rhizoma* (dan shen) and *Carthami Flos* (hong hua). In the treatment of abdominal masses, it is combined with *Cinnamomi Ramulus* (gui zhi) and *Poria* (fu ling). In the treatment of traumatic injury, it is combined with *Olibanum* (ru xiang) and *Myrrha* (mo yao).

（3）经闭痛经，癥瘕积聚，跌打损伤。本品辛行散血，能活血祛瘀。治瘀滞经闭、痛经，常配丹参、红花等同用。治癥瘕积聚，常与桂枝、茯苓等配伍。治跌打损伤，常配乳香、没药等同用。

(4) Carbuncle and ulcer, and acute appendicitis. The medicinal herb acts to cool blood, dissipate stagnation, clear heat and dissolve carbuncle. In the treatment of carbuncle and ulcer, it is combined with *Taraxaci Herba* (pu gong ying) and *Violae Herba* (zi hua di ding). In the treatment of acute appendicitis with abdominal pain, it is combined with *Rhei Radix et Rhizoma* (da huang) and *Persicae Semen* (tao ren), to form up Rhubarb and Moutan Bark Decoction (Da Huang Mu Dan Pi Tang).

（4）疮痈，肠痈。本品能凉血散瘀、清热消痈。治疮痈，可与蒲公英、紫花地丁等同用。治肠痈腹痛，常与大黄、桃仁等配伍，如大黄牡丹皮汤。

Usage and dosage Apply 6～15 g in decoction.

用法用量 煎服，6～15克。

Precautions for use It is cautious to apply for pregnant women and those with heavy blood flow in menstruation.

使用注意 孕妇及月经过多者慎用。

Paeoniae Radix Rubra (chi shao)

It is the dried product from the root of *Paeonia lactiflora* Pall, or the root of *Paeonia veitchii* Lynch, family Ranunculaceae. *Paeonia lactiflora* Pall is mainly produced in Inner Mongolia and northeast China, while *Paeonia veitchii* Lynch is mainly produced in Sichuan Province. The medicinal herb is collected in spring and autumn, applied in crude form or in fried form.

Features Flavor: bitter. Property: slight cold. Meridian tropism: the Liver Meridian.

Actions Clear heats, cool blood, dissipate stagnation and relieve pain.

Application

(1) Macula, hemoptysis and epistaxis due to heat in blood. The medicinal herb acts to cool blood and activate blood. In the treatment of heat entering Ying (Nutrient) and Xue (Blood) Phases manifested by general macula, it is combined with *Moutan Cortex* (mu dan pi) and *Scrophulariae Radix* (xuan shen). In the treatment of hemoptysis and epistaxis, it is combined with *Rehmanniae Radix* (sheng di huang) and *Imperatae Rhizoma* (bai mao gen).

(2) All types of pain due to stagnation and stasis. The medicinal herb acts to activate blood, dredge meridians, dissipate stagnation and relieve pain. In the treatment of amenorrhea and dysmenorrhea, it is combined with *Leonuri Herba* (yi mu cao) and *Cyperi Rhizoma* (xiang fu). In the treatment of abdominal masses, it is combined with *Cinnamomi Ramulus* (gui zhi) and *Carthami Flos* (hong hua). In the treatment of traumatic injury, it

赤芍

为芍药科植物芍药或川赤芍的干燥根。芍药主产于内蒙古和东北等地;川赤芍主产于四川。春、秋季采挖。生用或炒用。

性味归经 苦,微寒。归肝经。

功效 清热凉血,散瘀止痛。

应用

(1) 血热斑疹,吐衄。本品能凉血、活血。治热入营血,身发斑疹,常与牡丹皮、玄参等配伍。治血热所致吐衄,多与生地黄、白茅根等同用。

(2) 瘀滞诸痛证。本品功能活血通经、祛瘀止痛。治经闭痛经,常与益母草、香附等配伍。治癥瘕积聚,常配伍桂枝、红花等。治跌扑伤痛,常与乳香、没药等同用。

is combined with *Olibanum* (ru xiang) and *Myrrha* (mo yao).

Furthermore, the medicinal herb is bitter and attributive to the Liver Meridian, and acts to clear and reduce the liver fire, applied to treat redness of eyes due to heat in liver, or cataract.

此外,本品苦泄入肝,能清泄肝火,可治肝热目赤,或目生翳障。

Usage and dosage Apply 6～15 g in decoction.

用法用量 煎服,6～15克。

Precautions for use It is not advisable to apply for those with amenorrhea due to blood deficiency. The medicinal herb is incompatible with *Radix et Rhizoma Veratri Nigri* (li lu).

使用注意 血虚经闭不宜。反藜芦。

Arnebiae Radix (zi cao)

紫草

It is the dried product from the root of *Arnebia euchroma* (Royle) Johnst., or *Arnbia guttata* Bunge., family Boraginaceae. The medicinal herb is mainly produced in Xinjiang, Tibet and Inner Mongolia. It is collected in spring and autumn, applied in crude form.

为紫草科植物新疆紫草或内蒙紫草的干燥根。主产于新疆、西藏和内蒙古。春、秋季采挖。生用。

Features Flavor: sweet and salty. Property: cold. Meridian tropism: the Heart Meridian and the Liver Meridian.

性味归经 甘、咸,寒。归心、肝经。

Actions Clear heats, cool blood, activate blood, relieve toxin, promote eruption and dissipate macula.

功效 清热凉血,活血解毒,透疹消斑。

Application

(1) Macula in dark color and measles with unsmooth eruption. The medicinal herb acts to clear heat, cool blood, activate blood, relieve toxin and promote eruption. In the treatment of general macula in dark color due to heat-toxin in blood, it is combined with *Paeoniae Radix Rubra* (chi shao) and *Cimicifugae Rhizoma* (sheng ma). In the treat-

应用

(1) 斑疹紫黑,麻疹不透。本品功善清热凉血,活血解毒透疹。治血热毒盛,身发斑疹,色紫黑而不红活,常与赤芍、升麻等同用。治麻疹透发不畅,咽喉肿痛者,常与牛蒡子、连翘等同用。

ment of measles with unsmooth eruption and sore throat, it is combined with *Arctii Fructus* (niu bang zi) and *Forsythiae Fructus* (lian qiao).

(2) Carbuncle, abscess, furuncle and ulcer, eczema with itching, scalding by water and burning by fire. The medicinal herb applied externally acts to cool blood and relieve toxin. In the treatment of unhealed carbuncle and ulcer, it is applied singly or combined with *Angelicae Dahuricae Radix* (bai zhi) and *Angelicae Sinensis Radix* (dang gui), to form up Granulation-Promoting Rubin Ointment (Sheng Ji Yu Hong Gao). It is applied to treat eczema with itching, scalding by water and burning by fire in combining with other medicinal herbs.

（2）痈疽疮疡，湿疹瘙痒，水火烫伤。本品外用能凉血解毒。可单用，或配伍白芷、当归等同用，治疮痈溃不收口，如生肌玉红膏。并可通过配伍，治湿疹瘙痒和水火烫伤。

Usage and dosage Apply 5～10 g in decoction. Apply a proper amount for external use or make it into ointment or oil for external use.

用法用量 煎服，5～10克。外用适量，熬膏或油浸外涂。

Precautions for use It is prohibited to apply for those with loose fecess due to spleen deficiency.

使用注意 脾虚便溏者忌服。

Bubali Cornu **(shui niu jiao)**

水牛角

It is the product from the horn of *Bubalus bubalis* Linnaeus, family Bovidae. The buffalo horn is soaked and boiled in water, dried, cut into pieces or filed into powder.

为牛科动物水牛的角。取角后水煮，去角塞，干燥。镑片或锉粉用。

Features Flavor: bitter and salty. Property: cold. Meridian tropism: the Heart Meridian and the Liver Meridian.

性味归经 苦、咸，寒。归心、肝经。

Actions Clear heat, cool blood and relieve toxin.

功效 清热凉血，解毒。

Application

应用

(1) Heat entering Ying (Nutrient) and Xue (Blood) Phase pattern, hemoptysis and epistaxis due to heat in blood. The medicinal herb acts to

（1）热入营血证，血热吐衄。本品能清泄营血之热。治热入营血，高热不退，或身

clear heat from the Ying (Nutrient) and Xue (Blood) Phases. In the treatment of heat entering Ying (Nutrient) and Xue (Blood) Phase pattern manifested by high fever and general macula, it is combined with *Lonicerae Japonicae Flos* (jin yin hua) and *Scrophulariae Radix* (xuan shen). In the treatment of hemoptysis and epistaxis due to heat in blood, it is combined with *Rehmanniae Radix* (sheng di huang) and *Moutan Cortex* (mu dan pi).

发斑疹，常与金银花、玄参等配伍。治血热吐衄，常与生地黄、牡丹皮等同用。

(2) Carbuncle and ulcer, and throat impediment. The medicinal herb acts to clear heat, relieve toxin, cool blood and subside swell. In the treatment of carbuncle and ulcer with redness and swelling, or throat impediment and sore throat due to heat-toxin, it is combined with the heat-clearing and toxin-relieving herbs and swell-subsiding and pain-stopping herbs.

(2) 疮痈，喉痹。本品功能清热解毒、凉血消肿。治疮痈红肿或热毒喉痹咽痛，常与清热解毒、消肿止痛药同用。

Usage and dosage Apply 15～30 in decoction. It is decocted first, or filed into powder to infuse for oral administration. Apply a proper amount for external use.

用法用法 煎服，15～30 克，宜先煎。或锉末冲服。外用适量。

Precautions for use It is not advisable to apply for those with deficiency and cold of spleen and stomach.

使用注意 脾胃虚寒者不宜用。

Section 5 False heat-clearing herbs

第 5 节 清虚热药

Artemisiae Annuae Herba (qing hao)

青蒿

It is the dried product from the herb of *Artemisia annua* L., family Compositae. The medicinal herb is collected in autumn when it is fully flower-

为菊科植物黄花蒿的干燥地上部分。秋季花盛开时采割。生用。

ing, applied in crude form.

Features Flavor: bitter and pungent. Property: cold. Meridian tropism: the Liver Meridian and the Gallbladder Meridian.

性味归经 苦、辛，寒。归肝、胆经。

Actions Clear the false heat, relieve summer-heat and treat malaria.

功效 清虚热，解暑热，截疟。

Application

应用

(1) False heat pattern. The medicinal herb is bitter and pungent and acts to clear heat from blood and relieve feverish sensation. In the treatment of febrile disease with yin consumption and fever, it is combined with *Trionycis Carapax* (bie jia) and *Moutan Cortex* (mu dan pi), to form up Sweet Wormwood and Turtle Shell Decoction (Qing Hao Bie Jia Tang). In the treatment of yin deficiency manifested by feverish sensation and tidal fever, it is combined with *Gentianae Macrophyllae Radix* (qin jiao) and *Anemarrhenae Rhizoma* (zhi mu).

（1）虚热证。本品苦泄辛散，清透兼之，能凉血热、退骨蒸。治热病伤阴发热，常与鳖甲、丹皮等配伍，如青蒿鳖甲汤。治阴虚骨蒸潮热，可与秦艽、知母等配伍同用。

(2) Exogenous summer-heat attack pattern. The medicinal herb acts to clear heat and reduce summer-heat. In the treatment of exogenous summer-heat pattern, it is combined with *Pogostemonis Herba* (huo xiang).

（2）暑热外感。本品能清热解暑。配广藿香治暑热外感，发热头痛。

(3) Malaria. The medicinal herb acts to treat malaria. In the treatment of malaria, it is applied by taking juice from fresh herb.

（3）疟疾。本品有截疟之功。治疟疾，可用大量鲜青蒿绞汁服用。

Usage and dosage Apply 6～12 g in decoction. Or take juice from fresh herb.

用法用量 煎服，6～12克。或鲜品绞汁。

Precautions for use It is not advisable to decoct it for long time.

使用注意 不宜久煎。

Cynanchi Atrati Radix et Rhizoma (bai wei)

白薇

It is the dried product from the root and rhizome of *Cymanchum atratum* Bunge or *Cymanchum*

为萝藦科植物白薇或蔓生白薇的干燥根及根茎。

versicolor Bunge, family Asclepiadaceae. The medicinal herb is collected in spring and autumn, applied in crude form.

春、秋季采挖。生用。

Features Flavor: bitter and salty. Property: cold. Meridian tropism: the Stomach Meridian, the Liver Meridian and the Kidney Meridian.

性味归经 苦、咸，寒。归胃、肝、肾经。

Actions Clear false heat, clear heats, cool blood, promote urination, treat stranguria, relieve toxin and treat carbuncle.

功效 清虚热，清热凉血，利尿通淋，解毒疗疮。

Application

应用

(1) Fever due to yin deficiency and false heat pattern after delivery. The medicinal herb is attributive to the Xue (Blood) Phase and acts to clear false heat and relieve feverish sensation. In the treatment of feverish sensation and tidal fever due to yin deficiency, it is combined with *Anemarrhenae Rhizoma* (zhi mu) and *Trionycis Carapax* (bie jia). In the treatment of blood deficiency and low-grade fever after delivery, it is combined with *Angelicae Sinensis Radix* (dang gui) and *Ginseng Radix et Raizoma* (ren shen).

(1) 阴虚发热，产后虚热。本品入血分，善清虚热、除骨蒸。治阴虚骨蒸潮热，多与知母、鳖甲等同用。治产后血虚，低热不退，常与当归、人参等同用。

(2) Heat entering Ying (Nutrient) and Xue (Blood) Phases. The medicinal herb acts to clear pathogenic heat from Ying (Nutrient) Phase and Xue (Blood) Phase. In the treatment of heat entering Ying (Nutrient) and Xue (Blood) Phases manifested by high fever, restlessness, thirst and deep-red tongue, it is combined with *Rehmanniae Radix* (sheng di huang) and *Bubali Cornu* (shui niu jiao).

(2) 热入营血。本品能清营血邪热。治热入营血，高热烦躁，舌绛红者，常配伍生地黄、水牛角等同用。

(3) Stranguria with burning sensation and bleeding. The medicinal herb acts to clear heat, cool blood, promote urination and treat stranguria. In the treatment of stranguria with burning sensation and bleeding, it is combined with *Plantaginis Herba* (che

(3) 热淋，血淋。本品功能清热凉血、利尿通淋。治热淋、血淋，常与车前草、木通等同用。

qian cao) and *Akebiae Caulis* (mu tong).

(4) Carbuncle, ulcer, sore throat and poisonous snake bite. The medicinal herb is bitter and cold and acts to clear heat and relieve toxin. In the treatment of carbuncle and ulcer due to heat-toxin, it is applied by smashing into paste for external use, or combined with *Taraxaci Herba* (pu gong ying) and *Forsythiae Fructus* (lian qiao) for oral administration. In the treatment of sore throat, it is combined with *Belamecandae Rhizoma* (she gan) and *Arctii Fructus* (niu bang zi). In the treatment of poisonous snake bite, it is applied by smashing into paste for external use.

（4）疮痈咽痛，毒蛇咬伤。本品苦寒清热解毒。治热毒疮痈，可单味捣烂外敷，或配伍蒲公英、连翘等内服。治咽喉肿痛，可与射干、牛蒡子等同用。治毒蛇咬伤，可捣烂外敷。

Usage and dosage Apply 5～10 g in decoction. Apply a proper amount for external use.

用量用法 煎服，5～10克。外用适量。

Lycii Cortex (di gu pi)

地骨皮

It is the dried product from the root cortex of *Lycium chinensis* Mill, and *Lycium barbarum* L., family Solanaceae. The medicinal herb is collected in early spring or late autumn, applied in crude form.

为茄科植物枸杞或宁夏枸杞的干燥根皮。春初或秋后采挖，剥取根皮。生用。

Features Flavor: sweet. Property: cold. Meridian tropism: the Lung Meridian, the Liver Meridian and the Kidney Meridian.

性味归经 甘，寒。归肺、肝、肾经。

Actions Cool blood, relieve feverish sensation, purify lung and reduce fire.

功效 凉血除蒸，清肺降火。

Application

应用

(1) Fever due to yin deficiency. The medicinal herb acts to cool blood, clear false heat and relieve feverish sensation. In the treatment of yin deficiency and internal heat pattern manifested by feverish sensation and tidal fever, it is combined with *Stellariae Radix* (yin chai hu) and *Anemarrhenae*

（1）阴虚发热。本品具凉血热、清虚热、退骨蒸之功。治阴虚内热，骨蒸潮热，常配银柴胡、知母等同用，如清骨散。

Rhizoma (zhi mu), to form up Bone Heat-Clarifying Powder (Qing Gu San).

(2) Bleeding due to heat in blood. The medicinal herb acts to clear heat and cool blood. In the treatment of bleeding due to heat in blood, such as hemoptysis, epistaxis and bloody urine, it is applied singly or combined with other blood-cooling and bleeding-stanching herbs.

（2）血热出血。本品能清热凉血。治血热妄行的吐血、衄血、尿血诸证，可单味煎服，或配伍其他凉血止血药。

(3) Cough due to heat in lung. The medicinal herb acts to purify lung and reduce fire. In the treatment of up-reverse flow of qi due to heat in lung as coushing and panting, it is combined with *Cortex Mori Albae Radicis* (sang bai pi) and *Glycyrrhizae Radix et Rhizoma* (gan cao), to form up White Lung-Reducing Powder (Xie Bai San).

（3）肺热咳嗽。本品善清肺降火。治肺热气逆，咳嗽气喘，常与桑白皮、甘草等同用，如泻白散。

Furthermore, the medicinal herb acts to reduce heat and produce fluid, to treat diabetes.

此外，本品还能泄热生津，治消渴证。

Usage and dosage Apply 9～15 g in decoction.

用法用量 煎服，9～15克。

Stellariae Radix (yin chai hu)

银柴胡

It is the dried product from the root of *Stellaria dichotoma* L. var. *lanceolate* Bunge, family Caryophyllaceae. The medicinal herb is collected in spring and summer when it is sprouting or in autumn when it is withered, applied in crude form.

为石竹科植物银柴胡的干燥根。春、夏间植株萌发或秋后枝叶枯萎时采挖。生用。

Features Flavor: sweet. Property: slightly cold. Meridian tropism: the Liver Meridian and the Stomach Meridian.

性味归经 甘，微寒。归肝、胃经。

Actions Clear false heat and reduce fever in infantile malnutrition.

功效 清虚热，除疳热。

Application

应用

(1) Fever due to yin deficiency. The medicinal herb acts to clear false heat, as the special herb to

（1）阴虚发热。本品长于退虚热，为专治虚热之品。

treat false heat. In the treatment of yin deficiency and internal heat pattern manifested by feverish sensation and nocturnal sweats, it is combined with *Lycii Cortex* (di gu pi) and *Artemisiae Annuae Herba* (qing hao), to form up Bone Heat-Clarifying Powder (Qing Gu San).

治阴虚内热，骨蒸盗汗，常与地骨皮、青蒿等配伍，如清骨散。

(2) Fever in infantile malnutrition. The medicinal herb acts to reduce fever in infantile malnutrition. In the treatment of infantile malnutrition manifested by fever, bigbelly and emaciation, it is combined with *Codonopsis Radix Pilosulae* (dang shen) and *Galli Gigerii Endothelium Corneum* (ji nei jin).

（2）小儿疳热。本品善除疳热。治小儿疳积发热，腹大消瘦，常与党参、鸡内金等同用。

Usage and dosage Apply 3～10 g in decoction.

用法用量 煎服，3～10克。

Remarks *Bupleuri Radix* (chai hu) and *Stellariae Radix* (yin chai hu)

按语 柴胡与银柴胡

The two medicinal herbs are similar in names but different in actions. *Bupleuri Radix* (chai hu) is a plant of family Umbelliferae, while *Stellariae Radix* (yin chai hu) is a plant of family Caryophyllaceae. Chai hu acts to reduce fever, soothe liver, relieve depression and elevate yang qi, while yin chai hu acts to clear false heat and reduce fever in infantile malnutrition.

二药药名相近，功效迥异。柴胡为伞形科植物，银柴胡为石竹科植物。柴胡能疏散退热、疏肝解郁、升举阳气。银柴胡专清虚热，且除疳热。

Picrorhizae Rhizoma (hu huang lian)

胡黄连

It is the dried product from the rhizome of *Picrorhizae scrophulariiflora* Pennell, family Scrophulariaceae. The medicinal herb is mainly produced in Tibet. It is collected in autumn when it is withered, applied in crude form.

玄参科植物胡黄连的干燥根茎。主产于西藏。秋季地上部分枯萎时采挖。生用。

Features Flavor: bitter. Property: cold. Meridian tropism: the Liver Meridian, the Stomach

性味归经 苦，寒。归肝、胃、大肠经。

Meridian and the Large Intestine Meridian.

Actions Clear false heat, reduce fever in infantile malnutrition and eliminate damp and heat.

Application

(1) Fever due to yin deficiency. The medicinal herb acts to clear false heat. In the treatment of fever due to yin deficiency, it is combined with *Stellariae Radix* (yin chai hu) and *Lycii Cortex* (di gu pi).

(2) Fever in infantile malnutrition. The medicinal herb acts to reduce fever in infantile malnutrition. In the treatment of infantile malnutrition manifested by fever, abdominal distension and emaciation, it is combined with *Poria* (fu ling), *Massa Medicata Fermentata* (shen qu) and *Crataegi Fructus* (shan zha), to form up Baby-Fleshing Up Pills (Fei Er Wan).

(3) Diarrhea and dysentery due to damp-heat, and hemorrhoids with swelling and pain. The medicinal herb is bitter and cold and acts to clear heat and desiccate damp. In the treatment of diarrhea and dysentery due to damp-heat, it is combined with *Pulsatillae Radix* (bai tou weng). In the treatment of hemorrhoids with swelling and pain, it is applied by grinding into powder for oral administration or external use.

Usage and dosage Apply 3～10 g in decoction.

Remarks *Coptidis Rhizoma* (huang lian) and *Picrorhizae Rhizoma* (hu huang lian)

Both the medicinal herbs are bitter and cold and act to clear heat and desiccate damp. The difference is that *Coptidis Rhizoma* (huang lian) is a plant of family Ranunculaceae, while *Picrorhizae*

功效 清虚热，除疳热，清湿热。

应用

（1）阴虚发热。本品能清退虚热，常与银柴胡、地骨皮等同用，治阴虚发热。

（2）小儿疳热。本品亦除疳热。治小儿疳积，消瘦腹胀，为低热不退，常配伍茯苓、神曲、山楂等同用，如肥儿丸。

（3）湿热泻痢，痔疮肿痛。本品苦寒清热燥湿。治湿热泻痢，可单用，或与白头翁等配伍。治痔疮肿痛，可研末，内服外用皆宜。

用法用量 煎服，3～10克。

按语 黄连与胡黄连

二药均苦寒，能清热燥湿。不同的是黄连为毛莨科植物，胡黄连为玄参科植物。黄连为清实热药物，既可清

Rhizoma (hu huang lian) is a plant of family Scrophulariaceae. Besides, huang lian is a medicinal herb to clear true heat, acting to clear heat, reduce fire and relieve toxin, while hu huang lian acts to eliminate damp-heat and clear false heat as well, applied to treat fever due to yin deficiency and fever in infantile malnutrition.

热燥湿，还能清热泻火解毒。胡黄连既清湿热，亦清虚热，能治阴虚发热、小儿疳热。

Brief summary

1 Heat-clearing and fire-reducing herbs

Both *Gypsum Fibrosum* (shi gao) and *Anemarrhenae Rhizoma* (zhi mu), attributive to the Lung and Stomach Meridians, act to clear heat and reduce fire, applied to treat excess heat pattern in Qi (Energy) Phase. They are often applied in mutual reinforcement. Shi gao acts to clear true heat from lung and stomach, applied to treat cough due to heat in lung and toothache due to fire in stomach. Its crude form acts to clear heat and reduce fire for oral administration, while its calcined form acts to desiccate damp and astringe carbuncle for external use. Zhi mu is sweet and bitter in flavor and cold and moist in property and acts to moisturize lung and nourish stomach yin, applied to treat cough due to dryness in lung and diabetes due to internal heat. It also acts to nourish kidney yin and reduce false fire, applied to treat feverish sensation due to yin deficiency.

Both *Phragmitis Rhizoma* (lu gen) and *Trichosanthis Radix* (tian hua fen), attributive to the Lung and Stomach Meridians, act to clear heat and produce fluid, applied to treat febrile disease manifested by thirst due to consumption of fluid. Lu gen strongly acts to clear heat. It acts to clear heat from

小　结

1 清热泻火药

石膏、知母，均入肺胃经，功能清热泻火，治疗气分实热证，常相须为用。其中石膏重在清解，又善清肺胃实热，治肺热咳嗽、胃火牙痛；内服生用清热泻火，煅后外用收湿敛疮。知母甘苦性寒质润，清中有润，能润肺燥滋胃阴，治肺燥咳嗽、内热消渴；能滋肾阴、降虚火，治阴虚骨蒸。

芦根、天花粉，均入肺胃经，为清热生津之品，常治热病津伤口渴。其中芦根清热力强，既善清肺热、消痈，治肺热咳嗽、肺痈吐脓，又清胃热、止呕，治胃热呕吐；还能

lung and dissolve carbuncle, to treat cough due to heat in lung and purulent sputum due to pulmonary abscess, and it also acts to clear heat from stomach and relieve vomiting, to treat vomiting due to heat in stomach. It also acts to promote urination. Tian hua fen strongly acts to produce fluid. It acts to clear heat from lung and moisturize lung, applied to treat cough due to heat or dryness in lung. It also acts to subside swell and drain pus, as the major herb for carbuncle and ulcer in external medicine.

利尿。天花粉生津作用佳，既清肺热又润肺燥，治肺热或燥咳；又消肿排脓，为外科疮疡要药。

Both *Gardeniae Fructus* (zhi zi) and *Lophatheri Herba* (dan zhu ye), attributive to the Heart Meridian, act to clear heat and relieve restlessness, applied to treat febrile disease manifested by restlessness thirst. Zhi zi is attributive to the Triple Energizer Meridian and strongly acts to reduce fire. It acts to clear fire from triple energizer, as the major herb to treat febrile disease manifested by restlessness. It also acts to cool blood, relieve toxin and eliminate damp-heat, to treat bleeding due to heat in blood, carbuncle and ulcer due to heat-toxin and jaundice due to damp-heat. It acts to subside swell and relieve pain, to treat traumatic injuries for external use. Dan zhu ye acts to reduce fire from heart and small intestine, and to clear heat and promote urination, applied to treat heart transmitting to small intestine pattern manifested by restlessness, thirst, ulcers of mouth and tongue, and dark urine and difficult and painful urination.

栀子、淡竹叶，均入心经，有清热除烦之功，常用于热病心烦口渴。其中栀子入三焦经，泻火力强，既善清三焦之火而除烦，为治热病烦闷之要药，又凉血解毒、清利湿热，以治血热出血、热毒疮疡、湿热黄疸；外用消肿止痛，治跌打损伤。淡竹叶善清心与小肠之火，长于清热利尿，多用于心热移于小肠之烦渴、口舌生疮、尿赤涩痛。

Both *Prunellae Spica* (xia ku cao) and *Cassiae Semen* (jue ming zi), attributive to the Liver Meridian, act to purify liver and brighten eyes, to treat redness of eyes due to fire in liver. Xia ku cao strongly acts to purify liver and brighten eyes, as the major herb to treat pain of eyes. It also acts to

夏枯草、决明子，均入肝经，功能清肝明目，治肝火目赤。其中夏枯草清肝明目之力较强，为治目珠疼痛之要药；又散结消肿，为治瘰疬、瘿瘤多用。决明子质润，兼

dissipate stagnation and subside swell, to treat scrofula and goiter. Jue ming zi is moist and acts to moisturize intestines and promote defecation, to treat constipation due to dryness-heat.

能润肠通便而治燥热便秘。

2 Heat-clearing and damp-desiccating herbs

All *Scutellariae Radix* (huang qin), *Coptidis Rhizoma* (huang lian) and *Phellodendri Cortex Chiensis* (huang bo) are bitter and cold and act to clear heat, desiccate damp, reduce fire and relieve toxin. They are applied in mutual reinforcement, applied to treat damp-heat pattern and fire-toxin pattern. Huang qin acts to eliminate damp-heat from upper energizer and clear fire from lung, as the major herb to treat cough due to damp-heat, summer-heat or heat in lung. It acts to reduce fire and stanch bleeding, to treat bleeding due to heat in blood. It acts to clear heat and quiet fetus, applied to treat fetal irritability. Huang lian acts to clear fire from heart and eliminate damp-heat from middle energizer, as the major herb to treat diarrhea and dysentery due to damp-heat and vomiting due to heat in stomach, and also the major herb to treat febrile disease manifested by high fever and restlessness. It acts to reduce fire, relieve toxin and treat carbuncle, applied to treat all types of carbuncle, furuncle, ulcer and eruption due to toxin. Huang bo acts to eliminate damp-heat from lower energizer, as the major herb to treat morbid leucorrhea, stranguria, jaundice, and swelling and pain of foot and knee due to downward-infusion of damp-heat. It acts to reduce the Xiang (Premiere) Fire and clear false heat, applied to treat yin deficiency and fire hyperactivity pattern manifested by feverish sensation and tidal fever.

2 清热燥湿药

黄芩、黄连、黄柏均性味苦寒,具有清热燥湿、泻火解毒之功,常相须为用,治湿热、火毒之证。其中黄芩善清上焦湿热及肺火,为治湿温、暑温及肺热咳嗽之要药;还能泻火止血,治血热出血;清热安胎,治胎热胎动不安。黄连善清心火及中焦湿热,既是治湿热泻痢、胃热呕吐之要药,又为治热盛火炽、高热烦燥之良品;且善泻火解毒疗疮,常治痈疽疔毒诸证。黄柏善清下焦湿热,为治湿热下注之带下、淋浊、黄疸及足膝肿痛等证之良药;且善泻相火、清虚热,治阴虚火旺,骨蒸潮热。

Both *Gentianae Radix et Rhizoma* (long dan) and *Sophorae Flavescentis Radix* (ku shen) act to clear heat, desiccate damp and eliminate damp-heat from lower energizer, applied to treat jaundice, dark urine, swollen perineum, pruritus vulvae, eczema and morbid leucorrhea. Long dan acts to reduce true fire from liver and gallbladder, applied to treat headache due to fire in liver, and also treat excess heat in the Liver Meridian manifested by high fever and convulsion. Ku shen acts to kill worms and promote urination, applied to treat scabies, leprosy, and difficult and painful urination.

龙胆草、苦参，均能清热燥湿，尤善清下焦湿热，治黄疸尿赤、阴肿、阴痒、湿疹、带下等。其中龙胆草又长于泻肝胆实火，既治肝火头痛，又治肝经热盛，高热抽搐。苦参又能杀虫、利尿，治疥癣、麻风，以及小便涩痛。

3 Heat-clearing and toxin-relieving herbs

3 清热解毒药

Both *Lonicerae Japonicae Flos* (jin yin hua) and *Forsythiae Fructus* (lian qiao) act to clear heat, relieve toxin, and eliminate wind-heat, applied to treat carbuncle and ulcer in early stage with exterior symptoms or carbuncle and ulcer due to toxin, and also treat wind-heat pattern and febrile disease in any of Wei (Defense) Phase, Qi (Energy) Phase, Ying (Nutrient) Phase and Xue (Blood) Phase. Jin yin hua acts to relieve toxin, cool blood and stop dysentery, to treat dysentery with bleeding. Lian qiao acts to dissolve carbuncle and dissipate stagnation, as the major herb to treat carbuncle, scrofula and goiter.

金银花、连翘，均能清热解毒、疏散风热，治疮痈初起兼有表证或疮痈毒盛，以及外感风热或温热病卫、气、营、血各个阶段。其中金银花清透解毒力强，又凉血止痢，治疗血痢。连翘长于消痈散结，为疮家要药，又治瘰疬痰核。

Both *Isatidis Radix* (ban lan gen) and *Dryopteris Crassirhizomatis Rhizoma* (guan zhong) act to clear heat, relieve toxin and cool blood. Ban lan gen acts to clear heat, relieve toxin, cool blood and benefit throat, applied to treat heat-toxin pattern manifested by eruption, sore throat, carbuncle, furuncle, ulcer and mumps. Guan zhong acts to

板蓝根、贯众，均能清热解毒、凉血。其中板蓝根清热解毒、凉血利咽，常治温毒发斑、咽喉肿痛、疮痈肿毒、痄腮等证。贯众的清热解毒、凉血主要用于时疫感冒、外感风热、痄腮等；又能凉血

clear heat, relieve toxin and cool blood, applied to treat influenza, exogenous wind-heat and mumps. It acts to cool blood and stanch bleeding, applied to treat bleeding due to heat in blood, especially good for uterine bleeding due to heat in blood. It acts to kill worms, applied to treat various types of intestinal parasites.

止血,治血热出血,尤宜于血热崩漏;还能杀虫,用于多种肠道寄生虫病。

Both *Taraxaci Herba* (pu gong ying) and *Violae Herba* (zi hua di ding) act to clear heat and relieve toxin, applied to treat carbuncle and ulcer. Pu gong ying, the key herb to treat acute mastitis, also acts to treat acute appendicitis. It acts to dispel dampness, applied to treat stranguria due to heat and jaundice. Zi hua di ding acts to treat furuncle and abscess, to relieve toxin from snake, and subside swell and pain.

蒲公英、紫花地丁,均能清热解毒,善治疮痈。其中蒲公英为治乳痈要药,亦治肠痈;又利湿,治热淋、黄疸。紫花地丁尤为治疔疮要药,还能解蛇毒、消肿痛。

Both *Houttuyniae Herba* (yu xing cao) and *Andrographitis Herba* (chuan xin lian), attributive to the Lung Meridian, act to clear heat, relieve toxin and eliminate heat from lung, applied to treat pulmonary abscess, cough with purulent sputum and cough due to heat in lung. Yu xing cao, as the special herb for the Lung Meridian, acts to treat cough due to heat in lung. It acts to promote urination and treat stranguria, applied to treat difficult and painful urination due to heat. Chuan xin lian is bitter and cold and acts to clear heat and desiccate damp, applied to treat various types of damp-heat pattern, and also acts to dissolve carbuncle, subside swell and relieve toxin from snake.

鱼腥草、穿心莲,均入肺经,能清热解毒、清泄肺热,善治肺痈、咳吐脓血和肺热咳嗽。其中鱼腥草为肺经专药,为治肺热咳嗽要药;又利尿通淋,治热淋涩痛。穿心莲苦寒清热燥湿,治湿热诸证,还能散痈消肿、解蛇毒。

Herba Scutellariae Barbatae (ban zhi lian), pungent and bitter in flavor and cold in property, acts to clear heat, relieve toxin, dissolve stasis and promote urination, applied to treat carbuncle and

半枝莲,辛苦性寒,能清热解毒、化瘀利尿,治热毒疮痈、毒蛇咬伤,以及跌打损伤、水肿、黄疸。

ulcer due to heat-toxin, poisonous snake bite, traumatic injuries, edema and jaundice.

Both *Sargentodoxae Caulis* (da xue teng) and *Patriniae Herba* (bai jiang cao) act to clear heat and relieve toxin, applied to treat acute appendicitis, carbuncle and ulcer. Da xue teng acts to activate blood and relieve pain, applied to treat traumatic injuries and Bi (Obturation) Pattern due to wind-damp. Bai jiang cao acts to treat pulmonary abscess and to dissolve stasis and relieve pain, applied to treat abdominal pain due to blood stasis after delivery.

红藤、败酱草,均能清热解毒,均治肠痈、疮痈。其中红藤又能活血止痛,为跌打损伤、风湿痹痛所常用。败酱草亦治肺痈;且能祛瘀止痛,治产后瘀滞腹痛。

Both *Pulsatillae Radix* (bai tou weng) and *Fraxini Cortex* (qin pi) act to clear heat, relieve toxin and stop diarrhea, applied to treat diarrhea and dysentery due to heat-toxin. Bai tou weng is bitter and cold and attributive to the Large Intestine Meridian, and acts to cool blood, as the major herb to treat dysentery. Qin pi is pungent and astringent in flavor and cold in property, and acts to clear heat, desiccate damp and relieve toxin, applied to treat dysentery and morbid leucorrhea. It acts to clear heat from liver, applied to treat redness, swelling and pain of eyes due to heat in liver.

白头翁、秦皮,均能清热解毒、止痢,可用于热毒泻痢。其中白头翁且苦寒,专入大肠经,且能凉血,为治痢要药。秦皮苦涩性寒,兼能清热燥湿,既解毒止痢、止带,还能清泄肝热,治肝热目赤肿痛。

Rhizoma Belamecandae (she gan), attributive to the Lung Meridian, acts to clear heat, relieve toxin and benefit throat, applied to treat sore throat due to heat-toxin. It acts to dissolve phlegm, applied to treat cough and panting with excessive sputum.

射干,专入肺经,能清热解毒利咽,多用于热毒咽喉肿痛;兼能消痰涎,治喘咳痰多。

4 Heat-clearing and blood-cooling herbs

4 清热凉血药

Both *Rehmanniae Radix* (sheng di huang) and *Scrophulariae Radix* (xuan shen) are sweet in flavor and cold and moist in property, and act to clear heat, cool blood, nourish yin and produce fluid, ap-

生地黄、玄参,均味甘性寒质润,善能清热凉血、养阴生津,治热入营血证及阴伤津亏之证。其中生地黄功偏

plied to treat heat entering Ying (Nutrient) Phase and Xue (Blood) Phase pattern and yin deficiency and fluid depletion pattern. Sheng di huang acts to nourish yin and cool blood, applied to treat yin deficiency and heat in blood. It acts to cool blood and stanch bleeding, applied to treat bleeding due to heat in blood. Xuan shen acts to subdue fire, nourish yin, relieve toxin and dissipate stagnation, applied to fire excess and yin deficiency pattern manifested by sore throat, carbuncle, furuncle, ulcer, scrofula and goiter.

养阴凉血，阴虚血热多用；又凉血止血，治血热出血。玄参功偏降火滋阴，解毒散结，火盛阴亏之咽喉肿痛及痈疮肿毒、瘰疬痰核等证多用。

Both *Moutan Cortex* (mu dan pi) and *Paeoniae Radix Rubra* (chi shao) act to clear heat, cool blood, activate blood and dissipate stasis, applied to treat blood heat pattern and blood stasis pattern. Mu dan pi acts to clear heat and reduce false heat, applied to treat yin deficiency pattern manifested by fever, absence of sweating and feverish sensation. Chi shao acts to dissolve stasis and relieve pain, applied to treat various pains due to stagnation, and acts to clear heat from liver.

牡丹皮、赤芍，均能清热凉血、活血散瘀，治血热、血瘀病证。其中牡丹皮善清透阴分伏热，具退虚热之功，治阴虚发热、无汗骨蒸。赤芍则长于祛瘀止痛，用于多种瘀阻疼痛之证，且清肝热。

Both *Arnebiae Radix* (zi cao) and *Bubali Cornu* (shui niu jiao) act to clear heat, cool blood and relieve toxin, applied to treat eruption and macula due to heat-toxin. Zi cao acts to cool blood, activate blood and promote eruption, as the major herb to treat eruption and macula in deep color. It acts to treat scalding by water, burning by fire, eczema, carbuncle and ulcer. Shui niu jiao acts to clear heat from Ying (Nutrient) and Xue (Blood) Phases, applied to treat heat entering Ying (Nutrient) Phase and Xue (Blood) Phase pattern manifested by high fever, loss of consciousness, general macula, and treat hemoptysis, epistaxis and bleeding due to heat

紫草、水牛角，均能清热凉血解毒，治温毒斑疹。紫草长于凉血活血、透疹，为治疹毒内陷、斑疹紫黑要药，外用又治水火烫伤、湿疹疮痈。水牛角长于清营血之热，治热入营血、高热神昏、身发斑疹，以及血热吐衄出血。

in blood.

5 False heat-clearing herbs

All *Artemisiae Annuae Herba* (qing hao), *Cynanchi Atrati Radix et Rhizoma* (bai wei) and *Lycii Cortex* (di gu pi) act to clear false heat and to reduce true heat as well. Qing hao is pungent and acts to clear heat due to yin deficiency, applied to treat false heat in febrile disease due to consumption of yin. It also acts to treat malaria and relieve summer-heat, applied to treat chills and fever in malaria and restlessness and thirst due to summer-heat. Bai wei acts to cool blood and reduce heat, applied to treat fever due to yin deficiency and false heat after delivery, and also to treat heat entering Ying (Nutrient) and Xue (Blood) Phases manifested by high fever, restlessness and thirst. It acts to relieve heat-toxin and promote urination, applied to treat carbuncle, ulcer, sore throat, burning urination and bloody urine. Di gu pi acts to cool blood and clear false heat from liver and kidney, applied to treat sweating, feverish sensation, and bleeding due to heat in blood. It acts to purify lung and subdue fire, applied to treat cough due to heat in lung.

Both *Stellariae Radix* (yin chai hu) and *Picrorhizae Rhizoma* (hu huang lian) act to clear false heat and heat in infantile malnutrition, applied to treat fever due to yin deficiency and fever in infantile malnutrition. Yin chai hu, is the special herb for clearing false heat and fever in infantile malnutrition. Hu huang lian acts to eliminate damp-heat, applied to treat diarrhea, dysentery, and swelling and pain of hemorrhoids due to damp-heat.

5 清虚热药

青蒿、白薇、地骨皮，既善清虚热，又能泻实热。其中青蒿善辛散清透阴分伏热，多用于热病伤阴之虚热；又能截疟、解暑，治疟疾寒热、暑热烦渴。白薇凉血泄热力强，既治阴虚发热、产后虚热，又治热入营血、高热烦渴；且能解毒疗疮、利尿通淋，治疮痈咽痛、热淋、血淋。地骨皮则长于凉血退蒸，善清肝肾虚热，以除有汗骨蒸，并治血热出血；尚善清肺降火，治肺热咳嗽。

银柴胡、胡黄连，均能清虚热、除疳热，治阴虚发热、小儿疳热。其中银柴胡为清虚热、除疳热专药。胡黄连又善清湿热，常治湿热泻痢、痔疮肿痛。

Chapter 3 Reducing and Purging Herbs

第3章 泻下药

The Chinese medicinal herbs acting to make diarrhea, or to lubricate and moisturize large intestine to promote defecation are called the reducing and purging herbs.

According to their action characteristics and indications, the reducing and purging herbs are divided into the attacking-purging herbs, the moisturizing-purging herbs and the purging and water-eliminating herbs. The attacking-purging herbs are mostly bitter and cold and act to purge and promote defecation, applied to treat constipation and dry feces due to heat accumulation. The moisturizing-purging herbs are mostly the seeds and kernels of plants, sweet and moist, and act to moisturize intestines and promote defecation. They are moderate and mild, applied to treat constipation due to dryness in intestines for weak body in ageing, blood deficiency or body fluid deficiency. The purging and water-eliminating herbs are mostly bitter, cold and poisonous with strong purging action and capabk to promote urination, and act to eliminate water from defecation and urination, applied to treat water-rheum retention and accumulation pattern of excess type.

It is necessary to pay attention in application of this category of medicinal herbs that the attacking-

能引起腹泻，或滑润大肠，促进排便的药物，称为泻下药。

根据泻下药的作用特点及适应证的不同，有攻下药、润下药及峻下逐水药之分。攻下药性味大多苦寒，具较强的攻下通便之功，主要用于热结便秘、燥屎坚结的病证。润下药大多为植物种子或种仁，味甘质润，能润肠燥通便，药性和缓，主要用于年老体虚、血虚津枯的肠燥便秘。峻下逐水药大多苦寒有毒，药力峻猛，兼能利尿，可使水饮从二便排出，主要用于体内水饮停聚之实证。

使用本类药物需注意：应用本类药中的攻下药与峻

purging herbs and purging and water-eliminating herbs should not be applied in overdose or for long time, and it is necessary to stop administration of these medicinal herbs as soon as the disease is cured. It is not advisable to apply these medicinal herbs for people in old age or weak body constitution and for pregnant women.

下逐水药，当中病即止，不可多用久用。年老体弱以及孕妇不宜应用。

Section 1 Attacking-purging herbs

第1节 攻下药

Rhei Radix et Rhizoma (da huang)

大黄

It is the dried product from the root and rhizome of *Rheum palmatum* L., *Rheum tanguticum* Maxim. ex Balf. or *Rheum officinale* Baill., family Polygonaceae. The former is also called "bei da huang", while the latter is also called "nan da huang". The medicinal herb is collected in late autumn when it is withered or in early spring before it is sprouting, applied in crude form, stir-baking form with millet wine or carbonized form.

为蓼科草本植物掌叶大黄、唐古特大黄或药用大黄的干燥根及根茎。掌叶大黄、唐古特大黄习称"北大黄"。药用大黄习称"南大黄"。秋末茎叶枯萎时或次年春发芽前采挖。生用、酒炒、酒蒸或炒炭用。

Features Flavor: bitter. Property: cold. Meridian tropism: the Spleen Meridian, the Stomach Meridian, the Large Intestine Meridian, the Liver Meridian and the Pericardium Meridian.

性味归经 苦，寒。归脾、胃、大肠、肝、心包经。

Actions Reduce, purge and attack accumulation, clear heat, reduce fire, cool blood, relieve toxin, dissolve stasis, dredge meridians, eliminate damp and treat jaundice.

功效 泻下攻积，清热泻火，凉血解毒，逐瘀通经，利湿退黄。

Application

(1) Constipation due to excess heat accumulation. The medicinal herb is bitter, cold and descending, and acts to reduce, purge and attack accu-

应用

(1) 实热积滞便秘。本品苦寒沉降，泻下攻积力强，尤善治热结便秘，常与芒硝、

mulation. In the treatment of constipation due to heat accumulation, it is combined with *Natrii Sulfas* (mang xiao), *Magnoliae Officinalis Cortex* (hou po) and *Aurantii Fructus Immaturus* (zhi shi), to form up Major Purgative Decoction (Da Cheng Qi Tang), or it is combined with *Zingiberis Rhizoma* (gan jiang) and *Aconiti Radix Lateralis Praeparata* (fu zi), to treat constipation due to yang deficiency and cold accumulation, to form up Spleen-Warming Decoction (Wen Pi Tang).

厚朴、枳实同用，如大承气汤。亦或与干姜、附子等配伍，治阳虚冷积便秘，如温脾汤。

(2) Bleeding due to heat in blood, and pathogenic fire flaming-up pattern. The medicinal herb is bitter and acts to reduce and subdue fire, cool blood and clear heat. In the treatment of bleeding due to heat in blood, it is combined with *Coptidis Rhizoma* (huang lian) and *Scutellariae Radix* (huang qin), to form up Heart-Reducing Decoction (Xie Xin Tang). In the treatment of pathogenic fire flaming-up pattern manifested by redness of eyes, sore throat and ulcers of mouth and tongue, it is combined with the heat-clearing and fire-reducing herbs.

(2) 血热出血证，火邪上炎诸证。本品苦泄降火、凉血清热。治血热出血，常与黄连、黄芩等同用，如泻心汤。治火邪上炎所致的目赤、咽痛、口舌生疮等证，可与清热泻火药同用。

(3) Carbuncle and ulcer due to heat-toxin, burning and scalding wounds. The medicinal herb acts to reduce fire, relieve toxin, attack accumulation and clear heat. In the treatment of carbuncle and ulcer manifested by redness, swelling and pain, it is combined with the heat-clearing and toxin-relieving herbs. In the treatment of acute appendicitis, it is combined with *Moutan Cortex* (mu dan pi) and *Persicae Semen* (tao ren), to form up Rhubarb and Moutan Bark Decoction (Da Huang Mu Dan Pi Tang). It is applied by grinding into powder for external use to treat scalding by water and burning by fire.

(3) 热毒疮疡，烧烫伤。本品泻火解毒、攻积泄热。治疮痈红肿疼痛，常与清热解毒药同用。治肠痈，常与牡丹皮、桃仁等同用，如大黄牡丹皮汤。研末调敷，可治水火烫伤。

(4) Stagnant blood pattern. The medicinal herb is a commonly-used herb to treat stagnant blood pattern. In the treatment of amenorrhea, it is combined with the stasis-dissolving and meridian-dredging herbs. In the treatment of irregular menstruation and abdominal pain after delivery, it is combined with *Angelicae Sinensis Radix* (dang gui) and *Leonuri Herba* (yi mu cao). In the treatment of traumatic injury, it is combined with *Persicae Semen* (tao ren), *Carthami Flos* (hong hua), to form up Recovery and Blood-Activating Decoction (Fu Yuan Huo Xue Tang).

(4) 瘀血证。本品为瘀血证之常用药。治经闭不通，可与逐瘀通经药同用。治月经不调、产后腹痛，可与当归、益母草等同用。治跌打伤痛，可与桃仁、红花等同用，如复元活血汤。

(5) Jaundice and stranguria due to damp-heat. The medicinal herb acts to eliminate damp-heat and treat jaundice. In the treatment of jaundice due to damp-heat, it is combined with *Artemisiae Scopariae Herba* (yin chen) and *Gardeniae Fructus* (zhi zi), to form up Artemisia Decoction (Yin Chen Hao Tang). In the treatment of stranguria due to damp-heat, it is combined with *Akebiae Caulis* (mu tong) and *Plantaginis Semen* (che qian zi), to form up Eight Corrections Powder (Ba Zheng San).

(5) 湿热黄疸，淋证。本品能利湿热、退黄疸。治湿热黄疸，常与茵陈、栀子等同用，如茵陈蒿汤。治湿热淋证，常配木通、车前子等同用，如八正散。

Usage and dosage Apply 3～15 g in decoction. Apply a proper amount for external use. The medicinal herb acts to attack accumulation and promote defecation in crude form, applied in decoction by decocting later or taken after being infused in hot water. It acts to activate blood and ascend in prepared form with millet wine. It acts to stanch bleeding in carbonized form.

用法用量 煎服，3～15克。外用适量。生用攻积通便，入煎剂宜后下或泡服。酒制活血力强，且能上行。炒炭止血。

Precautions for use It is cautious to apply for those with spleen and stomach deficiency. It is prohibited to apply for women in pregnancy, menstruation or lactation period.

使用注意 脾胃虚弱者慎用。妇女妊娠期、月经期、哺乳期忌服。

Natrii Sulfas (mang xiao)

It is the refined crystalline sodium sulphate, usually made from natural sources, natrii sulfas as its chief component ($Na_2SO_4 \cdot 10H_2O$).

Features Flavor: salty and bitter. Property: cold. Meridian tropism: the Stomach Meridian and the Large Intestine Meridian.

Actions Reduce, purge and promote defecation, moisturize dryness, soften hardness, clear heat and subside swell.

Application

(1) Constipation due to excess heat accumulation. The medicinal herb is salty and cold, and acts to reduce heat, promote defecation, moisturize dryness and soften hardness. In the treatment of excess heat accumulation pattern manifested by dry feces, abdominal distension and pain, it is combined with *Rhei Radix et Rhizoma* (da huang), to form up Major Purgative Decoction (Da Cheng Qi Tang) or Stomach-Regulating Purgative Decoction (Tiao Wei Cheng Qi Tang).

(2) Ulcer in mouth, sore throat, redness of eyes, carbuncle and ulcer. The medicinal herb acts to clear heat and subside swell for external use. In the treatment of sore throat and ulcer in mouth, it is combined with *Borneolum Syntheticum* (bing pian) and *Borax* (peng sha) by grinding them into powder, to form up *Borneol* and *Borax* Powder (Bing Peng San). In the treatment of redness, swelling and pain of eyes, it is applied singly grinding into powder and mixed with water for eye drop. In the treatment of carbuncle and ulcer, it is combined

芒硝

为硫酸盐类矿物芒硝族芒硝经加工精制而成的结晶体。主要成分为含水硫酸钠。

性味归经 咸、苦，寒。归胃、大肠经。

功效 泻下通便，润燥软坚，清热消肿。

应用

（1）实热积滞便秘。本品苦咸性寒，具泻热通便，润燥软坚之功。治实热壅滞，大便燥结，腹满胀痛，常与大黄配伍同用，如大承气汤、调胃承气汤。

（2）口疮，咽痛，目赤，疮痈。本品外用能清热消肿。治咽痛、口疮，可与冰片、硼砂等研末，如冰硼散。治目赤肿痛，可单用玄明粉化水滴眼。治疮痈，可配冰片外敷。

with *Borneolum Syntheticum* (bing pian) for external use.

Furthermore, the medicinal herb acts to withdraw milk after delivery.

此外，本品外敷能回乳。

Usage and dosage Apply 6～12 g, by infusing into decoction or hot water for oral administration. Apply a proper amount for external use.

用法用量 6～12 克，冲入药汁内或开水溶化服。外用适量。

Precautions for use It is prohibited to apply for women in pregnancy or lactation period.

使用注意 孕妇及哺乳期妇女忌服。

Remarks *Natrii Sulfas* (mang xiao), *Mirabilitum Depuratum* (pu xiao) and *Natrii Sulfas Exsiccatus* (xuan ming fen)

按语 芒硝、朴硝与玄明粉

All the three herbs are different products of family Mirabilite, class sulphate, with similar actions. Mang xiao is a refined crystallometry with pure property, applied for oral administration. Pu xiao is a crude product with impure property, applied for external use. Xuan ming fen is a weathered and dried product from mang xiao with the purest property, applied for oral administration or made into powder for external use to treat sore throat and ulcer in mouth.

三者为硫酸盐类矿物芒硝族芒硝的不同加工品，功效相似。芒硝为精制而成的结晶体，质地较纯，可作内服。朴硝为粗制品，质地不纯，多作外敷之用。玄明粉为芒硝经风化干燥制得，质地最纯，除内服外，常制成散剂，作治疗咽痛、口疮之外用。

Sennae Folium (fan xie ye)

番泻叶

It is the dried product from the leaflet of *Cassia angustifolia* Vahl and *Cassia acutifolia* Delile, family Leguminosae. The former is produced in India, Egypt and Sudan, collected before it is flowering. The latter is produced in Egypt, collected in September when it is ripening. It is also cultivated in China, applied in crude form.

为豆科植物狭叶番泻或尖叶番泻的干燥小叶。前者主产于印度、埃及和苏丹，于花开前采摘。后者主产于埃及，于 9 月间果实将成熟时采摘。中国亦有栽培。生用。

Features Flavor: sweet and bitter. Property: cold. Meridian tropism: the Large Intestine Meridian.

性味归经 甘、苦，寒。归大肠经。

Actions Reduce, purge and promote defeca-

功效 泻下导滞通便，

tion, and promote waterflow.

Application

(1) Constipation due to heat accumulation. The medicinal herb is bitter, cold and descending, and acts to reduce, purge and promote defecation, and clear excess heat. In the treatment of constipation and abdominal pain due to heat accumulation or habitual constipation, it is applied singly by infusing in hot water, or combined with Cortex *Aurantii Fructus Immaturus* (zhi shi) and *Magnoliae Officinalis* (hou po).

(2) Edema with distension and fullness. The medicinal herb acts to promote waterflow and subside swell. In the treatment of edema with distension and fullness, it is applied singly by infusing into hot water or combined with *Pharbitidis Semen* (qian niu zi) and *Arecae Pericarpium* (da fu pi).

Usage and dosage Apply 2～6 g decoction by decocting later or by infusing in hot water.

Precautions for use It is prohibited to apply for women in lactation, menstruation or pregnancy period.

利水。

应用

(1) 热结便秘。本品苦寒降泄，具泻下导滞、清泄实热之功。治热结便秘腹痛或习惯性便秘等，可单味泡服，或与枳实、厚朴等配伍同用。

(2) 水肿胀满。本品泡服，或与牵牛子、大腹皮等同用，能泻下行水消胀，治水肿胀满。

用法用量 煎服，2～6克，后下。或开水泡服。

使用注意 妇女哺乳期、月经期及孕妇忌用。

Aloe (lu hui)

It is the dried product from the juice of the base of the leaf of a perennial evergreen plant, *Aloe barbadensis* Mill, family Liliaceae. The medicinal herb is collected all year round, applied in crude form.

Features Flavor: bitter. Property: cold. Meridian tropism: the Liver Meridian, the Stomach Meridian and the Large Intestine Meridian.

Actions Reduce, purge and promote defecation, purify liver, reduce fire, kill worms and treat infantile malnutrition.

芦荟

为百合科植物库拉索芦荟汁液的浓缩干燥物。全年可采收加工。生用。

性味归经 苦，寒。归肝、胃、大肠经。

功效 泻下通便，清肝泻火，杀虫疗疳。

Application

(1) Constipation due to heat accumulation. The medicinal herb is bitter and cold, and acts to reduce, purge and promote defecation and clear fire from liver. In the treatment of constipation due to heat accumulation and heart and liver fire flaming pattern manifested by restlessness and insomnia, it is combined with *Cinnabaris* (zhu sha), to form up Toillette Pills (Geng Yi Wan).

(2) Excess fire in the Liver Meridian. The medicinal herb acts to clear fire from liver. In the treatment of fire hyperactivity in the Liver Meridian manifested by dizziness, headache, restlessness, anger, epilepsy and convulsion, it is combined with *Angelicae Sinensis Radix* (dang gui), *Indigo Naturalis* (qing dai) and *Gentianae Radix et Rhizoma* (long dan cao), to form up Angelica, Gentian and Aloe Decoction (Dang Gui Long Hui Wan).

(3) Infantile malnutrition. The medicinal herb acts to kill worms, dissipate accumulation and treat infantile malnutrition. In the treatment of infantile malnutrition, it is combined with *Ginseng Radix et Raizoma* (ren shen), *Atractylodis Macrocephalae Rhizoma* (bai zhu) and *Picrorhizae Rhizoma* (hu huang lian), to form up Baby-Fleshing Up Pills (Fei Er Wan).

Usage and dosage It is applied to make pills or powder, take 2～5 g. Apply a proper amount for external use.

Precautions for use It is prohibited to apply for those with spleen and stomach deficiency manifested by poor appetite and loose feces and for pregnant women.

应用

（1）热结便秘。本品苦寒泻下通便，兼清肝火。尤善治热结便秘，兼见心肝火旺、烦躁失眠者，可与朱砂同用，即更衣丸。

（2）肝经实火证。本品善清肝火。治肝经火盛所致的头晕头痛、烦躁易怒、惊痫抽搐等证，常与当归、青黛、龙胆草等同用，如当归龙荟丸。

（3）小儿疳积。本品能杀虫消积、疗疳。治小儿疳积，常与人参、白术、胡黄连等同用，如肥儿丸。

用法用量 入丸散，2～5克。外用适量。

使用注意 脾胃虚弱，食少便溏及孕妇忌服。

Section 2 Moisturizing-purging herbs

第 2 节 润下药

Cannabis Fructus (huo ma ren)

It is the dried product from the fruits of *Cannabis sativa* L., family Moraceae. The medicinal herb is collected in autumn, applied in crude form or fried form.

Features Flavor: sweet. Property: neutral. Meridian tropism: the Spleen Meridian, the Stomach Meridian and the Large Intestine Meridian.

Actions Moisturize intestines and promote defecation.

Application

Constipation due to dryness in intestines. The medicinal herb is sweet, neutral and moist, and acts to moisturize intestines, promote defecation and nourish body. In the treatment of constipation due to dryness in intestines for those with ageing, weak body constitution, blood deficiency or body fluid deficiency, it is applied singly or made porridge. In the treatment of dryness and heat in intestines and stomach, it is combined with *Rhei Radix et Rhizoma* (da huang) and *Magnoliae Officinalis Cortex* (hou po), to form up Hemp Seed Decoction (Ma Zi Ren Wan).

Usage and dosage Apply 10～15 g in decoction.

火麻仁

为桑科植物大麻的干燥成熟种实。秋季采收。生用或炒用。

性味归经 甘，平。归脾、胃、大肠经。

功效 润肠通便。

应用

肠燥便秘。本品甘平质润，功善润肠通便，略兼滋养之功。治年老体弱、血虚津亏之肠燥便秘，可单用或煮粥食用。若肠胃燥热，可与大黄、厚朴等同用，如麻子仁丸。

用法用量 煎服，10～15 克。

Pruni Semen (yu li ren)

It is the dried product from the seeds of *Prumus humilis* or *Prumus japonica* Thunb., *Drunus pedunculata Maxim*., family Rosaceass. The medicinal herb is collected in summer and autumn, ap-

郁李仁

为蔷薇科植物欧李、郁李或长柄扁桃的干燥成熟种子。夏、秋季采摘。生用。

plied in crude form.

Features Flavor: pungent, bitter and sweet. Property: neutral. Meridian tropism: the Large Intestine Meridian and the Small Intestine Meridian.

性味归经 辛、苦、甘，平。归大肠、小肠经。

Actions Moisturize intestines, promote defecation, subdue qi and promote waterflow.

功效 润肠通便，下气利水。

Application

应用

(1) Constipation due to dryness in intestines. The medicinal herb acts to moisturize intestines, promote defecation and dissipate qi stagnation in intestines. In the treatment of constipation due to qi stagnation or dryness in intestines, it is combined with *Platycladi Semen* (bai zi ren) and *Armeniacae Amarum Semen* (ku xing ren), to form up Five Seeds Pills (Wu Ren Wan). In the treatment of constipation due to blood deficiency or dryness in intestines, it is combined with *Angelicae Sinensis Radix* (dang gui) and *Polygoni Multiflori Radix* (he shou wu).

（1）肠燥便秘。本品功能润肠通便，兼行肠中气滞，可用于气滞肠燥便秘之证，常与柏子仁、杏仁等同用，如五仁丸。治血虚肠燥便秘，可与当归、何首乌等同用。

(2) Edema and difficult urination. The medicinal herb acts to subdue qi, promote waterflow and subside swell. In the treatment of edema and difficult urination, it is combined with *Cortex Mori Albae Radicis* (sang bai pi) and *Polyporus Umbellatus* (zhu ling).

（2）水肿，小便不利。本品能下气利水消肿。治水肿、小便不利，常与桑白皮、猪苓等同用。

Usage and dosage Apply 6～10 g in decoction.

用法用量 煎服，6～10克。

Precautions for use It is cautious to apply for pregnant women.

使用注意 孕妇慎用。

Section 3 Purging and water-eliminating herbs

第3节 峻下逐水药

Kansui Radix (gan sui)

甘遂

It is the dried product from the root tuber of

为大戟科植物甘遂的干

Euphorbia Kansui T.N. Liou ex T.P. Wang, family Euphorbiaceae. The medicinal herb is collected in spring before it is flowering or in late autumn when it is withered, applied in stir-baking form with vinegar.

燥块根。春季开花前或秋末茎叶枯萎后采挖。醋炙后用。

Features Flavor: bitter. Property: cold and poisonous. Meridian tropism: the Lung Meridian, the Kidney Meridian and the Large Intestine Meridian.

性味归经 苦,寒;有毒。归肺、肾、大肠经。

Actions Reduce water, eliminate rheum, subside swell and dissipate stagnation.

功效 泻水逐饮,消肿散结。

Application

应用

(1) Edema, hydrothorax and ascites. The medicinal herb is bitter and cold, and acts to reduce the lower and eliminate rheum. In the treatment of edema, hydrothorax and ascites, it is applied singly by grinding into powder for oral administration, or combined with *Euphorbiae Pekinensis Radix* (da ji) and *Genkwa Flos* (yuan hua) by grinding them into powder for oral administration together with jujube soup, to form up Ten Jujubes Decoction (Shi Zao Tang).

(1) 水肿,胸腹积水。本品苦寒泻下,逐饮力峻。治水肿、胸腹积水,可单用研末服,或与大戟、芫花为末,枣汤送服,如十枣汤。

(2) Epilepsy. The medicinal herb acts to reduce water and eliminate phlegm and rheum. In the treatment of epilepsy due to wind-phlegm, it is applied by roasting with pork heart, mixing with *Cinnabaris* (zhu sha) and grinding them into powder, then making into pills.

(2) 癫痫。本品能泻水逐痰涎。治风痰癫痫,可用甘遂末入猪心煨过,与朱砂末为丸服。

(3) Carbuncle, furuncle and ulcer. The medicinal herb is applied to grinding into powder and mixing with water for external use to treat carbuncle and ulcer.

(3) 痈肿疮毒。本品研末水调外敷,治疮痈。

Usage and dosage It is applied make into pills or powder, 0.5～1.5 g. It is prepared with vinegar for oral administration, while applied in crude form

用法用量 入丸散服,0.5～1.5 克;内服宜醋制。外用适量,生用。

for external use.

Precautions for use It is prohibited to apply for pregnant women. The medicinal herb is incompatible to *Glycyrrhizae Radix et Rhizoma* (gan cao).

使用注意 孕妇忌服。反甘草。

Euphorbiae Pekinensis Radix (jing da ji)

京大戟

It is the dried product from the root of *Euphorbia pekinensis* Rupr., family Euphorbiaceae. The medicinal herb is collected in autumn and winter, applied in crude form or prepared form with vinegar.

为大戟科植物大戟的干燥根。秋、冬季采挖。生用或醋制。

Features Flavor: bitter. Property: cold and poisonous. Meridian tropism: the Lung Meridian, the Spleen Meridian and the Kidney Meridian.

性味归经 苦,寒;有毒。归肺、脾、肾经。

Actions Reduce water, eliminate rheum, subside swell and dissipate stagnation.

功效 泻水逐饮,消肿散结。

Application

应用

(1) Edema, hydrothorax and ascites. The medicinal herb acts to reduce water and eliminate rheum. In the treatment of edema and ascites, it is combined with *Fructus Ziziphi Jujubae* (da zao), or combined with *Kansui Radix* (gan sui) and *Genkwa Flos* (yuan hua). In the treatment of hydrothorax due to rheum retention manifested by hypochondriac pain and thick sputum, it is combined with gan sui and *Sinapis Semen Albae* (bai jie zi), to form up Saliva-Controlling Elixer (Kong Xian Dan).

(1) 水肿,胸腹积水。本品具泻水逐饮之功。治水肿、腹水,可与枣同煮,食枣,或与甘遂、芫花等同用。治胸胁停饮、胁痛、痰稠,可与甘遂、白芥子同用,即控涎丹。

(2) Carbuncle, ulcer, furuncle, scrofula and goiter. In the treatment of carbuncle, ulcer and furuncle, it is applied to smashing the fresh herb into paste for external use. In the treatment of scrofula and goiter, it is applied by boiling with eggs which are taken.

(2) 痈疮肿毒,瘰疬痰核。治痈肿疮毒,鲜品捣烂外敷。治瘰疬痰核,与鸡蛋同煮,食鸡蛋。

Usage and dosage Apply 1.5～3 g in decoction. Apply 1 g of pills or powder. It is advisable to prepare it with vinegar for oral administration, while applied a proper amount for external use in crude form.

用法用量 煎服，1.5～3 克；入丸散服，每次 1 克；内服宜醋制。外用适量，生用。

Precautions for use It is prohibited to apply for those with weak body constitution and pregnant women. The medicinal herb is incompatible to *Glycyrrhizae Radix et Rhizoma* (gan cao).

使用注意 体弱及孕妇忌用。反甘草。

Genkwa Flos (yuan hua)

芫花

It is the dried product from the flower bud of *Daphne genkwa* Sieb. et Zucc, family Thymelaeaceae. The medicinal herb is collected in spring before it is flowering, applied in crude form or prepared form with vinegar.

为瑞香科植物芫花的干燥花蕾。春季花未开放前采摘。生用或醋制。

Features Flavor: bitter and pungent. Property: warm and poisonous. Meridian tropism: the Lung Meridian, the Spleen Meridian and the Kidney Meridian.

性味归经 苦、辛，温；有毒。归肺、脾、肾经。

Actions Reduce water, eliminate rheum, kill worms and treat sores.

功效 泻水逐饮，杀虫疗疮。

Application

应用

(1) Edema, hydrothorax and ascites. The medicinal herb acts to reduce water and eliminate rheum. In the treatment of hydrothorax due to water-rheum in chest and hypochondria, it is combined with *Kansui Radix* (gan sui) and *Euphorbiae Pekinensis Radix* (jing da ji).

(1) 水肿，胸腹积水。本品功能泻水逐饮，尤多用于泻胸胁之水饮，常与甘遂、京大戟等配伍同用。

(2) Coughing and panting due to phlegm accumulation. The medicinal herb acts to reduce rheum, dissolve phlegm and stop coughing. In the treatment of coughing and panting due to phlegm-rheum accumulation or due to up-reverse flow of qi, it is com-

(2) 咳嗽痰喘。本品能泻饮祛痰止咳。治痰饮壅滞、气逆咳喘，可与桑白皮、葶苈子等同用。或配伍干姜、细辛等温肺化饮药同用。

bined with *Cortex Mori Albae Radicis* (sang bai pi) and *Semen Descurainiae* (ting li zi), or combined with the lung-warming and rheum-dissolving herbs, as *Zingiberis Rhizoma* (gan jiang) and *Asari Radix et Rhizoma* (xi xin).

(3) Carbuncle, furuncle, tinea favosa, psoriasis and chilblain. The medicinal herb acts to kill worms and treat sores for external use. It is applied singly by grinding into powder and daubing, or applied by decocting and washing externally.

(3) 痈疽,秃疮,顽癣,冻疮。本品外用能杀虫疗疮。可单用研末,外涂;或水煎外洗。

Usage and dosage Apply 1.5～3 g in decoction, apply 0.6 g of powder. It is applied in prepared form with vinegar for oral administration, while applied in crude form for external use.

用法用量 煎服,1.5～3 克;入散剂,每次 0.6 克;内服宜醋制。外用适量,生用。

Precautions for use It is prohibited to apply for those with weak body constitution and pregnant women. The medicinal herb is incompatible to *Glycyrrhizae Radix et Rhizoma* (gan cao).

使用注意 体虚者及孕妇忌服。反甘草。

Pharbitidis Semen (qian niu zi)

牵牛子

It is the dried product from the seed of *Pharbitis nil* (L.) Choisy or *Pharbitis prupurea* (L.) voigt, family Convolvulaceae. The medicinal herb is collected in late autumn when its fruits are ripening while the nut shells are not cracking. It is applied in crude form or fried form.

为旋花科植物牵牛或圆叶牵牛的干燥成熟种子。秋末果实成熟、果壳未开裂时采收。生用或炒用。

Features Flavor: bitter. Property: cold and poisonous. Meridian tropism: the Lung Meridian, the Kidney Meridian and the Large Intestine Meridian.

性味归经 苦,寒;有毒。归肺、肾、大肠经。

Actions Reduce water, promote defecation, dissolve phlegm, eliminate rheum, kill worms and attack accumulation.

功效 泻水通便,消痰逐饮,杀虫攻积。

Application

应用

(1) Edema with distension and fullness. The

(1) 水肿胀满。本品既

medicinal herb acts to attack accumulation, promote defecation, eliminate water and promote urination, so as to remove water-damp by promoting defecation and urination. In the treatment of edema, difficult defecation and urination, it is applied singly by grinding into powder, or combined with *Kansui Radix* (gan sui) and *Euphorbiae Pekinensis Radix* (jing da ji).

攻积通便,又逐水利尿,善通利二便以除水湿。治水肿、二便不利者,可单用研末服,或与甘遂、京大戟等同用。

(2) Constipation and food retention. The medicinal herb acts to reduce, purge and promote defecation, and eliminate accumulation and stagnation. In the treatment of constipation due to heat or dysentery due to damp-heat, it is applied singly or combined with *Rhei Radix et Rhizoma* (da huang) and *Arecae Semen* (bing lang). In the treatment of food retention and indigestion, it is combined with *Raphani Semen* (lai fu zi).

(2) 大便秘结,食积停滞。本品能泻下通便、消除积滞。治热结便秘或湿热痢疾,单用即效,或与大黄、槟榔同用。治食积不消,可与莱菔子同用。

(3) Coughing and panting due to phlegm accumulation. The medicinal herb acts to reduce lung, dissolve phlegm and eliminate rheum. In the treatment of coughing and panting due to phlegm accumulation and puffy face, it is combined with *Semen Descurainiae* (ting li zi), *Armeniacae Amarum Semen* (ku xing ren) and *Magnoliae Officinalis Cortex* (hou po).

(3) 痰壅喘咳。本品能泻肺消痰逐饮。治痰饮咳喘,面目浮肿,常与葶苈子、杏仁、厚朴等同用。

(4) Abdominal pain due to parasites. The medicinal herb acts to kill worms and promote defecation. In the treatment of abdominal pain due to parasites, it is combined with bing lang.

(4) 虫积腹痛。本品既杀虫又通便。可治虫积腹痛,常配槟榔等同用。

Usage and dosage Apply 3～6 g in decoction, or apply 1.5～3 g of pills or powder. Its property can be moderated after frying.

用法用量 煎服,3～6克;入丸散服,每次1.5～3克。炒用药性减缓。

Precautions for use It is prohibited to apply for pregnant women. It is not advisable to apply it

使用注意 孕妇忌服。不宜与巴豆、巴豆霜同用。

together with *Fructus Crotonis* (ba dou) and *Semen Crotonis Preparata* (ba dou shuang).

Brief summary

1 Attacking-purging herbs

Both *Rhei Radix et Rhizoma* (da huang) and *Natrii Sulfas* (mang xiao) are bitter and cold and act to reduce heat and promote defecation, applied to treat constipation due to heat accumulation in mutual reinforcement. Da huang is bitter, cold and descending, and acts to reduce fire, cool blood and relieve toxin, applied to treat carbuncle and ulcer due to heat-toxin, all fire-heat flaming-up patterns, and bleeding due to heat in blood. It acts to dissolve damp and clear heat, applied to treat jaundice due to damp-heat. It is attributive to the Xue (Blood) Phase and acts to dissolve stasis and dredge meridian, applied to treat blood stasis patterns. Mang xiao is salty and cold, and acts to moisturize dryness, soften hardness and clear the lower, applied to treat constipation with dry feces. It acts to clear heat and subside swell for external use, applied to treat carbuncle and ulcer, redness of eyes, sore throat and mouth ulcer.

Both *Sennae Folium* (fan xie ye) and *Aloe* (lu hui) are cold and act to clear the lower and promote defecation, applied to treat constipation due to heat accumulation. Fan xie ye is stronger in reducing and purging, applied to treat constipation due to heat accumulation or habitual constipation. It acts to promote waterflow, applied to treat edema with distension and fullness. Lu hui acts to reduce liver fire, applied to treat heart and liver fire hyperactivity

小　结

1 攻下药

大黄、芒硝，均具苦寒泻热通便之功，治热结便秘常相须为用。其中大黄苦寒清降，能泻火凉血解毒，治热毒疮痈，火热上炎诸证，以及血热出血；还能利湿热、退黄疸，治湿热黄疸；入血分，善逐瘀通经，以治瘀血证。芒硝咸寒润燥软坚泻下，尤宜于燥屎坚结难下者，外用清热消肿，可治疮痈、目赤、咽痛、口疮。

番泻叶、芦荟，均性寒能泻下通便，治热结便秘。其中番泻叶泻下力较强，善治热结便秘或习惯性便秘；且能利水，治水肿胀满。芦荟兼能清肝火，故常用于热结便秘兼见心肝火旺、烦躁失眠者，亦治肝经实火证；且能杀虫疗疳，治小儿疳积。

pattern manifested by restlessness and insomnia, and to treat excess fire in the Liver Meridian. It acts to kill worms, applied to treat infantile malnutrition.

2 Moisturizing-purging herbs

Both *Cannabis Fructus* (huo ma ren) and *Pruni Semen* (yu li ren) are the kernels of plants and containing vegetable fat, act to moisturize intestines and promote defecation, applied to treat constipation caused by blood deficiency, body fluid deficiency or dryness in intestines in those with ageing, weak body constitution, chronic disease or delivery. Huo ma ren is sweet and moist and acts to reinforce body, applied to treat constipation due to body fluid deficiency, blood deficiency or dryness in intestines. Yu li ren is moist, bitter and descending and acts to promote defecation, subdue qi and promote urination, applied to treat edema and difficult urination.

2 润下药

火麻仁、郁李仁，均为植物种仁，富含油脂，善于润肠通便，凡年老、体弱、久病，产后血虚津枯肠燥便秘均可应用。其中火麻仁甘润兼能补虚，津血不足的肠燥便秘用之效佳。郁李仁质润苦降，通便力较强，且能下气利尿，又治水肿、小便不利。

3 Purging and water-eliminating herbs

All *Kansui Radix* (gan sui), *Euphorbiae Pekinensis Radix* (jing da ji) and *Genkwa Flos* (yuan hua) are poisonous products and act to reduce water and eliminate rheum, applied to treat edema, hydrothorax and ascites. Both gan sui and jing da ji are cold and act to subside swell and dissipate stagnation, applied to treat carbuncle and ulcer due to heat-toxin for external use. As for the action to reduce water and eliminate rheum, gan sui is the strongest, jing da ji is the next, while yuan hua is the weakest. Gan sui acts to dissolve phlegm and rheum, applied to treat epilepsy due to phlegm misting heart aperture. Yuan hua is warm and acts to eliminate rheum, dis-

3 峻下逐水药

甘遂、京大戟、芫花，均为有毒之品，善泻水逐饮，治水肿、胸腹积水。甘遂、京大戟均性寒，还能消肿散结，外用治疮痈肿毒。三药中泻水逐饮力最强者为甘遂，京大戟次之，芫花最弱。其中甘遂还能泻痰饮，治痰迷癫痫；芫花性温，还能泻饮祛痰止咳，杀虫疗疮，治咳嗽痰喘、痈疽、顽癣等。

solve phlegm and relieve cough, and to kill worms as well, applied to treat cough and panting due to phlegm, carbuncle, ulcer and psoriasis.

Pharbitidis Semen (qian niu zi) is bitter, cold and poisonous and applied to reduce water, eliminate rheum, attack accumulation and promote defecation, as the good product to promote defecation and urination. It acts to dissolve phlegm, eliminate rheum and kill worms, applied to treat panting and cough due to phlegm accumulation and abdominal pain due to parasites.

牵牛子,苦寒有毒,能泻水逐饮、攻积通便,为通利二便之品。还能消痰逐饮、杀虫,治痰壅喘咳、虫积腹痛。

Chapter 4 Wind-Damp-Eliminating Herbs

第4章 祛风湿药

The medicinal herbs acting to eliminate wind-damp and relieve pain in Bi (Obturation) Pattern are called the wind-damp-eliminating herbs.

以祛除风湿、解除痹痛为主要作用的药物，称祛风湿药。

This type of medicinal herbs, mostly pungent, bitter, dry and dispersing, are different in cold or warm property, and act to eliminate pathogenic wind-damp locating in muscles, meridians and joints, to relieve pain in Bi (Obturation) Pattern, dredge meridians and strengthen tendons and bones. They are applied to treat Bi (Obturation) Pattern due to wind-damp, spasm and cramp of tendons and vessels, numbness, hemiplegia, aching and pain at low back and knee, and paralysis and weakness of lower limbs.

本类药物多辛散苦燥，药性寒温不一。功善祛除停留于肌表、经络、关节间的风湿之邪，还兼有止痹痛、通经络、强筋骨等作用。主要用于风湿痹痛、筋脉拘挛、麻木不仁、半身不遂、腰膝酸痛、下肢痿弱等证。

Bi (Obturation) Pattern is caused by different pathogens of wind, cold, damp and heat with various symptoms and signs. In the application of the wind-damp-eliminating herbs, it is advisable to combine the relevant herbs according to the preponderant pathogens. For the condition due to preponderant wind, it is advisable to combine the medicinal herbs acting to eliminate wind and dredge meridians. For the condition due to preponderant damp, it is advisable to combine the medicinal herbs acting to desiccate damp, dissolve damp and strengthen spleen. For the condition due to prepon-

引起痹证的风、寒、湿或热邪各有偏胜，症状表现不同，使用祛风湿药时当根据邪之偏胜，酌情配伍相关药物。风胜者，可配伍祛风通经之品；湿胜者，配伍燥湿利湿、健脾药同用；寒胜者，配伍散寒温阳通络之品；热胜者，宜与清热药同用。若风湿日久，肝肾虚损者，除选择兼能强筋骨的祛风湿药外，当与补肝肾强腰膝之品同用。

derant cold, it is advisable to combine the medicinal herbs acting to dispel cold, warm yang and dredge meridians. For the conditional due to preponderant heat, it is advisable to combine the medicinal herbs acting to clear heat. For the chronic condition in which pathogenic wind-damp attacks for long time and liver and kidney are deficient, it is advisable to combine the medicinal herbs acting to reinforce liver and kidney and strengthen low back and knees, at the same time when applying the wind-damp-eliminating herbs.

Some of the medicinal herbs are pungent, fragrant, bitter and dry, and easy to consume the yin and blood. Therefore, it is cautious to apply for those with yin deficiency or blood deficiency.

本类部分药物辛香苦燥,易耗伤阴血,故阴虚血亏者应慎用。

Angelicae Pubescentis Radix (du huo)

独活

It is the dried product from the root of *Angelica pubescens* Maxim. f. *biserrata* Shan. et Yuan, family Umbelliferae. The medicinal herb is collected in late autumn or early spring, applied in crude form.

为伞形科植物重齿毛当归的干燥根。秋末或春初采挖。生用。

Features Flavor: pungent and bitter. Property: slightly warm. Meridian tropism: the Kidney Meridian and the Bladder Meridian.

性味归经 辛、苦,微温。归肾、膀胱经。

Actions Eliminate wind, remove damp, treat Bi (Obturation) Pattern, stop pain and relieve exterior pattern.

功效 祛风除湿,通痹止痛,解表。

Application

应用

(1) Pain in Bi (Obturation) Pattern and headache. The medicinal herb is pungent and bitter in flavor and dry and warm in property, acting to descend, to eliminate wind-damp, remove cold, treat Bi (Obturation) Pattern and stop pain. In the treatment of cold-damp Bi (Obturation) Pattern with

(1) 风湿痹痛,头痛。本品辛散苦燥温通,性下行,善祛风湿散寒、通痹止痛,尤善治下部寒湿痹痛。常与附子、乌头、防风等同用。与桑寄生、杜仲、熟地黄等补肝肾

pain in lower part, it is combined with *Aconiti Radix* Praeparata (fu zi), *Aconiti Radix* (wu tou) and *Radix Ledebouriellae* (fang feng). In the treatment of chronic Bi (Obturation) Pattern involving liver and kidney manifested by cold and pain at low back and knees, it is combined with the liver and kidney-reinforcing herbs, as *Ramulus Loranthi* (sang ji sheng), *Eucommiae Cortex* (du zhong) and *Rehmanniae Radix Praeparata* (shu di huang), to form up Lovage and Angelica Decoction (Du Huo Ji Sheng Tang).

药同用，亦治久痹肝肾两虚，腰膝冷痛等证，如独活寄生汤。

(2) Exterior pattern of wind, cold and damp. The medicinal herb acts to relieve exterior pattern. In the treatment of headache due to exterior pattern of wind, cold and damp, it is combined with *Rhizoma seu Radix Notopterygii* (qiang huo) and *Radix Ledebouriellae* (fang feng).

（2）风寒夹湿表证。本品兼能解表。治风寒夹湿表证头痛，常与羌活、防风等同用。

Usage and dosage Apply 3～10 g in decoction.

用法用量 煎服，3～10克。

Remarks *Rhizoma seu Radix Notopterygii* (qiang huo) and *Angelicae Pubescentis Radix* (du huo)

按语 羌活与独活

It did not make a distinction between qiang huo and du huo in ancient times. It is said in *Shen Nong's Herbal Canon* (Shen Nong Ben Cao Jing) that du huo is also called qiang huo. Since Song (960—1279) and Yuan (1271—1368) Dynasties, qiang huo is identified from du huo in classics and clinical practice.

羌活、独活，古时不分。《神农本草经》记载只有独活，并谓独活一名羌活。自宋元以后，本草记载及临床应用才将羌活从独活中分出另列。

Both the medicinal herbs are the plants of family Umbelliferae, acting to eliminate wind and damp and relieve exterior pattern. Qiang huo is pungent, warm, dry and ascending, and acts to relieve exterior pattern and treat wind-damp Bi (Obturation)

二药均为伞形科植物，均能祛风湿、解表。不同的是羌活辛散温燥，性善上行，发散力强，善解表且治上半身风湿痹痛。独活药性较

Pattern with pain in upper part. Du huo is moderate and descending, and acts to eliminate wind-damp and treat wind-damp Bi (Obturation) Pattern with pain in lower part.

缓，性善下行，善祛风湿，治下半身风湿痹痛。

Aconiti Radix (chuan wu)

川乌

It is the dried product from the parent root of *Aconitum carmichaeli* Debx., family Ranunculaceae. The medicinal herb is collected in summer and autumn, removed its daughter root and applied in crude form or prepared form.

为毛茛科植物乌头的干燥母根。夏、秋季采挖，除去子根。生用或制用。

Features Flavor: pungent and bitter. Property: hot and extremely poisonous. Meridian tropism: the Heart Meridian, the Spleen Meridian, the Liver Meridian and the Kidney Meridian.

性味归经 辛、苦，热，有大毒。归心、脾、肝、肾经。

Actions Eliminate wind, remove damp, dispel cold and stop pain.

功效 祛风除湿，散寒止痛。

Application

应用

(1) Bi (Obturation) Pattern due to wind, cold and damp. The medicinal herb is hot in property and acts to eliminate wind, to dispel cold and to stop pain. In the treatment of Bi (Obturation) Pattern due to wind, cold and damp manifested by joint pain, it is combined with *Ephedrae Herba* (ma huang), *Paeoniae Radix Alba* (bai shao) and *Astragali Radix* (huang qi), to form up Monkshood Decoction (Wu Tou Tang).

（1）风寒湿痹。本品性热，功善祛风散寒止痛。治风寒湿痹，关节疼痛，常与麻黄、白芍、黄芪等同用，如乌头汤。

(2) Pains due to cold-damp. The medicinal herb acts to dispel cold and stop pain. In the treatment of various pains due to cold-damp, it is applied singly in honeyed decoction, to form up Greater Monkshood Decoction (Da Wu Tou Jian). It is also applied for anesthesia.

（2）寒湿诸痛。本品散寒止痛力强。可治各种寒湿疼痛，可单用，浓煎加蜜服，即大乌头煎。亦用于麻醉止痛。

Usage and dosage Apply 1.5～3 g in decoc-

用法用量 煎服，1.5～

tion. It is advisable to decoct first and for long time. It is poisonous in crude form, so it is applied in prepared form for oral administration.

3克。应先煎、久煎。生用有毒,内服多制用。

Precautions for use It is prohibited to apply for pregnant women. The medicinal herb is incompatible to *Pinelliae Rhizoma* (ban xia), *Trichosanthis Fructus* (gua lou), *Fritillariae Cirrhosae Bulbus* (chuan bei mu), *Bulbus Fritillariae Thunbergii* (zhe bei mu), *Bletillae Rhizoma* (bai ji) and *Radix Ampelopsis* (bai lian).

使用注意 孕妇忌用。反半夏、瓜蒌、川贝母、浙贝母、白及、白蔹。

Clematidis Radix et Rhizoma (wei ling xian)

威灵仙

It is the dried product from the root and rhizome of the perennial trailing shrub, *Clematis chinensis* Osbeck. or *Clematis hexapetala* Pall. or *Clematis manshurica* Rupr., family Ranunculaceae. The medicinal herb is collected in autumn, applied in crude form.

为毛茛科植物威灵仙、棉团铁线莲或东北铁线莲的干燥根及根茎。秋季采挖。生用。

Features Flavor: pungent and salty. Property: warm. Meridian tropism: the Bladder Meridian.

性味归经 辛、咸,温。归膀胱经。

Actions Eliminate wind-damp, dredge meridians, dissolve phlegm-rheum and treat fishbone lodging in throat.

功效 祛风湿,通经络,消痰水,治骨鲠。

Application

应用

(1) Bi (Obturation) Pattern due to wind-damp. The medicinal herb acts to dredge meridians, as the major herb to treat Bi (Obturation) Pattern due to wind-damp. It is applied singly by grinding it into powder and taking with warm wine, or combined with *Radix Notopterygii* (qiang huo), *Radix Ledebouriellae* (fang feng) and *Rhizoma Ligustici Chuanxiong* (chuan xiong).

(1) 风湿痹痛。本品性善通利,为治风湿痹痛之要药。可单用为末,温酒调服;或与羌活、防风、川芎等配用。

(2) Accumulation of phlegm and rheum. The

(2) 痰饮积聚。本品能

medicinal herb acts to dissolve phlegm and rheum, applied with *Pinelliae Rhizoma* (ban xia) and *Zingiberis Rhizoma Recens* (sheng jiang).

消痰水，常多与半夏、姜汁等同用。

(3) Fishbone lodging in throat. The medicinal is applied to treat fishbone lodging in throat. It is applied singly or decocted with vinegar and taken slowly.

（3）诸骨鲠喉。本品为治诸骨鲠喉所常用。可单用或醋煎汤，缓慢咽下。

Usage and dosage Apply 6～10 g in decoction, or 30～50 g in the treatment of fishbone lodging in throat.

用法用量 煎服，6～10克。治骨鲠可用30～50克。

Stephaniae Tetrandrae Radix (fang ji)

防己

It is the dried product from the tuberous root of a perennial trailing vine, *Stephania tetrandra* S. Moore, family Menispermaceae. The medicinal herb is collected in autumn, applied in crude form.

为防己科植物粉防己的干燥根。秋季采挖。生用。

Features Flavor: bitter. Property: cold. Meridian tropism: the Bladder Meridian and the Lung Meridian.

性味归经 苦，寒。归膀胱、肺经。

Actions Eliminate wind, stop pain, promote waterflow and subside swell.

功效 祛风止痛，利水消肿。

Application

应用

(1) Bi (Obturation) Pattern due to wind-damp. The medicinal herb is cold in property. In the treatment of Bi (Obturation) Pattern due to heat manifested by redness, swelling and motor impairment of joint, it is combined with *Coicis Semen* (yi yi ren) and *Talcum* (hua shi), to form up Bi (Obturation) Pattern-Alleviating Decoction (Xuan Bi Tang). In the treatment of Bi (Obturation) Pattern due to wind, cold and damp, it is combined with the wind-eliminating and cold-dispelling herbs.

（1）风湿痹痛。本品性寒，善治热痹，症见关节红肿、屈伸不利，常与薏苡仁、滑石等同用，如宣痹汤。治风寒湿痹，可与祛风散寒药同用。

(2) Edema and difficult urination. The medicinal herb acts to promote waterflow, subside swell

（2）水肿，小便不利。本品能利水消肿、清下焦湿热。

and remove damp-heat from lower energizer. In the treatment of edema, abdominal fullness and difficult defecation and urination, it is combined with *Semen Zanthoxyli* (jiao mu), *Semen Descurainiae* (ting li zi) and *Rhei Radix et Rhizoma* (da huang), to form up Tetrandra, Zanthoxylum, Pepperweed Seed and Rhubarb Pills (Ji Jiao Li Huang Wan). In the treatment of edema due to spleen deficiency, it is combined with *Astragali Radix* (huang qi).

治水肿腹满，二便不利，常与椒目、葶苈子、大黄同用，即己椒苈黄丸。治脾虚水肿，可与黄芪等同用。

Usage and dosage Apply 5～10 g in decoction.

用法用量 煎服，5～10克。

Precautions for use It is cautious to apply for those with yin deficiency, weak body constitution or deficiency and cold in spleen and stomach.

使用注意 阴虚体弱、脾胃虚寒者慎用。

Remarks *Saposhnikoviae Radix* (fang feng) and *Stephaniae Tetrandrae Radix* (fang ji)

按语 防风与防己

Both the medicinal herbs act to eliminate wind and damp. Fang ji is a plant of family Menispermaceae, while fang feng is a plant of family Umbelliferae. Fang feng is pungent and sweet in flavor, slightly warm in property, and acts to eliminate wind and relieve exterior pattern, and also to dissolve damp and stop convulsion, applied to treat exterior pattern, Bi (Obturation) Pattern due to wind and damp, and tetanus. Fang ji is bitter in flavor, cold in property, and acts to eliminate wind-damp and stop pain, and also to promote waterflow and subside swell, applied to treat Bi (Obturation) Pattern due to wind, damp and heat, edema and difficult urination.

二药均能祛风湿。不同的是防风为伞形科植物，防己为防己科植物。防风辛甘微温，既祛风解表，又胜湿、止痉，善治表证、风湿痹痛、破伤风。防己苦寒，既祛风湿止痛，又利水消肿，善治风湿热痹、水肿小便不利。

Gentianae Macrophyllae Radix (qin jiao)

秦艽

It is the dried product from the root of a perennial herb, *Gentiana macrophylla* Pall. or *Gentiana*

为龙胆科植物秦艽、麻花秦艽、粗茎秦艽或小秦艽

straminea Maxim. or *Gentiana crassicaulis Duchie ex* Burk. or *Gentiana dahurica* Fisch., family Gentianaceae. The medicinal herb is collected in spring and autumn, applied in crude form.

的干燥根。春、秋季采挖。生用。

Features Flavor: bitter and pungent. Property: slightly cold. Meridian tropism: the Stomach Meridian, the Liver Meridian and the Gallbladder Meridian.

性味归经 苦、辛，微寒。归胃、肝、胆经。

Actions Eliminate wind-damp, stop pain in Bi (Obturation) Pattern, remove damp-heat and reduce false heat.

功效 祛风湿，止痹痛，清湿热，退虚热。

Application

应用

(1) Bi (Obturation) Pattern and numbness of hands and feet. The medicinal herb, as the major herb to treat Bi (Obturation) Pattern, is applied to acute or chronic Bi (Obturation) Pattern due to cold or heat. It also acts to clear heat, so it is more applied to treat Bi (Obturation) Pattern due to heat, and combined with *Stephaniae Tetrandrae Radix* (fang ji), *Anemarrhenae Rhizoma* (zhi mu) and *Lonicerae Japonicae Caulis* (ren dong teng). In the treatment of Bi (Obturation) Pattern due to wind, cold and damp, it is combined with *Aconiti Radix* (chuan wu), *Rhizoma seu Radix Notopterygii* (qiang huo) and *Radix Ledebouriellae* (fang feng).

（1）风湿痹痛，手足不遂。本品为治痹痛所常用，无论新久、寒热痹痛皆可应用。因兼能清热，故对热痹更为适宜，常与防己、知母、忍冬藤等同用。若治风寒湿痹，可与川乌、羌活、防风等同用。

(2) Jaundice due to damp-heat. The medicinal herb acts to clear heat and dissolve damp. In the treatment of jaundice due to damp-heat, it is applied singly or combined with *Artemisiae Scopariae Herba* (yin chen hao) and *Gardeniae Fructus* (zhi zi).

（2）湿热黄疸。本品能清利湿热。治湿热黄疸，可单用，或与茵陈、栀子等同用。

(3) Feverish sensation, tidal fever and infantile malnutrition with fever. The medicinal herb acts to reduce false heat and relieve feverish sensation. In the treatment of feverish sensation and tidal fever, it is combined with zhi mu, *Lycii Cortex* (di gu pi)

（3）骨蒸潮热，小儿疳热。本品能退虚热，除骨蒸。治骨蒸潮热，常与知母、地骨皮、鳖甲等同用，如秦艽鳖甲散。治小儿疳热，兼湿热者，

and *Trionycis Carapax* (bie jia), to form up Large-Leaved Gentian and Turtle Shell Powder (Qin Jiao Bie Jia San). In the treatment of infantile malnutrition with fever due to damp-heat, it is combined with *Lycii Cortex* (di gu pi) and *Rhizoma Picrorhizae* (hu huang lian).

常与地骨皮、胡黄连等同用。

Usage and dosage Apply 3～10 g in decoction.

用法用量 煎服,3～10克。

Chaenomelis Fructus (mu gua)

木瓜

It is the dried product from the fruit of *Chaenomeles speciosa* (Sweet) Nakai, family Rosaceae. The medicinal herb produced in Xuancheng, Anhui Province is called "xuan mu gua". It is collected in summer and autumn when its fruits are green and yellow, applied in crude form.

为蔷薇科植物贴梗海棠的干燥近成熟果实。安徽宣城产者称"宣木瓜"。夏、秋两季果实绿黄时采摘。生用。

Features Flavor: sour. Property: warm. Meridian tropism: the Liver Meridian and the Spleen Meridian.

性味归经 酸,温。归肝、脾经。

Actions Soothe tendons, activate meridians, eliminate damp and harmonize stomach.

功效 舒筋活络,除湿和胃。

Application

应用

(1) Bi (Obturation) Pattern due to damp, spasm and beriberi with swelling and pain. The medicinal herb acts to soothe tendons, activate meridians, dissolve damp and relieve Bi (Obturation) Pattern, as the major herb for Bi (Obturation) Pattern manifested by spasm. It is combined with *Olibanum* (ru xiang), *Myrrha* (mo yao) and *Rehmanniae Radix* (sheng di huang), to form up Papaya Decoction (Mu Gua Jian). In the treatment of beriberi, it is combined with *Euodiae Fructus* (wu zhu yu) and *Arecae Semen* (bing lang), to form up Cock Crowing Powder (Ji Ming San).

(1) 湿痹拘挛,脚气肿痛。本品功善舒筋活络、化湿利痹,为治痹痛见筋脉拘急之要药。常与乳香、没药、生地黄等同用,如木瓜煎。治脚气,常与吴茱萸、槟榔等同用,如鸡鸣散。

(2) Vomiting, diarrhea and cramp. The medicinal herb acts to dissolve damp, soothe tendons and stop vomiting and diarrhea. In the treatment of vomiting, diarrhea and abdominal pain cramp due to damp, it is combined with wu zhu yu, *Pinelliae Rhizoma* (ban xia) and *Coptidis Rhizoma* (huang lian).

（2）吐泻转筋。本品能化湿浊、舒筋络、止吐泻。治湿浊所致的呕吐泄泻、腹痛转筋，常与吴茱萸、半夏、黄连等同用。

Usage and dosage Apply 6～9 g in decoction.

用法用量 煎服，6～9克。

Agkistrodon (qi she)

蕲蛇

It is the dried product from the eviscerated body of *Agkistrodon acutus* (Guenther), family Grotalidae. The medicinal herb is caught in summer and autumn, eviscerated and dried, and then prepared in millet wine.

为蝰科动物五步蛇除去内脏的干燥全体。夏、秋季捕捉，除去内脏，干燥后以黄酒润透。

Features Flavor: sweet and salty. Property: warm and poisonous. Meridian tropism: the Liver Meridian.

性味归经 甘、咸，温；有毒。归肝经。

Actions Eliminate wind, dredge meridians and relieve spasm.

功效 祛风通络，止痉。

Application

应用

(1) Bi (Obturation) Pattern due to wind-damp, deviation of mouth and hemiplegia. The medicinal herb acts to "penetrate bone and catch wind", and to eliminate wind and dredge meridians. In the treatment of Bi (Obturation) Pattern due to wind-damp manifested by muscle spasm, wind stroke manifested by deviation of mouth and hemiplegia, it is combined with *Radix Ledebouriellae* (fang feng), *Angelicae Pubescentis Radix* (du huo) and *Gastrodiae Rhizoma* (tian ma), in prepared form with millet wine or made into pills for oral administration.

（1）风湿顽痹，口眼㖞斜，半身不遂。本品能"透骨搜风"，祛风通络，善治风湿顽痹所致的筋脉拘挛，以及中风所致的口眼㖞斜、半身不遂，可与防风、独活、天麻等同用，浸酒或制丸服用。

(2) Leprosy, scabies and itching skin. The medicinal herb acts to eliminate wind and stop itching. In the treatment of various skin diseases, it is com-

（2）麻风，疥癣，皮肤瘙痒。本品能祛风止痒。治各类皮肤病证，可与祛风、杀虫

bined with the wind-eliminating and worm-killing herbs, for oral administration or external use.

等药同用，内服外用皆宜。

(3) Acute or chronic convulsion in infants, and tetanus. The medicinal herb acts to eliminate wind, relieve convulsion and stop spasm, as the major herb for convulsion and spasm. In the treatment of acute convulsion in infants, it is combined with the heat-clearing and wind-removing herbs, as *Bovis Calculus* (niu huang). In the treatment of chronic convulsion, it is combined with *Atractylodis Macrocephalae Rhizoma* (bai zhu) and *Dioscoreae Rhizoma* (shan yao). In the treatment of tetanus, it is combined with *Scolopendra subspinipes* (wu gong) and prepared by grinding into powder, and then taken with millet wine, to form up Life-Rescuing Powder (Ding Ming San).

(3) 小儿急慢惊风，破伤风。本品能祛风、定惊、止抽搐，为治惊风抽搐之要药。治小儿急惊风，常与牛黄等清热息风药同用。治慢惊风，常与白术、山药等同用。治破伤风，可配蜈蚣等研末，煎酒调服，即定命散。

Usage and dosage Apply 3～9 g in decoction. Grind it into powder and take 1～1.5 g each time, 2～3 times a day.

用法用量 煎服，3～9克。研末服，每次 1～1.5 克。每日 2～3 次。

Precautions for use It is prohibited to apply for those with yin deficiency or heat in blood.

使用注意 阴虚血热者忌服。

Acanthopanacis Cortex (wu jia pi)

五加皮

It is the dried product from the root cortex of *Acanthopanax gracilistylus* W. W. Smith, family Araliaceae. The medicinal herb is collected in summer and autumn and then peeled, applied in crude form.

为五加科植物细柱五加的干燥根皮。夏、秋季采挖，剥取根皮。生用。

Features Flavor: pungent and bitter. Property: warm. Meridian tropism: the Liver Meridian and the Kidney Meridian.

性味归经 辛、苦，温。归肝、肾经。

Actions Eliminate wind-damp, reinforce liver and kidney, strengthen tendons and bones, and promote waterflow.

功效 祛风湿，补肝肾，强筋骨，利水。

Application

应用

(1) Bi (Obturation) Pattern due to wind-damp.

(1) 风湿痹痛。本品既

The medicinal herb acts to eliminate wind-damp, and also to reinforce liver and kidney and strengthen tendons and bones as well. It is applied to treat Bi (Obturation) Pattern due to wind-damp, and also to treat liver and kidney deficiency due to chronic Bi (Obturation) Pattern. It is applied singly by preparing with millet wine, or combined with other medicinal herbs.

祛风湿，又补肝肾、强筋骨。既治风湿痹痛，又治久痹肝肾虚者，可单用浸酒服，亦可与其他药物配伍同用。

(2) Weakness at low back and knees, and retarded walking ability in children. The medicinal herb acts to reinforce liver and kidney and strengthen tendons and bones. In the treatment of weakness at low back and knees due to liver and kidney deficiency, it is combined with *Achyranthis Bidentatae Radix* (huai niu xi), *Eucommiae Cortex* (du zhong) and *Epimedium davidii* (yin yang huo). In the treatment of retarded walking ability in children, it is combined with *Plastrum Testudinis* (gui jia) and huai niu xi.

（2）腰膝软弱，小儿行迟。本品能补肝肾，强筋骨。治肝肾虚所致腰膝软弱，常与怀牛膝、杜仲、淫羊藿等同用。治小儿行迟，常与龟甲、牛膝等同用。

(3) Edema and beriberi. The medicinal herb acts to promote waterflow. In the treatment of edema, it is combined with *Poriae Cutis* (fu ling pi), *Citri Reticulatae Pericarpium* (chen pi) and *Arecae Pericarpium* (da fu pi), to form up Five Cortices Drink (Wu Pi Yin). In the treatment of beriberi and edema, it is combined with *Arecae Pericarpium* (da fu pi) and *Chaenomelis Fructus* (mu gua).

（3）水肿，脚气。本品尚能利水。治水肿，常与茯苓皮、陈皮、大腹皮等同用，如五皮饮。治脚气浮肿，可与大腹皮、木瓜等同用。

Usage and dosage Apply 5～10 g in decoction.

用法用量 煎服，5～10克。

Precautions for use It is cautious to apply for those with yin deficiency and fire hyperactivity, dry tongue or bitter taste in mouth.

使用注意 阴虚火旺、舌干口苦者慎服。

Taxilli Herba (sang ji sheng)

桑寄生

It is the dried product from the stem and

为桑寄生科植物桑寄生

branch of *Taxillus chinensis* (DC.) Danser, family Loranthaceae. The medicinal herb is collected from winter to next spring, applied in crude form.

的干燥带叶茎枝。冬季至次春采割。生用。

Features Flavor: bitter and sweet. Property: neutral. Meridian tropism: the Liver Meridian and the Kidney Meridian.

性味归经 苦、甘,平。归肝、肾经。

Actions Eliminate wind-damp, reinforce liver and kidney, strengthen tendons and bones, and quiet fetus.

功效 祛风湿,补肝肾,强筋骨,安胎。

Application

应用

(1) Bi (Obturation) Pattern due to wind-damp. The medicinal herb acts to eliminate wind-damp and relax tendons, and also to reinforce liver and kidney and strengthen tendons and bones as well. In the treatment of chronic Bi (Obturation) Pattern due to wind-damp and aching and weakness at low back and knees due to liver and kidney deficiency, it is combined with *Angelicae Pubescentis Radix* (du huo), *Achyranthis Bidentatae Radix* (niu xi) and *Eucommiae Cortex* (du zhong), to form up Lovage and Angelica Decoction (Du Huo Ji Sheng Tang).

(1) 风湿痹痛。本品既祛风湿、舒筋络,又长于益肝肾、强筋骨,尤适用于风湿久痹,肝肾亏虚所致的腰膝酸软,可与独活、牛膝、杜仲等配伍同用,如独活寄生汤。

(2) Threatened miscarriage with vaginal bleeding, and fetal irritability. The medicinal herb acts to reinforce liver and kidney, nourish blood and quiet fetus. In the treatment of threatened miscarriage and fetal irritability caused by liver and kidney deficiency, it is combined with *Asini Corii Colla* (e jiao), *Radix Dipsaci* (xu duan) and *Cuscutae Semen* (tu si zi).

(2) 胎漏下血,胎动不安。本品能补肝肾、养血安胎。治肝肾亏虚之胎漏、胎动不安,常与阿胶、续断、菟丝子等药同用。

Usage and dosage Apply 9～15 g in decoction.

用法用量 煎服,9～15克。

Cibotii Rhizoma (gou ji)

狗脊

It is the dried product from the rhizome of *Cibotium barometz* (L.) J. Sm., family Dicksonlaceae. The medicinal herb is collected in autumn

为蚌壳蕨科植物金毛狗脊的干燥根茎。秋、冬二季采挖。生用或砂烫制用。

and winter, applied in crude form or prepared form by stir-baking with sand.

Features Flavor: bitter and sweet. Property: warm. Meridian tropism: the Liver Meridian and the Kidney Meridian.

性味归经 苦、甘，温。归肝、肾经。

Actions Eliminate wind-damp, reinforce liver and kidney, and strengthen back and knees.

功效 祛风湿，补肝肾，强腰膝。

Application

Bi (Obturation) Pattern due to wind-damp lack of strength in the lumbus and knees. The medicinal herb is bitter, sweet and warm, and acts to eliminate pathogenic wind, cold and damp from spine and back, and to reinforce liver and kidney and strengthen low back and knees as well. In the treatment of Bi (Obturation) Pattern complicated by kidney deficiency manifested by low back pain, spinal stiffness and failure to bend forward and backward, it is combined with *Angelicae Pubescentis Radix* (du huo), *Ramulus Loranthi* (sang ji sheng) and *Acanthopanacis Cortex* (wu jia pi). Aching and weakness at low back and kness. In the treatment of kidney deficiency mainfested by aching and weakness at low back and kness, and weakness in lower limbs, it is combined with *Semen Cuscutae* (tu si zi), *Cortex Eucommiae* (du zhong) and *Radix Dipsaci* (xu duan).

应用

风湿痹痛，腰膝软弱。本品苦甘性温，善能祛脊背风寒湿邪，又能补肝肾、强腰膝。治风湿痹痛兼肾虚的腰痛脊强、不能俯仰，常与独活、桑寄生、五加皮等同用。治肾虚腰膝酸软，下肢无力，常与菟丝子、杜仲、续断等同用。

Usage and dosage Apply 6～12 g in decoction. The medicinal herb is dry in property in crude form, while its dry property is modified in prepared form.

用法用量 煎服，6～12克。生用性燥，制用燥性得缓。

Precautions for use It is prohibited to apply for those with kidney deficiency and false heat.

使用注意 肾虚有热者忌用。

Brief summary

小　结

Both *Angelicae Pubescentis Radix* (du huo) and *Aconiti Radix* (chuan wu) are warm and hot, and act to eliminate wind, remove damp and stop pain, applied to treat Bi (Obturation) Pattern due to wind, cold and damp. Du huo is warm and descending, applied to treat Bi (Obturation) Pattern due to wind-damp in lower body. It also acts relieve exterior pattern, applied to treat exterior pattern of wind, cold and damp. Chuan wu is hot and poisonous, and acts to eliminate wind and remove damp, and also to dispel cold and stop pain, as the major herb for all pains caused by cold and damp.

独活、川乌，均性温热，善祛风除湿、止痛，治风寒湿痹。其中独活性温，性善下行，善治下半身的风湿痹痛，且能解表，治风寒夹湿之表证。川乌性热有毒，除祛风除湿外，其散寒止痛力甚佳，为治寒湿诸痛之要药。

Clematidis Radix et Rhizoma (wei ling xian) is pungent, salty and warm, and acts to eliminate wind-damp and dredge meridians. As the major herb to treat Bi (Obturation) Pattern due to wind-damp, it acts to dissolve phlegm and rheum, applied to treat diseases due to phlegm or rheum accumulation, and fishbone lodging in throat.

威灵仙，味辛咸性温，具有祛风湿、通经络的作用，尤性善通利。为治风湿痹痛之要药；且能消痰水、治骨鲠，用于痰饮积聚、诸骨哽喉。

Both *Stephaniae Tetrandrae Radix* (fang ji) and *Gentianae Macrophyllae Radix* (qin jiao) are cold and cool in property, and act to clear heat, eliminate wind and remove damp, applied to treat Bi (Obturation) Pattern due to heat manifested by swelling and pain of joints. Fang ji acts to promote waterflow and subside swell, applied to treat edema and difficult urination. Qin jiao is cool but not cold, applied to treat acute or chronic Bi (Obturation) Pattern due to cold or heat. It also acts to eliminate damp and heat, applied to treat jaundice, and to reduce false heat, applied to treat feverish sensation and tidal fever.

防已、秦艽，均药性寒凉，具清热祛风除湿之功，善治热痹关节肿痛，其中防已又能利水消肿，治水肿、小便不利。秦艽性凉不寒，无论新久、寒热痹痛皆宜；且能清湿热，治黄疸；退虚热，治骨蒸潮热。

Both *Chaenomelis Fructus* (mu gua) and *Agkistrodon* (qi she) are warm in property, and act to treat Bi (Obturation) Pattern due to wind-damp manifested by spasm and cramp. Mu gua is sour and warm, and acts to relax tendons, activate meridians, dissolve damp and stop pain, as the major herb to treat Bi (Obturation) Pattern manifested by muscle spasm. It also acts to remove damp and harmonize stomach, applied to treat vomiting, diarrhea and cramp. Qi she, an animal-type herb, is good at moving and acts to penetrate bone and catch wind and to eliminate wind and dredge meridians, applied to treat Bi (Obturation) Pattern due to wind-damp manifested by muscle spasm. It also acts to relieve convulsion, as the major herb to treat convulsion, applied to treat acute or chronic convulsion in infants, and also to treat tetanus with spasm.

木瓜、蕲蛇，均性温，均治风湿痹痛见筋脉拘急。其中木瓜酸温，功善舒筋活络、化湿利痹，为治痹痛见筋脉拘急之要药；且能除湿和胃，治吐泻转筋。蕲蛇为动物药，性善走窜，能透骨搜风，善祛风通络，善治风湿顽痹之筋脉拘急；且能止痉，为治惊风抽搐之要药，既治小儿急慢惊风，又治破伤风抽搐。

All *Acanthopanacis Cortex* (wu jia pi), *Taxilli Herba* (sang ji sheng) and *Cibotii Rhizoma* (gou ji) act to eliminate wind-damp, reinforce liver and kidney, and strengthen tendons and bones, and act to treat aching and weakness at low back and knees due to Bi (Obturation) Pattern complicated by liver and kidney deficiency. Wu jia pi acts to promote waterflow, applied to treat edema and difficult urination. Sang ji sheng acts to nourish blood, reinforce liver and kidney and quiet fetus by nourishing blood, applied to treat threatened miscarriage with vaginal bleeding and fetal irritability. Gou ji acts to reinforce liver and kidney and strengthen back and knees, applied to treat kidney deficiency manifested by stiffness and pain at low back and spine, failure to bend forward and backward, aching and weakness at low back and knees.

五加皮、桑寄生、狗脊，均能祛风湿、补肝肾、强筋骨，善治风湿痹痛兼肝肾不足腰膝酸软者。其中五加皮还能利水，可治水肿、小便不利。桑寄生则长于养血、补肝肾，还能养血安胎，治胎漏下血及胎动不安。狗脊尤善补肝肾、强腰膝，既治肾虚腰脊强痛、俯仰不利，还治腰膝酸软无力。

Chapter 5 Damp-Dissolving Herbs

第5章 化湿药

The medicinal herbs, fragrant and warm in property and acting to dissolve damp, wake up spleen, desiccate damp and strengthen spleen are called the damp-dissolving herbs.

This type of medicinal herbs are mostly pungent, fragrant and warm in property, or bitter, warm and dry in property, and act to dissolve damp and wake up spleen or act to desiccate damp and strengthen spleen, applied to treat damp blocking spleen which fails to dominate transportation and transformation, manifested by distension and fullness in epigastria or abdomen, poor appetite, fatigue and white-sticky tongue coating, or applied to treat damp-heat blocking spleen manifested by sweet taste in mouth and excessive saliva. Some of the medicinal herbs act to reduce summer heat, applied to treat summer heat-damp pattern and damp-heat pattern.

It is necessary to notice in application of this type of medicinal herbs that the damp accumulation is often complicated by qi stagnation, and qi-promoting method is helpful to dissolve damp, therefore the qi-promoting herbs are combined. In the condition of damp caused by spleen deficiency, it is necessary to combine the spleen-reinforcing herbs. This type of medicinal herbs, mostly pungent, warm,

凡气香性温，以化湿醒脾、燥湿运脾为主要作用的药物，称为化湿药。

本类药物大多气辛香性偏温，或味苦性温燥，善于化湿醒脾或燥湿健脾。适用于脾为湿困、运化失常所致的脘腹痞满、食少体倦、舌苔白腻，或湿热困脾之口甘多涎等。部分药物兼能解暑，治暑湿、湿温等证。

使用本类药物需注意：湿阻常兼气滞，行气有助于化湿，可配伍行气药同用。若脾虚生湿者，当配伍补脾药同用。本类药物辛温香燥，易耗气伤阴，阴虚血燥、气虚者宜慎用。其气芳香，入汤剂不宜久煎。

fragrant and dry in property, often consume qi and exhaust yin, therefore it is cautious to apply for those with yin deficiency, dryness in blood or qi deficiency. Due to their fragrant property, it is not advisable to decoct the medicinal herbs for long time.

Pogostmonis Herba (guang huo xiang)

广藿香

It is the dried product from the aerial parts of a perennial herb, *Pogostemon cablin* (Blanco) Benth., family Labiatae. The medicinal herb is mainly produced in Guangdong Province, collected when the twigs and leaves are flouring, and applied in crude form.

为唇形科植物广藿香的干燥地上部分。主产于广东。枝叶茂盛时采割。生用。

Features Flavor: pungent. Property: slightly warm. Meridian tropism: the Spleen Meridian, the Stomach Meridian and the Lung Meridian.

性味归经 辛,微温。归脾、胃、肺经。

Actions Dissolve damp, reduce summer heat and stop vomiting.

功效 化湿,解暑,止呕。

Application

应用

(1) Damp blocking middle energizer pattern. The medicinal herb is fragrant in flavor and acts to dissolve damp-turbidity and wake up spleen and stomach. In the treatment of damp-turbidity blocking middle energizer manifested by distension and fullness in epigastria or abdomen, poor appetite, nausea and vomiting, it is combined with *Atractylodis Rhizoma* (cang zhu), *Magnoliae Officinalis Cortex* (hou po) and *Pinelliae Rhizoma* (ban xia).

(1) 湿阻中焦证。本品气味芳香,善化湿浊、醒脾胃。治湿浊阻于中焦,症见脘腹痞闷、食欲不振、恶心呕吐,常与苍术、厚朴、半夏等同用。

(2) Summer heat-damp pattern and early stage of damp-heat pattern. The medicinal herb is warm and fragrant, but not dry, and acts to dissolve damp, reduce summer heat and relieve exterior pattern. In the treatment of external attack of wind-

(2) 暑湿证,湿温初起。本品性温不燥,能芳香化湿、解暑发表。治暑月外感风寒、内伤生冷的恶寒发热、头痛脘闷、呕吐泄泻,常与紫

cold or internal damage of cold in summer, manifested by aversion to cold, fever, headache, distension in epigastria, vomiting and diarrhea, it is combined with *Perillae Folium* (zi su ye), hou po and ban xia, to form up Agastache Vital Force Powder (Huo Xiang Zheng Qi San). In the treatment of early stage of damp-heat pattern, it is combined with *Scutellariae Radix* (huang qin), *Talcum* (hua shi) and *Artemisiae Scopariae Herba* (yin chen hao), to form up Sweet Dew Toxin-Dispersing Elixir (Gan Lu Xiao Du Dan).

苏、厚朴、半夏等同用，如藿香正气散。治湿温初起，湿热并重者，可与黄芩、滑石、茵陈等同用，如甘露消毒丹。

(3) Vomiting. The medicinal herb acts to dissolve damp, harmonize middle energizer and stop vomiting. In the treatment of vomiting caused by damp-turbidity, it is applied singly or combined with ban xia.

（3）呕吐。本品功善化湿和中、止呕。治湿浊所致呕吐，可单用，或与半夏等同用。

Usage and dosage Apply 3～10 g in decoction. Apply double dose in fresh form.

用法用量 煎服，3～10克。鲜品加倍。

Precautions for use It is prohibited to apply for those with yin deficiency and fire hyperactivity.

使用注意 阴虚火旺者忌用。

Eupatorii Herba (pei lan)

佩兰

It is the dried product from the aerial part of a perennial herb, *Eupatorium fortunei* Turcz., family Compositae. The medicinal herb is collected in summer and autumn, applied in crude form.

为菊科植物佩兰的干燥地上部分。夏、秋季分次采割。生用。

Features Flavor: pungent. Property: neutral. Meridian tropism: the Spleen Meridian, the Stomach Meridian and the Lung Meridian.

性味归经 辛，平。归脾、胃、肺经。

Actions Dissolve damp and reduce summer heat.

功效 化湿，解暑。

Application

应用

(1) Damp blocking middle energizer pattern. The medicinal herb is fragrant and acts to dissolve

（1）湿阻中焦证。本品气香化湿，能醒脾开胃。治

damp, wake up spleen and promote appetite. In the treatment of damp blocking middle energizer, it is combined with *Pogostmonis Herba* (guang huo xiang) in mutual reinforcement, or combined with *Atractylodis Rhizoma* (cang zhu) and *Magnoliae Officinalis Cortex* (hou po). It is also applied to treat damp-heat in Spleen Meridian manifested by sweet taste or stickiness in mouth, excessive saliva and foul breath.

湿阻中焦，常与广藿香相须为用；或与苍术、厚朴等配伍。亦治脾经湿热的口中甜腻、多涎、口臭等证。

(2) External attack of summer heat-damp. The medicinal herb acts to dissolve damp and reduce summer heat. In the treatment of summer heat-damp pattern, it is combined with guang huo xiang and *Moslae Herba* (xiang ru). In the treatment of early stage of damp-heat pattern, it is combined with *Talcum* (hua shi) and *Coicis Semen* (yi yi ren).

（2）外感暑湿，湿温初起。本品既化湿，又解暑。治暑湿证，常与藿香、香薷等同用。治湿温初起，可与滑石、薏苡仁等同用。

Usage and dosage Apply 3～10 g in decoction.

用法用量 煎服，3～10克。

Atractylodis Rhizoma (cang zhu)

苍术

It is the dried product from the rhizome of *Atractylodes lancea* (Thunb.) DC. or *Atractylodes chinensis* (DC.) koidz., family Compositae. The former is produced in Mao Mountain, Jiangsu Province in high quality, also called "mao cang zhu" or "mao zhu" or short. It is collected in spring and autumn. It is applied in crude form or prepared form by frying with wheat bran.

为菊科植物茅苍术或北苍术的干燥根茎。前者产于江苏茅山，质佳，名茅苍术，简称茅术。春、秋季采挖。生用或者麸炒用。

Features Flavor: pungent and bitter. Property: warm. Meridian tropism: the Spleen Meridian, the Stomach Meridian and the Liver Meridian.

性味归经 辛、苦，温。归脾、胃、肝经。

Actions Desiccate damp, strengthen spleen, eliminate wind-damp and brighten eyes.

功效 燥湿健脾，祛风湿，明目。

Application

(1) Damp blocking middle energizer pattern. The medicinal herb is pungent, bitter, warm and dry in property and acts to desiccate damp and strengthen spleen. In the treatment of damp blocking middle energizer pattern manifested by distension and fullness in epigastria or abdomen, poor appetite, nausea, vomiting and turbid-sticky tongue coating, it is combined with *Magnoliae Officinalis Cortex* (hou po) and *Citri Reticulatae Pericarpium* (chen pi), to form up Stomach-Calming Powder (Ping Wei San).

(2) Bi (Obturation) Pattern due to wind-damp, swelling and pain at foot and knee. The medicinal herb acts to eliminate wind-damp. In the treatment of Bi (Obturation) Pattern due to wind-damp in which damp is prominent, it is combined with *Notopterygii Rhizoma et Radix* (qiang huo) and *Angelicae Pubescentis Radix* (du huo). In the treatment of damp-heat downward infusion manifested by swelling and pain at foot and knee, it is combined with *Phellodendri Cortex Chiensis* (huang bo), to form up Two Wonderful Herbs Powder (Er Miao San).

(3) Night blindness and blurred vision. In the treatment of night blindness or blurred vision, the medicinal herb is applied singly or combined with lamb liver or pork liver by boiling or steaming.

Usage and dosage Apply 3～9 g in decoction. The medicinal herb is dry in property in crude form, and its dry property is modified in prepared form by frying.

Precautions for use It is prohibited to apply for those of yin deficiency and internal heat, and those of qi deficiency with profuse sweating.

应用

(1) 湿阻中焦证。本品辛苦温燥，功善燥湿健脾。治寒湿阻于中焦所致的脘腹痞闷、食欲不振、恶心呕吐、舌苔浊腻，常与厚朴、陈皮等配伍，如平胃散。

(2) 风湿痹痛，足膝肿痛。本品能祛风湿。治风寒湿痹，以湿胜者尤宜，常与羌活、独活等同用。治湿热下注之足膝肿痛，可与黄柏同用，即二妙散。

(3) 夜盲，眼目昏涩。本品单用，或与羊肝、猪肝蒸煮同食，治夜盲，眼目昏涩。

用法用量 煎服，3～9克。生用性燥，炒用燥性得缓。

使用注意 阴虚内热、气虚多汗者忌用。

Magnoliae Officinalis Cortex (hou po)

厚朴

It is the dried product from the bark and bark of branch and root of *Magnolia officinalis* Rehd. et Wils. or *Magnolia officinalis* Rehd. et Wils. var. *biloba* Rehd. et Wils., family Magnoliaceae. The medicinal herb is collected from April to June, applied in crude form or prepared form by stir-frying with ginger juice.

为木兰科植物厚朴或凹叶厚朴的干燥干皮、根皮及枝皮。4～6月剥取。生用，或姜汁炙用。

Features Flavor: bitter and pungent. Property: warm. Meridian tropism: the Spleen Meridian, the Stomach Meridian, the Lung Meridian and the Large Intestine Meridian.

性味归经 苦、辛，温。归脾、胃、肺、大肠经。

Actions Desiccate damp, dissolve phlegm, subdue qi and soothe panting.

功效 燥湿消痰，下气平喘。

Application

应用

(1) Damp blocking middle energizer pattern. The medicinal herb acts to desiccate damp and promote qi flow. In the treatment of damp blocking middle energizer or qi stagnation in spleen and stomach manifested by distension and fullness in epigastria or abdomen and poor appetite, it is combined with *Atractylodis Rhizoma* (cang zhu) and *Citri Reticulatae Pericarpium* (chen pi), to form up Stomach-Calming Powder (Ping Wei San).

(1) 湿阻中焦证。本品功善燥湿、行气。善治湿阻中焦、脾胃气滞的脘腹胀满、不思饮食，常与苍术、陈皮等同用，如平胃散。

(2) Accumulation and stagnation in intestines and stomach. The medicinal herb acts to subdue qi, dilate middle energizer, dissolve accumulation and relieve stagnation. In the treatment of food retention or qi stagnation manifested by abdominal distension and constipation, it is combined with *Aurantii Fructus Immaturus* (zhi shi) and *Rhei Radix et Rhizoma* (da huang), to form up Magnolia Bark and Three Agents Decoction (Hou Po San Wu Tang).

(2) 肠胃积滞。本品能下气宽中、消积导滞。治食积气滞、腹胀便秘，常与枳实、大黄配伍同用，即厚朴三物汤。

(3) Panting and cough due to phlegm-rheum. The medicinal herb acts to subdue lung qi, dissolve phlegm and rheum and soothe panting and cough. In the treatment of panting and cough due to phlegm-rheum, it is combined with *Cinnamomi Ramulus* (gui zhi) and *Armeniacae Amarum Semen* (ku xing ren), or combined with *Perillae Folium* (zi su zi), *Exocarpium Citri Leiocarpae* (ju pi) and *Angelicae Sinensis Radix* (dang gui).

(3) 痰饮喘咳。本品能下肺气、消痰涎、平咳喘。治痰饮咳喘,可与桂枝、杏仁等同用,或与紫苏子、陈皮、当归等同用。

Usage and dosage Apply 3～10 g in decoction. The medicinal herb is dry in property in crude form, and its dry property is modified in prepared form by stir-frying with ginger juice.

用法用量 煎服,3～10克。生用性燥,姜汁炙燥性得减。

Precautions for use It is cautious to apply for those with weak body constitutions or pregnant women.

使用注意 体虚及孕妇慎用。

Amomi Fructus (sha ren)

砂仁

It is the dried product from the ripe fruit of *Amomum villosum* lour. (*Yangchunsha*), *Amomnm villosum Amomum longiligulare* T.L. Wu. var. *xanthioides* T. L. Wu et Senjen, family Zingiberaceae (*Leukesha* or *Hainansha*). The former is mainly produced in Guangdong and Guangxi Provinces in China in high quality. The medicinal herb is collected in summer and autumn when the fruits are ripe, applied in crude form.

为姜科植物阳春砂、绿壳砂或海南砂的干燥成熟果实。阳春砂主产于我国广东、广西等地,质量为优。于夏秋间果实成熟时采收。生用。

Features Flavor: pungent. Property: warm. Meridian tropism: the Spleen Meridian and the Stomach Meridian.

性味归经 辛、温。归脾、胃经。

Actions Dissolve damp, promote appetite, warm spleen, stop diarrhea, regulate qi flow, and quiet fetus.

功效 化湿开胃,温脾止泻,理气安胎。

Application

(1) Damp blocking middle energizer and qi stagnation in spleen and stomach. The medicinal herb acts to dissolve damp and wake up spleen, and to promote qi flow and warm middle energizer as well. In the treatment of disharmony between spleen and stomach due to damp blockage or qi stagnation, it is combined with *Magnoliae Officinalis Cortex* (hou po), *Citri Reticulatae Pericarpium* (chen pi) and *Aurantii Fructus Immaturus* (zhi shi). In the treatment of spleen deficiency causing qi stagnation, it is combined with *Codonopsis Radix* (dang shen), *Atractylodis Macrocephalae Rhizoma* (bai zhu) and *Poria* (fu ling), to form up Costus Root and Amomum with Six Nobles Decoction (Xiang Sha Liu Jun Zi Tang).

(2) Vomiting and diarrhea due to deficiency and cold. The medicinal herb acts to promote appetite, stop vomiting, warm middle energizer and stop diarrhea. In the treatment of deficiency and cold in spleen and stomach manifested by vomiting and diarrhea, it is applied singly or combined with *Zingiberis Rhizoma* (gan jiang) and *Aconiti Lateralis Radix Praeparata* (fu zi).

(3) Morning sickness in pregnancy and fetal irritability. The medicinal herb acts to promote qi flow, harmonize middle energizer, stop vomiting and quiet fetus. In the treatment of morning sickness in pregnancy and fetal irritability, it is combined with *Perillae Caulis* (zi su geng) and bai zhu.

Usage and dosage Apply 3～6 g in decoction and decoct later.

Precautions for use It is prohibited to apply

应用

（1）湿阻中焦，脾胃气滞。本品既化湿醒脾，又行气温中。治湿阻或气滞所致脾胃不和诸证，常与厚朴、陈皮、枳实等同用。治脾虚气滞者，可与党参、白术、茯苓等同用，如香砂六君子汤。

（2）虚寒吐泻。本品能开胃止呕、温中止泻。治脾胃虚寒之呕吐、泄泻，可单用，或与干姜、附子等同用。

（3）妊娠恶阻，胎动不安。本品能行气和中、止呕安胎。治妊娠恶阻的呕吐及胎动不安，可与紫苏梗、白术等同用。

用法用量 煎服，3～6克。宜后下。

使用注意 阴虚有热者

for those of yin deficiency with heat.

Amomi Fructus Rotundus (bai dou kou)

It is the dried product from the ripe fruit of *Amomum kravanh* Pierre ex Gagnep or *Amonum compactum* Soland. ex Maton, family Zingiberaceae. The medicinal herb is collected in autumn, applied in crude form.

Features　Flavor: pungent. Property: warm. Meridian tropism: the Lung Meridian, the Spleen Meridian and the Stomach Meridian.

Actions　Dissolve damp, promote qi flow, warm middle energizer, stop vomiting, promote appetite and digest food.

Application

(1) Damp blocking middle energizer and qi stagnation in spleen and stomach. The medicinal herb acts to dissolve damp, promote qi flow and warm middle energizer. In the treatment of damp blocking middle energizer or qi stagnation in spleen and stomach manifested by distension and fullness at epigastria or abdomen, and poor appetite, it is combined with *Magnoliae Officinalis Cortex* (hou po) and *Citri Reticulatae Pericarpium* (chen pi). In the treatment of early stage of damp-heat pattern manifested by stuffy chest, loss of appetite and turbid-sticky tongue coating, it is combined with *Talcum* (hua shi), *Coicis Semen* (yi yi ren) and *Armeniacae Amarum Semen* (ku xing ren), to form up Three Seeds Decoction (San Ren Tang).

(2) Vomiting. The medicinal herb acts to warm middle energizer, dispel cold and stop vomiting. In the treatment of cold-damp or qi stagnation manifested by vomiting and regurgitation, it is ap-

忌服。

白豆蔻

为姜科植物白豆蔻或爪哇白豆蔻的干燥成熟果实。秋季采收。生用。

性味归经　辛，温。归肺、脾、胃经。

功效　化湿行气，温中止呕，开胃消食。

应用

（1）湿阻中焦，脾胃气滞。本品功善化湿、行气、温中。治湿阻中焦或脾胃气滞所致的脘腹胀满、不思饮食等，常与厚朴、陈皮等配伍同用。治湿温初起的胸闷不饥、舌苔浊腻者，可与滑石、薏苡仁、杏仁等同用，如三仁汤。

（2）呕吐。本品能温中、散寒、止呕，治寒湿气滞的呕吐反胃，可单用为末服，或配伍藿香、半夏、生姜等同用。

plied singly or combined with *Pogostmonis Herba* (guang huo xiang), *Pinelliae Rhizoma* (ban xia) and *Zingiberis Rhizoma Recens* (sheng jiang).

Usage and dosage Apply 3～6 g in decoction and decoct later.

用法用量 煎服,3～6克。宜后下。

Brief summary

小结

Both *Pogostmonis Herba* (guang huo xiang) and *Eupatorii Herba* (pei lan) are fragrant and attributive to the Spleen Meridian and the Stomach Meridian, and act to dissolve damp and reduce summer heat, applied to treat damp blocking middle energizer, early stage of damp-heat pattern and summer heat-damp pattern, in mutual reinforcement. Guang huo xiang is slightly warm and acts to dissolve damp, harmonize middle energizer and stop vomiting, as the major herb to treat vomiting due to damp-turbidity. Pei lan is neutral, slightly cool and moderate in property and acts to treat damp-heat in Spleen Meridian manifested by sweet taste or stickiness in mouth, excessive saliva or bitter taste in mouth.

广藿香、佩兰,均气味芳香,入脾胃经,善化湿、解暑,治湿阻中焦、湿温初起及暑湿证等,常相须为用。其中藿香性微温,尤善化湿和中止呕,为治湿浊所致呕吐之要药。佩兰性平偏凉,药力平和,又善治脾经湿热之口中甜腻、多涎或口苦等证。

Both *Atractylodis Rhizoma* (cang zhu) and *Magnoliae Officinalis Cortex* (hou po) are pungent, bitter, warm and dry in property and act to treat damp blocking middle energizer pattern. Cang zhu acts to strengthen spleen, applied to treat damp blockage and spleen deficiency manifested by poor appetite and loose feces. It also acts to eliminate wind-damp and brighten eyes, applied to treat Bi (Obturation) Pattern, swelling and pain of foot and knee, night blindness and blurred vision. Hou po acts to promote qi flow, applied to treat damp

苍术、厚朴,均辛苦温燥,治湿阻中焦诸证。其中苍术兼能健脾,湿阻兼脾虚食少便溏者多用;且能祛风湿、明目,善治风湿痹痛或足膝肿痛,以及夜盲、眼目昏涩。厚朴兼能行气,湿阻兼气滞胀满者宜之,并下气宽中、消积导滞,治肠胃积滞;且能下肺气平喘,治痰饮喘咳。

blockage and qi stagnation manifested by distension and fullness. It acts to subdue qi, dilate middle energizer, dissolve accumulation and relieve stagnation, applied to treat accumulation and stagnation in intestines and stomach. It also acts to subdue lung qi and soothe panting, applied to treat panting and cough due to phlegm-rheum.

Both *Amomi Fructus* (sha ren) and *Amomi Fructus Rotundus* (bai dou kou) are fragrant, pungent and warm in property and act to dissolve damp, promote qi flow, warm middle energizer and stop vomiting, applied to treat damp blocking middle energizer, qi stagnation in spleen and stomach and vomiting due to cold in stomach. Sha ren is attributive to spleen and stomach in middle energizer and strongly acts to stop diarrhea and quiet fetus, applied to treat diarrhea due to damp blockage or deficiency and cold, and also to treat morning sickness due to qi stagnation in pregnancy, and fetal irritability. Bai dou kou is attributive to the Spleen Meridian, the Stomach Meridian and the Lung Meridian, with moderate action, applied to treat early stage of damp-warm pattern.

砂仁、白豆蔻，均芳香辛温，善化湿行气、温中止呕，治湿阻中焦、脾胃气滞及胃寒呕吐等证。其中砂仁入中焦脾胃而力稍强，兼止泻、安胎，可治湿滞或虚寒泄泻，以及妊娠气滞恶阻、胎动不安等证。白豆蔻入脾胃肺经，药力稍缓，亦治湿温初起证。

Chapter 6 Waterflow-Promoting and Damp-Dissolving Herbs

第6章 利水渗湿药

The medicinal herbs acting to dredge water passage and to dissolve and eliminate water-damp, applied to treat internal retention of water-damp are called the waterflow-promoting and damp-dissolving herbs.

以通利水道，渗除水湿，治疗水湿内停病证为主要作用的药物，称利水渗湿药。

According to their different actions, characteristics and clinical applications, the medicinal herbs are divided into the waterflow-promoting and swell-subsiding herbs, the urine-promoting and urinary disturbance-treating herbs and the damp-dissolving and jaundice-relieving herbs.

根据其性能特点及临床应用的区别，相应分为利水消肿药、利尿通淋药和利湿退黄药。

The waterflow-promoting and swell-subsiding herbs are mostly sweet, bland and neutral in property and act to promote waterflow, dissolve damp and subside swell, applied to treat internal retention of water-damp manifested by edema, difficult urination, diarrhea, phlegm and rheum.

利水消肿药大多味甘淡性平，具有渗利水湿、利水消肿的作用。主要用于水湿内停而引起的水肿、小便不利，以及泄泻、痰饮等证。

The urine-promoting and urinary disturbance-treating herbs are bitter and cold in property, or sweet, bland and cold in property, and act to promote defecation, reduce damp-heat in lower energizer, promote urination and treat urinary disturbance, applied to treat damp-heat accumulating in bladder manifested by scanty and dark urine, burning urination, bloody urine, urinary stones, pro-

利水通淋药味苦性寒，或甘淡性寒，功能苦寒泄利，清下焦湿热。以利尿通淋为主要功效，主要用于湿热蕴结膀胱所致的小便短赤，热淋、血淋、石淋及膏淋、小便混浊等病证。

teinuria and turbid urine.

The damp-dissolving and jaundice-relieving herbs are mostly bitter and cold, and act to reduce damp-heat in liver and gallbladder, eliminate damp-heat, benefit gallbladder and treat jaundice, applied to treat jaundice due to damp-heat, also to treat furuncle, eczema and damp-heat pattern.

利湿退黄药性味多苦寒，善清肝胆湿热，以清利湿热，利胆退黄为主要功效。主要用于湿热黄疸，亦可治湿疮、湿疹、湿温等证。

It is necessary to notice in the application of this type of medicinal herbs that if qi moves, the water moves, and if qi stagnates, the water remains. Therefore, it is advisable to combine the qi-promoting herbs in the application of this type of medicinal herbs. Furthermore, the medicinal herbs are easy to consume body fluid, so it is cautious to apply for those of yin deficiency and fluid consumption.

使用本类药物需注意：气行则水行，气滞则水停，使用本类药物可与行气药同用。本类药易耗伤津液，阴虚津伤者应慎用。

Section 1 Waterflow-promoting and swell-subsiding herbs

第1节 利水消肿药

Poria (fu ling)

茯苓

It is the dried product from the sclerotium of *Poria cocos* (schw) Wolf, family Polyporaceae. The sclerotium mostly parasitizes on the root of Japanese red pine and *Pinus massamiana* Lamb., family Pinaceae. The medicinal herb, wild or cultivated, is collected from July to September, applied in crude form.

为多孔菌科真菌茯苓的干燥菌核。多寄生于松科植物赤松或马尾松等根上。野生或栽培。7～9月采挖。生用。

Features Flavor: sweet and bland. Property: neutral. Meridian tropism: the Heart Meridian, the Lung Meridian, the Spleen Meridian and the Kidney Meridian.

性味归经 甘、淡，平。归心、肺、脾、肾经。

Actions Promote waterflow, dissolve damp, strengthen spleen and quiet heart.

功效 利水渗湿，健脾，宁心。

Application

(1) Edema and difficult urination. The medicinal herb is bland in property and acts to promote waterflow, and sweet in property and acts to strengthen spleen, with a moderate action. In the treatment of all types of edema, it is combined with *Polyporus* (zhu ling), *Atractylodis Macrocephalae Rhizoma* (bai zhu) and *Alismatis Rhizoma* (ze xie), to form up Poria Five Powder (Wu Ling San). It is advisable to combine other medicinal herbs according to different causes of edema.

(2) Spleen deficiency pattern. The medicinal herb acts to strengthen spleen and reinforce middle energizer. In the treatment of spleen deficiency pattern manifested by poor appetite and loose feces, it is combined with *Ginseng Radix et Raizoma* (ren shen), bai zhu and *Glycyrrhizae Radix et Rhizoma* (gan cao), to form up Four Nobles Decoction (Si Jun Zi Tang). In the treatment of rheum retention due to spleen deficiency manifested by stuffiness at chest and hypochondria, blurred vision and palpitation, it is combined with *Cinnamomi Ramulus* (gui zhi), *Atractylodis Macrocephalae Rhizoma* (bai zhu) and gan cao, to form up Poria, Cinnamon, Atractylodes and Liquorice Decoction (Ling Gui Zhu Gan Tang).

(3) Palpitation and insomnia. The medicinal herb acts to quiet heart and calm mind. In the treatment of palpitation and insomnia, it is combined with *Ziziphi Spinosae Semen* (suan zao ren), *Angelicae Sinensis Radix* (dang gui) and *Polygalae Radix* (yuan zhi), to form up Angelica Splenic Decoction (Gui Pi Tang).

Usage and dosage Apply 10～15 in decoction.

应用

（1）水肿、小便不利。本品淡渗利水，味甘健脾，药性平和，可治各种水肿。常与猪苓、白术、泽泻等同用，如五苓散。亦可根据水肿不同原因，随证配伍。

（2）脾虚诸证。本品能健脾补中。治脾胃食少，纳呆便溏，常与人参、白术、甘草同用，即四君子汤。治脾虚停饮，胸胁支满，目眩心悸，常与桂枝、白术、甘草等同用，如苓桂术甘汤。

（3）心悸，失眠。本品能宁心安神。治心悸失眠，常与酸枣仁、当归、远志等同用，如归脾汤。

用法用量 煎服，10～15克。

Appendix

(1) *Poriae Cutis* (fu ling pi)

It is the dried product from the peel of the sclerotium of *Poria cocos* (schw) Wolf. The medicinal herb is sweet and bland in flavor, neutral in property, and attributive to the Lung Meridian, the Spleen Meridian and the Kidney Meridian. It acts to promote waterflow and subside swell, applied to treat edema and difficult urination. Apply 15～30 g in decoction.

(2) *Poria cum Ligno Hospite* (fu shen)

It is the product from the white-colored part of the pine root inside the sclerotium of *Poria cocos* (schw) Wolf. The medicinal herb is sweet and bland in flavor, neutral in property, and attributive to the Heart Meridian and the Spleen Meridian. It acts to quiet heart and calm mind, applied to treat palpitation, insomnia and poor memory. Apply 10～15 g in decoction.

附药

(1) 茯苓皮

为茯苓菌核的干燥外皮。性味甘、淡，平。归肺、脾、肾经。功能利水消肿。适用于水肿、小便不利。煎服，15～30 克。

(2) 茯神

为茯苓菌核中抱有松根的白色部分。性味甘、淡，平。归心、脾经。功能宁心安神，用于心悸、失眠、健忘等症。煎服，10～15 克。

Polyporus (zhu ling)

It is the dried product from the sclerotium of *Polyporus Umbellatus* (Pers.) Fries, family Polyporaceae. The sclerotium mostly parasitizes on the rotten root of birch, maple, oak tree, etc. The medicinal herb is collected in spring and autumn, applied in crude form.

Features Flavor: sweet and bland. Property: neutral. Meridian tropism: the Kidney Meridian and the Bladder Meridian.

Actions Promote waterflow and dissolve damp.

Application

Edema and difficult urination. The medicinal

猪苓

为多孔菌科真菌猪苓的干燥菌核。寄生于桦树、枫树、柞树等的腐朽根上。春、秋季采挖。生用。

性味归经 甘、淡，平。归肾、膀胱经。

功效 利水渗湿。

应用

水肿、小便不利，泄泻，

herb acts to promote waterflow. In the treatment of edema, it is applied singly or combined with *Poria* (fu ling) and *Atractylodis Macrocephalae Rhizoma* (bai zhu), to form up Poria Four Powder (Si Ling San). In the treatment of difficult urination due to accumulation of water and heat, it is combined with fu ling, *Alismatis Rhizoma* (ze xie) and *Asini Corii Colla* (E Jiao), to form up Umbelate Pore Decoction (Zhu Ling Tang). In the treatment of diarrhea, it is combined with *Codonopsis Radix* (dang shen), bai zhu and ze xie. In the treatment of stranguria, it is combined with *Akebiae Caulis* (mu tong) and *Phellodendri Cortex Chiensis* (huang bo). In the treatment of morbid leucorrhea, it is combined with *Angelicae Dahuricae Radix* (bai zhi).

淋浊,带下。本品利水力强,可单用,或与茯苓、白术等同用,如四苓散。治水热互结的小便不利,常配伍茯苓、泽泻、阿胶等同用,如猪苓汤;治泄泻,常与党参、白术、泽泻等同用。治淋浊,可与木通、黄柏等同用。治带下,可与白芷等同用。

Usage and dosage Apply 6～12 g in decoction.

用法用量 煎服,6～12克。

Precautions for use It is prohibited to apply for those who have no water-damp.

使用注意 无水湿者忌服。

Alismatis Rhizoma (ze xie)

泽泻

It is the dried product from the stem tuber of *Alisma orientale* (Sam) Juzep., family Alismataceae. The medicinal herb is collected in winter, applied in crude form or prepared form by frying with salty solution.

为泽泻科植物泽泻的干燥块茎。冬季采挖。生用或盐水炒用。

Features Flavor: sweet and bland. Property: cold. Meridian tropism: the Kidney Meridian and the Bladder Meridian.

性味归经 甘、淡,寒。归肾、膀胱经。

Actions Promote waterflow, dissolve damp, reduce heat, dissolve turbidity and decrease lipid.

功效 利水渗湿,泄热,化浊降脂。

Application

应用

(1) Edema, difficult urination, phlegm-rheum and diarrhea. The medicinal herb is bland in prop-

(1) 水肿、小便不利,痰饮,泄泻。本品淡渗利水。

erty and acts to promote waterflow. In the treatment edema and difficult urination, it is combined with *Poria* (fu ling), *Polyporus* (zhu ling) and *Atractylodis Macrocephalae Rhizoma* (bai zhu), to form up Poria Four Powder (Si Ling San). In the treatment of dizziness and blurred vision due to phlegm-rheum, it is combined with *Atractylodis Macrocephalae Rhizoma* (bai zhu) to form up Oriental Water Plantain Decoction (Ze Xie Tang). In the treatment of diarrhea due to water-damp, it is combined with the spleen-strengthening herbs.

治水肿、小便不利，常与茯苓、猪苓、白术同用，即四苓散。治痰饮眩晕，常与白术同用，即泽泻汤。治水湿泄泻，可与健脾药同用。

(2) Morbid leucorrhea and stranguria. The medicinal herb is cold in property and acts to reduce heat, especially to reduce damp-heat in lower energizer. In the treatment of morbid leucorrhea and stranguria due to damp-heat, it is combined with *Gentianae Radix et Rhizoma* (long dan), *Plantaginis Semen* (che qian zi) and *Akebiae Caulis* (mu tong), to form up Gentian Liver-Draining Decoction (Long Dan Xie Gan Tang).

(2) 带下，淋浊。本品性寒泄热，尤善泄下焦湿热。治湿热带下、淋浊，常与龙胆、车前子、木通等同用，如龙胆泻肝汤。

(3) Hyperlipemia. The medicinal herb acts to dissolve turbidity and decrease lipid. It is combined with other medicinal herbs according to patterns.

(3) 高脂血症。本品能降脂化浊。可根据证型配伍应用。

Furthermore, the medicinal herb is combined with the yin-nourishing herbs, for the purpose to reduce the Xiang (Premiere) Fire and protect the true yin, to form up Rehmannia Pills with Six Ingredients (Liu Wei Di Huang Wan).

此外，本品与滋阴药同用，能泻相火、保真阴，如六味地黄丸。

Usage and dosage Apply 6～10 g in decoction. The medicinal herb acts to promote waterflow and reduce heat in crude form, while acts to reduce the Xiang (Premiere) Fire in prepared form by salty solution.

用法用量 煎服，6～10克。生用利水、泄热，盐水制用能泻相火。

Coicis Semen (yi yi ren)

It is the dried product from the ripe seed of *Coix lacryma-jobi* L. var. ma-yuan (Roman.) stapf, family Gramineae. The medicinal herb is collected in autumn, applied in crude form or prepared form by frying.

Features Flavor: sweet and bland. Property: slightly cold. Meridian tropism: the Spleen Meridian, the Stomach Meridian and the Lung Meridian.

Actions Promote waterflow, dissolve damp, strengthen spleen, stop diarrhea, drain pus and relieve Bi (Obturation) Pattern.

Application

(1) Edema and difficult urination. The medicinal herb is sweet and bland in property and acts to promote waterflow, dissolve damp and strengthen spleen. In the treatment of edema and difficult urination due to spleen deficiency, it is combined with *Poria* (fu ling), *Alismatis Rhizoma* (ze xie) and *Astragali Radix* (huang qi).

(2) Diarrhea due to spleen deficiency. The medicinal herb acts to strengthen spleen and stop diarrhea. In the treatment of poor appetite and diarrhea due to spleen deficiency, it is combined with *Codonopsis Radix* (dang shen), *Atractylodis Macrocephalae Rhizoma* (bai zhu) and *Dioscoreae Rhizoma* (shan yao), to form up Ginseng, Poria and Atractylodes Powder (Shen Ling Bai Zhu San).

(3) Pulmonary abscess and acute appendicitis. The medicinal herb acts to clear heat and drain pus. In the treatment of pulmonary abscess manifested by cough with purulent sputum, it is combined with *Phragmitis Rhizoma* (lu gen), *Semen Benincasae*

薏苡仁

为禾本科植物薏苡的干燥成熟种仁。秋季采收。生用或炒用。

性味归经 甘、淡，微寒。归脾、胃、肺经。

功效 利水渗湿，健脾止泻，排脓，除痹。

应用

(1) 水肿、小便不利。本品甘淡渗利，功能利水渗湿，兼能健脾。治脾虚水肿、小便不利，常与茯苓、泽泻、黄芪等同用。

(2) 脾虚泄泻。本品能健脾止泻。治脾虚食少泄泻，常配伍党参、白术、山药等同用，如参苓白术散。

(3) 肺痈，肠痈。本品能清热排脓。治肺痈咳吐脓痰，常与芦根、桃仁同用，如苇茎汤；治肠痈腹痛，可与附子、败酱草等同用。

(dong gua ren) and *Persicae Semen* (tao ren), to form up Reed Stem Decoction (Wei Jing Tang). In the treatment of acute appendicitis manifested by abdominal pain, it is combined with *Aconiti Lateralis Radix Praeparata* (fu zi) and *Patriniae Herba* (bai jiang cao).

(4) Bi (Obturation) Pattern due to damp manifested by spasm. The medicinal herb acts to dissolve damp and relieve Bi (Obturation) Pattern, and it is cold in property and acts to clear heat, applied to treat Bi (Obturation) Pattern due to damp-heat. In the treatment of Bi (Obturation) Pattern manifested by muscle spasm, it is combined with *Cinnamomi Ramulus* (gui zhi), *Atractylodis Rhizoma* (cang zhu) and *Angelicae Sinensis Radix* (dang gui), or applied singly by cooking into porridge.

(4) 湿痹拘挛。本品能渗湿、除痹,性寒清热,善治湿热痹痛。治湿痹筋脉拘挛,常配伍桂枝、苍术、当归等同用,或以本品单味为末煮粥。

Furthermore, the medicinal herb acts to relieve toxin and dissipate stagnation, applied to treat wart and cancer.

此外,本品能解毒散结,治赘疣、癌肿。

Usage and dosage Apply 9～30 g in decoction. The medicinal herb acts to promote waterflow, relieve Bi (Obturation) Pattern and drain pus in crude form, while acts to strengthen spleen and stop diarrhea in prepared form by frying.

用法用量 煎服,9～30克。生用利水、除痹、排脓,炒用健脾止泻。

Section 2 Urine-promoting and Stranguria-relieving Herbs

第2节 利尿通淋药

Plantaginis Semen (che qian zi)

It is the dried product from the ripe seed of the perennial herb, *Plantago asiatica* L. or *Plantago depressa* Willa., family Plantaginaceae. The medicinal herb is collected in summer and autumn when

车前子

为车前科植物车前或平车前的干燥成熟种子。夏秋季种子成熟时采收。生用或盐水炙用。

the seeds are ripe, applied in crude form or prepared form by stir-frying with salty solution.

Features Flavor: sweet. Property: cold. Meridian tropism: the Liver Meridian, the Kidney Meridian, the Lung Meridian and the Small Intestine Meridian.

性味归经 甘,寒。归肝、肾、肺、小肠经。

Actions Clear heat, promote urination, relieve stranguria, dissolve damp, stop diarrhea, brighten eyes and eliminate phlegm.

功效 清热利尿通淋,渗湿止泻,明目,祛痰。

Application

(1) Stranguria due to heat and edema. The medicinal herb is lubricant, cold and cool in property, and acts to clear heat, promote urination and relieve stranguria. In the treatment of stranguria due to heat manifested by difficult and painful urination, it is combined with *Akebiae Caulis* (mu tong), *Talcum* (hua shi) and *Gardeniae Fructus* (zhi zi), to form up Eight Corrections Powder (Ba Zheng San). In the treatment of edema and difficult urination, it is combined with the waterflow-promoting and swell-subsiding herbs.

(2) Diarrhea due to summer heat and damp. The medicinal herb acts to promote waterflow, dissolve damp and stop diarrhea. In the treatment of watery diarrhea due to summer heat-damp, it is applied singly by cooking into porridge, or combined with the spleen-strengthening, waterflow-promoting and diarrhea-stopping herbs.

(3) Redness, swelling and pain of eyes. The medicinal herb is cold in property and acts to purify liver, reduce heat and brighten eyes. In the treatment of redness, swelling and pain of eyes due to heat in liver, it is combined with *Chrysanthemi Flos* (ju hua), *Cassiae Semen* (jue ming zi) and

应用

(1) 热淋,水肿。本品性滑利,药性寒凉,具清热利尿通淋之功。治热淋涩痛,常与木通、滑石、栀子等同用,如八正散。治水肿、小便不利,可与利水消肿药同用。

(2) 暑湿泄泻。本品能利水湿、止泄泻。治暑湿水泻,可单味研末,米饮送服,或与健脾利水止泻药同用。

(3) 目赤肿痛。本品性寒清肝,泄热明目。治肝热目赤肿痛,可与菊花、决明子、夏枯草等同用。

Prunellae Spica (xia ku cao).

(4) Cough due to phlegm-heat. The medicinal herb acts to purify lung and dissolve phlegm. In the treatment of cough with excessive sputum due to heat in lung, it is combined with *Trichosanthis Fructus* (gua lou) and *Scutellariae Radix* (huang qin).

（4）痰热咳嗽。本品能清肺化痰。治肺热咳嗽痰多，常与瓜蒌、黄芩等同用。

Usage and dosage Apply 9～15 g in decoction. It is advisable to decoct it wrapping.

用法用量 煎服，9～15克。宜布包煎。

Appendix *Plantaginis Herba* (che qian cao)

It is the product from the herb of Asiatic plantain, *Plantago asiatica* L., or *Plantago depressa* Willd., family Plantaginaceae. Its flavor and property are same as those of *Plantaginis Semen* (che qian zi). The medicinal herb also acts to clear heat, relieve toxin and stanch bleeding, applied to treat carbuncle, ulcer and furuncle due to heat-toxin, dysentery due to heat, and bleeding due to heat in blood. Apply 10～20 g in decoction. Apply double dose in fresh form, and apply a proper amount for external use.

附药 车前草

为车前或平车前的全草。性味功用同车前子，且能清热解毒，止血。用于治痈疮肿毒，热痢，以及血热出血等。煎服，10～20克。鲜品加倍。外用适量。

Talcum (hua shi)

滑石

It is the product from a kind of stone, mainly composed of hydrous magnesium silicate [$Mg_3(Si_4O_{10})(OH)_2$]. The medicinal herb is collected all over the year, applied in prepared form by grinding into powder or powder-refining with water.

为硅酸盐类矿物滑石族滑石，主要成分为含水硅酸镁[$Mg_3(Si_4O_{10})(OH)_2$]。全年可采。研粉或水飞用。

Features Flavor: sweet and bland. Property: cold. Meridian tropism: the Bladder Meridian, the Lung Meridian and the Stomach Meridian.

性味归经 甘、淡，寒。归膀胱、肺、胃经。

Actions Promote urination, relieve stranguria, clear heat and relieve summer heat. Dissolve damp and astringe sores for external use.

功效 利尿通淋，清热解暑，外用祛湿敛疮。

Application

(1) Stranguria due to heat or with stones. The

应用

（1）热淋，石淋。本品甘

medicinal herb is cold, sweet, bland, heavy and lubricant in property, and acts to clear heat, promote urination and relieve stranguria. In the treatment stranguria due to heat manifested by difficult and painful urination, it is combined with *Plantaginis Semen* (che qian zi) and *Akebiae Caulis* (mu tong). In the treatment of stranguria with stones, it is combined with *Lygodii Spora* (hai jin sha) and *Lysimachiae Herba* (jin qian cao).

淡性寒,质重滑利,具清热利尿通淋之功。治热淋涩痛,常与车前子、木通等同用。治石淋,可与海金沙、金钱草等配伍同用。

(2) Summer heat pattern manifested by restlessness and thirst. The medicinal herb acts to clear heat and relieve summer heat, and also to promote urination as well. In the treatment of summer heat pattern manifested by restlessness and thirst, it is combined with *Glycyrrhizae Radix et Rhizoma* (gan cao), to form up Six-One Powder (Liu Yi San).

(2)暑热烦渴。本品既清热解暑,又渗利小便。治暑热烦渴、小便不利,常与甘草同用,即六一散。

(3) Eczema, furuncle and miliaria. The medicinal herb acts to clear heat, dissolve damp and astringe sores for external use. In the treatment of eczema, furuncle and miliaria, it is applied singly or combined with dried *Alumen* (bai fan) and *Phellodendri Cortex Chiensis* (huang bo).

(3)湿疹,湿疮,痱子。本品外用具清热祛湿、敛疮之功。治湿疮、湿疹、痱子,可单用,或与枯矾、黄柏等配伍同用。

Usage and dosage Apply 10～20 g in decoction and decoct it first. Apply a proper amount for external use.

用法用量 煎服,10～20克。先煎。外用适量。

Akebiae Caulis (mu tong)

木通

It is the dried product from the stem of the deciduous woody liana, *Akebia quinata* (Thunb.) Decne., and *Akebia trifoliate* (Thunb.) Koidz., and *Akebia trifoliate* (Thunb.) Koidz. var. *australis* (Diels) Rehd. , family Akebia. The medicinal herb is collected in autumn, applied in crude form.

为木通科植物木通、三叶木通或白木通的干燥藤茎。秋季采收。生用。

Features Flavor: bitter. Property: cold. Me-

性味归经 苦,寒。归

ridian tropism: the Heart Meridian, the Small Intestine Meridian and the Bladder Meridian.

心、小肠、膀胱经。

Actions Promote waterflow, relieve stranguria, purify heart, relieve restlessness, stimulate menstrual flow and promote lactation.

功效 利水通淋，清心除烦，通经下乳。

Application

应用

(1) Stranguria due to heat and edema. The medicinal herb is bitter and cold in property and acts to promote urination and relieve stranguria. In the treatment of stranguria due to heat manifested by difficult and painful urination, it is combined with *Plantaginis Semen* (che qian zi) and *Talcum* (hua shi).

(1) 热淋，水肿。本品苦泄寒清、利尿通淋。治热淋涩痛，常与车前子、滑石等同用。治水肿，与利水消肿药同用。

(2) Mouth ulcer, restlessness and dark urine. The medicinal herb acts to clear heart fire, promote urination and guide fire to move downwards. In the treatment of mouth ulcer due to heart fire hyperactivity or restlessness and dark urine due to heart fire transmitting downwards to small intestine, it is combined with *Rehmanniae Radix* (sheng di huang), *Glycyrrhizae Radix et Rhizoma* (gan cao) and *Lophatheri Herba* (dan zhu ye), to form up Heat-Abducting Powder (Dao Chi San).

(2) 口舌生疮，心烦尿赤。本品具清心火、利小便之功，可引热下行。治心火上炎的口舌生疮，或心火下移小肠的心烦尿赤等证，可与生地黄、甘草、竹叶等同用，即导赤散。

(3) Amenorrhea and lactation deficiency. The medicinal herb acts to stimulate menstrual flow and promote lactation. In the treatment of amenorrhea, it is combined with *Carthami Flos* (hong hua) and *Salviae Miltiorrhizae Radix et Rhizoma* (dan shen). In the treatment of lactation blockage or lactation deficiency, it is combined with made soup with pork trotter.

(3) 经闭乳少。本品具通经、下乳之功。治经闭，可与红花、丹参等同用。治产后乳汁不通或乳少，可与猪蹄炖汤服。

(4) Bi (Obturation) Pattern due to damp-heat. The medicinal herb is bitter, cold and lubricant in property. In the treatment of Bi (Obturation) Pat-

(4) 湿热痹痛。本品苦寒通利，善治湿热痹痛，可与防己、秦艽等同用。

tern due to damp-heat, it is combined with *Stephaniae Tetrandrae Radix* (fang ji) and *Gentianae Macrophyllae Radix* (qin jiao).

Usage and dosage Apply 3～6 g in decoction.

用法用量 煎服，3～6克。

Precautions for use It is cautious to apply for those with deficiency and cold in spleen and stomach.

使用注意 脾胃虚寒者慎用。

Dianthi Herba (qu mai)

瞿麦

It is the dried product from the herb of fringed Pink, *Dianthus superbus* L. or *Dianthus chinensis* L., family Caryophyllaceae. The medicinal herb is collected in summer and autumn when it is flowering and fruitful, applied in crude form.

为石竹科植物瞿麦或石竹的干燥地上部分。夏、秋季花果期采割。生用。

Features Flavor: bitter. Property: cold. Meridian tropism: the Heart Meridian and the Small Intestine Meridian.

性味归经 苦，寒。归心、小肠经。

Actions Promote urination, relieve stranguria, activate blood and stimulate menstrual flow.

功效 利尿通淋，活血通经。

Application

(1) Stranguria. The medicinal herb is bitter, cold and descending in property, and acts to clear heat, promote urination and relieve stranguria, good at treating various types of stranguria. In the treatment of stranguria due to heat, it is combined with *Akebiae Caulis* (mu tong) and *Plantaginis Semen* (che qian zi), to form up Eight Corrections Powder (Ba Zheng San). In the treatment of stranguria manifested by bloody urine, it is combined with *Imperatae Rhizoma* (bai mao gen) and *Cirsii Herba* (xiao ji). In the treatment of stranguria with stones, it is combined with *Lygodii Spora* (hai jin sha) and *Lysimachiae Herba* (jin qian cao).

应用

(1) 淋证。本品苦寒降泄，能清热利尿通淋，善治各种淋证。治热淋，可与木通、车前子等同用，如八正散。治血淋，可与白茅根、小蓟等同用。治石淋，可与海金沙、金钱草等同用。

(2) Amenorrhea and dysmenorrhea. The medicinal herb acts to dissolve stasis, activate blood and stimulate menstrual flow. In the treatment of amenorrhea or dysmenorrhea due to blood stasis, it is combined with *Carthami Flos* (hong hua) and *Salviae Miltiorrhizae Radix et Rhizoma* (dan shen).

(2) 经闭痛经。本品能行散瘀滞、活血通经。常用于瘀滞经闭痛经,可与红花、丹参等同用。

Usage and dosage Apply 10～15 g in decoction.

用法用量 煎服,10～15克。

Precautions for use It is prohibited to apply for pregnant women.

使用注意 孕妇忌服。

Kochiae Fructus (di fu zi)

地肤子

It is the dried product from the ripe fruit of *Kochia scoparia* (L.) Schrad., family Chenopodiaceae. The medicinal herb is collected in autumn when the fruits are ripe, applied in crude form.

为藜科植物地肤的干燥成熟果实。秋季果实成熟时割取全草,晒干,打下果实。生用。

Features Flavor: bitter. Property: cold. Meridian tropism: the Bladder Meridian.

性味归经 苦,寒。归膀胱经。

Actions Clear heat, dissolve damp and stop itching.

功效 清热利湿,止痒。

Application

应用

(1) Stranguria due to heat. The medicinal herb acts to clear heat, dissolve damp and relieve stranguria. In the treatment of damp-heat in bladder manifested by difficult urination, dribbling urine and painful urination, it is combined with *Akebiae Caulis* (mu tong) and *Dianthi Herba* (qu mai).

(1) 热淋。本品有清热利湿、通淋作用。治膀胱湿热的小便不利,淋沥涩痛,常配伍木通、瞿麦等同用。

(2) Eczema, urticaria, skin itch and pruritus vulvae. The medicinal herb acts to clear heat, dissolve damp, eliminate wind and stop itching. In the treatment of eczema, urticaria and skin itch, it is combined with *Phellodendri Cortex Chiensis* (huang bo), *Schizonepetae Herba* (jing jie). In the treatment of damp-heat in lower energizer manifested by

(2) 湿疹,风疹,皮肤瘙痒,外阴瘙痒。本品能清热利湿、祛风止痒。治湿疹、风疹、皮肤瘙痒,常与黄柏、荆芥等配伍同用。治下焦湿热,外阴瘙痒,可与苦参、蛇床子、龙胆等煎汤外洗。

pruritus vulvae, it is combined with *Sophorae Flavescentis Radix* (ku shen), *Cnidii Fructus* (she chuang zi) and *Gentianae Radix et Rhizoma* (long dan), by decocting for external use.

Usage and dosage Apply 10～15 g in decoction. Apply a proper amount for external use.

用法用量 煎服，10～15克。外用适量。

Lygodii Spora (hai jin sha)

海金沙

It is the dried product from the ripe spore of the perennial climbing fern. *Lygodium japonicum* (Thunb.) Sw., family Lygodiaceae. The medicinal herb is collected in autumn when the spore has not been detached, applied in crude form.

为海金沙科植物海金沙的干燥成熟孢子。秋季孢子未脱落时采收。生用。

Features Flavor: sweet. Property: cold. Meridian tropism: the Bladder Meridian and the Small Intestine Meridian.

性味归经 甘，寒。归膀胱、小肠经。

Actions Clear heat, dissolve damp, relieve stranguria and stop pain.

功效 清热利湿，通淋止痛。

Application

Stranguria. The medicinal herb is cold in property and acts to clear heat, promote urination, relieve stranguria and stop pain, treating urethra pain. In the treatment of stranguria with stones or bloody urine, or painful urination, it is combined with *Plantaginis Semen* (che qian zi), *Lysimachiae Herba* (jin qian cao) and *Imperatae Rhizoma* (bai mao gen).

应用

各种淋证。本品性寒，功专清热利尿，通淋止痛，尤善治尿道疼痛。虽治各种淋证，但尤以治石淋、血淋效果为佳。可与车前子、金钱草、白茅根等同用。

Usage and dosage Apply 6～12 g in decoction by wrapping.

用法用量 煎服，6～12克。宜布包煎。

Dioscoreae Spongiosae Rhizoma (bi xie)

萆薢

It is the dried product from the rhizome of *Dioscorea Spongiosa* J. Q. Xi. M. Mizuno et W. L. Zhao, or *Dioscorea futschauensis* Uline ex R. Knuth, or *Dioscorea hypoglauca* Palibin, family Di-

为薯蓣科植物绵萆薢或福州薯蓣、粉背薯蓣的干燥根茎。秋、冬季采挖。生用。

oscoreaceae. The medicinal herb is collected in autumn and winter, applied in crude form.

Features Flavor: bitter. Property: neutral. Meridian tropism: the Kidney Meridian and the Stomach Meridian.

性味归经 苦，平。归肾、胃经。

Actions Dissolve damp, eliminate turbidity, dispel wind and treat Bi (Obturation) Pattern.

功效 利湿去浊，祛风除痹。

Application

应用

(1) Stranguria with turbid urine. The medicinal herb is the major herb to treat stranguria with turbid urine. In the treatment of stranguria with turbid urine in white color, it is combined with *Alpiniae Oxyphyllae Fructus* (yi zhi), *Linderae Radix* (wu yao) and *Acori Tatarinowii Rhizoma* (shi chang pu), to form up Sealwort Clear-Separating Drink (Bi Xie Fen Qing Yin).

（1）膏淋。本品为治膏淋要药。治膏淋，症见小便混浊、色白如米泔，可与益智仁、乌药、石菖蒲等同用，如萆薢分清饮。

(2) Bi (Obturation) Pattern due to wind-damp. The medicinal herb acts to eliminate wind-damp and treat Bi (Obturation) Pattern. In the treatment of Bi (Obturation) Pattern due to wind-cold, it is combined with *Aconiti Lateralis Radix Praeparata* (fu zi) and *Cinnamomi Ramulus* (gui zhi). In the treatment of Bi (Obturation) Pattern due to damp-heat, it is combined with *Phellodendri Cortex Chiensis* (huang bo) and *Stephaniae Tetrandrae Radix* (fang ji).

（2）风湿痹痛。本品能祛风湿、除痹痛。治风寒痹痛，可与附子、桂枝等同用。治湿热痹痛，则与黄柏、防己等同用。

Usage and dosage Apply 9～15 g in decoction.

用法用量 煎服，9～15克。

Section 3 Damp-dissolving and jaundice-relieving herbs

第3节 利湿退黄药

Artemisiae Scopariae Herba (yin chen)

It is the dried product from the whole herb of *Artemisia scoparia* Waldst. et kit. or *Artemisia Capillaris* Thunb., family Compositae. The medicinal herb is collected in spring when the young plant is 6～10 cm high or in autumn when the bud has grown up, applied in crude form.

Features Flavor: bitter and pungent. Property: slightly cold. Meridian tropism: the Spleen Meridian, the Stomach Meridian, the Liver Meridian and the Gallbladder Meridian.

Actions Clear heat, dissolve damp, benefit gallbladder and relieve jaundice.

Application

(1) Jaundice. The medicinal herb acts to clear heat, dissolve damp, benefit gallbladder and relieve jaundice, as the major herb to treat jaundice. In the treatment of jaundice due to damp-heat, it is applied singly or combined with *Gardeniae Fructus* (zhi zi) and *Rhei Radix et Rhizoma* (da huang), to form up Artemisia Decoction (Yin Chen Hao Tang). In the treatment of yin-type jaundice due to cold-damp, it is combined with *Aconiti Lateralis Radix Praeparata* (fu zi) and *Zingiberis Rhizoma* (gan jiang), to form up Artemisia Counterflow Cold Decoction (Yin Chen Si Ni Tang).

(2) Damp-heat pattern or summer heat-damp pattern, furuncle and eczema. In the treatment of damp-heat pattern or summer heat-damp pattern

茵陈

为菊科植物滨蒿或茵陈蒿的干燥地上部分。春季幼苗6～10厘米或秋季花蕾长成时采割。生用。

性味归经 苦、辛，微寒。归脾、胃、肝、胆经。

功效 清利湿热，利胆退黄。

应用

（1）黄疸。本品功善清利湿热，利胆退黄，为治黄疸之要药。治湿热黄疸，可单用，或与栀子、大黄配伍，即茵陈蒿汤。治寒湿阴黄，常与附子、干姜等同用，如茵陈四逆汤。

（2）湿温暑湿，湿疮湿疹。治湿温暑湿，小便短赤，常与黄芩、滑石等同用。治

manifested by scanty and dark urine, it is combined with *Scutellariae Radix* (huang qin) and *Talcum* (hua shi). In the treatment of furuncle and eczema, it is combined with *Phellodendri Cortex Chiensis* (huang bo), *Sophorae Flavescentis Radix* (ku shen) and *Cnidii Fructus* (she chuang zi), by decocting for external use.

湿疮、湿疹,可与黄柏、苦参、蛇床子配伍,煎汤外洗。

Usage and dosage Apply 6～15 g in decoction. Apply a proper amount for external use.

用法用量 煎服,6～15克。外用适量。

Precautions for use It is cautious to apply for those with blood deficiency and yellow-sallow complexion.

使用注意 血虚萎黄者慎用。

Lysimachiae Herba **(jin qian cao)**

金钱草

It is the dried product from the whole plant of *Lysimachia christinae* Hance, family Primulaceae. The medicinal herb is mainly produced in Sichuan Province. It is collected in summer and autumn, applied in crude form.

为报春花科植物过路黄的干燥全草。主产于四川。夏、秋季采收。生用。

Features Flavor: sweet and bland. Property: slightly cold. Meridian tropism: the Liver Meridian, the Gallbladder Meridian, the Kidney Meridian and the Bladder Meridian.

性味归经 甘、淡,微寒。归肝、胆、肾、膀胱经。

Actions Dissolve damp, relieve jaundice, promote urination, relieve stranguria, relieve toxin and subside swell.

功效 利湿退黄,利尿通淋,解毒消肿。

Application

(1) Jaundice due to damp-heat. The medicinal herb acts to eliminate damp-heat in liver and gallbladder, benefit gallbladder and relieve jaundice. In the treatment of jaundice due to damp-heat, it is combined with *Artemisiae Scopariae Herba* (yin chen hao) and *Gardeniae Fructus* (zhi zi).

应用

(1) 湿热黄疸。本品善清肝胆湿热、利胆退黄。治湿热黄疸,常与茵陈、栀子等同用。

(2) Stranguria with stones or due to heat. The

(2) 石淋、热淋。本品能

medicinal herb acts to promote urination, relieve stranguria and discharge stones. In the treatment of stranguria with stones, it is applied singly in large dose and taken as tea, or combined with *Lygodii Spora* (hai jin sha), *Galli Gigerii Endothelium Corneum* (ji nei jin) and *Talcum* (hua shi). In the treatment of stranguria due to heat, it is combined with *Plantaginis Semen* (che qian zi) and *Talcum* (hua shi).

(3) Carbuncle, ulcer and furuncle, and snake-bite or insect-bite. The medicinal herb acts to relieve toxin and subside swell. In the treatment of diseases, it is applied singly by smashing the fresh product to take the juice for oral administration and to take dregs for external use, or combined with the heat-clearing and toxin-relieving herbs.

Usage and dosage Apply 15～60 g in decoction. Apply a proper amount for external use.

利尿通淋、排石。治石淋，可单味大剂量煎汤代茶，或与海金沙、鸡内金、滑石等同用。治热淋，可与车前子、滑石等同用。

（3）痈肿疔毒，蛇虫咬伤。本品能解毒消肿。多以单味鲜品捣烂取汁内服，药渣外敷，或与清热解毒药同用。

用法用量 煎服，15～60 克。外用适量。

Polygoni Cuspidati Rhizoma et Radix (hu zhang)

It is the dried product from the rhizome of Giant or Japanese Knotweed, *Polygonum cuspidatum* Sieb. et Zucc., family Polygonaceae. The medicinal herb is collected in spring and autumn, applied in crude form.

Features Property: bitter. Property: slightly cold. Meridian tropism: the Liver Meridian, the Gallbladder Meridian and the Lung Meridian.

Actions Dissolve damp, relieve jaundice, clear heat, relieve toxin, dissipate stasis, stop pain, stop cough and dissolve phlegm.

Application

(1) Jaundice due to damp-heat, stranguria with turbid urine and morbid leucorrhea. The medicinal herb acts to clear heat, dissolve damp, benefit gall-

虎杖

为蓼科植物虎杖的干燥根茎和根。春、秋季采挖。生用。

性味归经 苦，微寒。归肝、胆、肺经。

功效 利湿退黄，清热解毒，散瘀止痛，止咳化痰。

应用

（1）湿热黄疸，淋浊，带下。本品能清利湿热、利胆退黄。治湿热黄疸，常与茵

bladder and relieve jaundice. In the treatment of jaundice due to damp-heat, it is combined with *Artemisiae Scopariae Herba* (yin chen hao), *Lysimachiae Herba* (jin qian cao) and *Gardeniae Fructus* (zhi zi). In the treatment of stranguria with turbid urine and morbid leucorrhea, it is combined with *Phellodendri Cortex Chiensis* (huang bo) and *Coicis Semen* (yi yi ren).

陈、金钱草、栀子等同用。治淋浊、带下，可与黄柏、薏苡仁等同用。

(2) Carbuncle, ulcer and furuncle, or scalding by water or burning by fire. The medicinal herb is bitter and cold in property and acts to clear heat and relieve toxin. In the treatment of carbuncle, ulcer and furuncle, or scalding by water or burning by fire, it is applied singly by decocting for oral administration or by grinding into powder for external use.

（2）痈疮肿毒，水烧烫伤。本品苦寒泄热，清热解毒。治痈疮肿毒或水火烫伤，可单用煎汤内服，或研末外敷。

(3) Amenorrhea, dysmenorrhea, traumatic injury and abdominal masses. The medicinal herb acts to activate blood, dissipate stasis, stimulate menstrual flow and stop pain. In the treatment amenorrhea or dysmenorrhea due to blood stasis, it is combined with *Leonuri Herba* (yi mu cao) and *Salviae Miltiorrhizae Radix et Rhizoma* (dan shen). In the treatment of traumatic injury, it is combined with *Olibanum* (ru xiang), *Myrrha* (mo yao) and *Carthami Flos* (hong hua). In the treatment of abdominal masses, it is combined with *Sparganii Rhizoma* (san leng) and *Curcumae Rhizoma* (e zhu).

（3）经闭痛经，跌打损伤，癥瘕积聚。本品有活血散瘀、通经止痛之功。治瘀滞经闭痛经，可与益母草、丹参同用。治跌打损伤，可与乳香、没药、红花等同用。治癥瘕积聚，可与三棱、莪术等配伍。

(4) Cough due to heat in lung. The medicinal herb acts to purify lung, dissolve phlegm and stop cough. In the treatment of cough due to heat in lung, it is combined with *Scutellariae Radix* (huang qin), *Eriobotryae Folium* (pi pa ye) and *Trichosanthis Fructus* (gua lou).

（4）肺热咳嗽。本品能清肺、祛痰、止咳。可与黄芩、枇杷叶、瓜蒌等同用。

Furthermore, the medicinal herb acts to reduce the lower and promote defecation, applied to treat constipation due to heat accumulation.

此外，本品还能泻下通便，可用于热结便秘。

Usage and dosage Apply 9～15 g in decoction. Apply a proper amount for external use.

用法用量 煎服，9～15克。外用适量。

Precautions for use It is prohibited to apply for pregnant women. It is cautious to apply for those with spleen deficiency manifested by loose feces.

使用注意 孕妇忌服。脾虚便溏者慎用。

Brief summary

小 结

1 Waterflow-promoting and swell-subsiding herbs

1 利水消肿药

Both *Poria* (fu ling) and *Coicis Semen* (yi yi ren) act to promote waterflow, dissolve damp and strengthen spleen, applied to treat edema and difficult urination due to internal retention of water-damp. Fu ling is moderate in property, so it promotes waterflow without damaging the Zheng (Anti-Pathogenic) Qi, as the major herb to promote waterflow and dissolve damp to treat various types of edema and spleen deficiency pattern. It also acts to calm mind, applied to treat palpitation and insomnia. Yi yi ren is cool in property and weaker than *Poria* (fu ling) in promoting waterflow and strengthening spleen. It acts to strengthen spleen, stop diarrhea, treat Bi (Obturation) Pattern and drain pus, applied to treat diarrhea due to spleen deficiency, Bi (Obturation) Pattern due to wind-damp, pulmonary abscess and acute appendicitis.

茯苓、薏苡仁，均能利水渗湿、健脾，治水湿内停所致的水肿、小便不利。其中茯苓药性平和，利水而不伤正气，为利水渗湿要药，可治各种水肿和脾虚诸证；又能安神，为心悸失眠所常用。薏苡仁性凉，利水、健脾之力逊于茯苓；又能健脾止泻、除痹、排脓，治脾虚泄泻、风湿痹痛，以及肺痈、肠痈等。

Both *Polyporus* (zhu ling) and *Alismatis Rhizoma* (ze xie) are attributive to the Kidney and Bladder Meridians and act to promote waterflow and dissolve damp, applied to treat edema and difficult urination due to internal retention of water-

猪苓、泽泻，均入肾、膀胱经，能利水渗湿，治水湿内停所致水肿、小便不利。其中猪苓性平，利水力强。泽泻性寒，兼能泄热，善治下焦

damp. Zhu ling is neutral in property and strongly acts to promote waterflow. Ze xie is cold in property and acts to reduce heat, applied to treat damp-heat pattern in lower energizer. It also acts to reduce the Xiang (Premiere) Fire, protect the true yin, decrease lipid and dissolve turbidity.

湿热证；还能泻相火、保真阴，降脂化浊。

2 Urine-promoting and stranguria-relieving herbs

2 利尿通淋药

Both *Plantaginis Semen* (che qian zi) and *Talcum* (hua shi) are cold in property and act to promote urination and relieve stranguria. Che qian zi is cold and lubricant in property, as the major herb to clear heat, promote waterflow and relieve stranguria. It acts to dissolve damp and stop diarrhea for the purpose to promote waterflow and separate the clear from the turbid, applied to treat watery diarrhea caused by excessive damp. It also acts to purify liver, brighten eyes, purify lung and dissolve phlegm, applied to treat redness of eyes due to fire in liver, and cough with sputum due to heat in lung. Hua shi is heavy and lubricant in property and acts to dissolve damp and open aperture, applied to relieve stranguria with stones or due to heat. It acts to clear heat and relieve summer heat, as the major herb to treat restlessness and thirst due to summer heat-damp, damp-heat or summer heat. It also acts to dissolve damp and astringe sores for external use, applied to treat furuncle and eczema.

车前子、滑石，均性寒，功能利尿通淋，均治淋证。其中车前子性寒滑利，为清热利水通淋要药；且能渗湿止泻，以利水湿、分清浊，治湿盛引起的水泻；并能清肝明目、清肺化痰，治肝火目赤，肺热痰咳。滑石质重滑利，渗湿利窍，善治石淋、热淋；且善清热解暑，为治暑湿、湿温、暑热烦渴之要药；外用又可收湿敛疮，治湿疮、湿疹。

Both *Akebiae Caulis* (mu tong) and *Dianthi Herba* (qu mai) are bitter and cold in property and act to clear heat, promote urination and treat stranguria, applied to treat stranguria due to damp-heat. Mu tong acts to purify heart, relieve restlessness,

木通、瞿麦，均性味苦寒，均能清热利尿通淋，治湿热淋证。其中木通且能清心除烦，上清心火，下泄小肠之热，善治心火上炎、下移小肠

clear the heart fire in the upper and reduce the small intestine heat in the lower, applied to treat heart fire flaming upwards or transmitting downwards to small intestines, manifested by mouth ulcer, restlessness and dark urine. It also acts to stimulate menstrual flow, promote lactation and treat Bi (Obturation) Pattern, applied to treat amenorrhea, lactation deficiency and Bi (Obturation) Pattern due to damp-heat. Qu mai acts to treat various types of stranguria. It is also attributive to the Xue (Blood) Phase and acts to activate blood and stimulate menstrual flow, applied to treat amenorrhea and dysmenorrhea.

之口舌生疮，以及心烦尿赤；且能通经下乳、通痹，治闭经乳少、湿热痹痛。瞿麦善治各种淋证；入血分能活血通经，治经闭痛经。

Both *Kochiae Fructus* (di fu zi) and *Lygodii Spora* (hai jin sha) act to clear heat, dissolve damp and relieve stranguria, applied to treat stranguria due to damp-heat. Di fu zi is weaker in clearing heat, promoting urination and relieving stranguria, but it acts to clear heat, dissolve damp, eliminate wind and stop itching, applied to treat eczema and skin itch. Hai jin sha acts to clear heat, promote urination, relieve stranguria and stop pain, applied to treat painful urination and stranguria with stones.

地肤子、海金沙，均能清热利湿、通淋，治湿热淋证。其中地肤子清热利尿通淋力较弱；且能清热利湿、祛风止痒，尤善治湿疹、皮肤瘙痒诸证。海金沙功专清热利尿、通淋止痛，尤善治尿道疼痛，且善治石淋。

Dioscoreae Rhizoma Spongiosae (bi xie) is bitter and neutral in property and acts to dissolve damp and eliminate turbidy, as the major herb to treat stranguria with turbid urine. It also acts to eliminate wind and dissolve damp, applied to treat Bi (Obturation) Pattern.

萆薢，性味苦平，善利湿去浊，为治膏淋之要药。且能祛风除湿，善治风湿痹痛。

3 Damp-dissolving and jaundice-relieving herbs

3 利湿退黄药

All *Artemisiae Scopariae Herba* (yin chen),

茵陈、金钱草、虎杖，均

Lysimachiae Herba (jin qian cao) and *Polygoni Cuspidati Rhizoma et Radix* (hu zhang) are cold in property and act to dissolve damp and relieve jaundice, applied to treat damp-heat type jaundice caused by damp-heat accumulating in liver and gallbladder. Yin chen is pungent, bitter and slightly cold in property and acts to eliminate damp-heat in liver and gallbladder, as the major herb to treat jaundice, applied to treat yang-type jaundice and yin-type jaundice. It also acts to treat furuncle and eczema. Jin qian cao is sweet, bland and slightly cold in property and acts to relieve jaundice caused by damp-heat in liver and gallbladder, and also acts to promote urination, relieve stranguria and discharge stones, as the major herb to treat stranguria with stones. It also acts to relive toxin and subside swell, applied to treat carbuncle, ulcer, snake-bite and insect-bite. Hu zhang is bitter and slightly cold in property and acts to dissipate stasis and stop pain, applied to treat amenorrhea, dysmenorrhea and traumatic injury. It acts to clear heat, relieve toxin, purify lung, stop cough and dissolve phlegm, applied to treat carbuncle, ulcer and cough due to heat in lung. It also acts to reduce heat and promote defecation, applied to treat constipation due to heat accumulation.

性寒,具有利湿退黄作用,治湿热蕴结肝胆所致湿热黄疸。其中茵陈辛苦微寒,功专利清肝胆湿热,为退黄疸要药,治黄疸,无论阳黄、阴黄,均可配伍应用;且治湿疮、湿疹。金钱草甘淡微寒,既除湿退黄以治肝胆湿热,又利尿通淋、排除结石,为治石淋之要药;且能解毒消肿,治疮痈肿毒、蛇虫咬伤。虎杖味苦微寒,又能散瘀止痛,治经闭痛经,跌打伤痛;且能清热解毒、清肺止咳化痰,治疮痈肿毒、肺热咳嗽;尚能泻热通便,治热结便秘。

Chapter 7 Interior-Warming Herbs

第7章 温里药

The medicinal herbs acting to warm the interior and eliminate cold, applied to treat interior cold pattern are called the interior-warming herbs.

The medicinal herbs are warm and hot in property and act to warm middle energizer, eliminate cold and strengthen spleen and stomach, or act to eliminate cold and warm liver, or act to bring back yang and rescue from the collapse. They are applied to treat inward attack of pathogenic cold and beleagued spleen yang manifested by cold pain at epigastria and abdomen, vomiting and diarrhea, or to treat cold congealing in the Liver Meridian manifested by cold pain at lower abdomen, headache and abdominal pain due to hernia, or to treat yang decline in heart and kidney and internal excess of yin cold manifested by counterflow cold and extremely minute pulse in yang collapse. Furthermore, they are also applied to treat chest Bi (Obturation) Pattern manifested by cardiac pain, panting and cough due to cold in lung.

It is necessary to pay attention in application of interior-warming herbs that the medicinal herbs are mostly pungent, hot and dry in property, so they are easy to consume yin and produce fire. It is prohibited to apply for those with heat pattern of excess, yin deficiency and fire hyperactivity pattern,

以温里祛寒,治疗里寒证为主要作用的药物,称为温里药。

本类药物大多药性温热,功能温中散寒、健运脾胃,或散寒暖肝,或回阳救逆。主要用于寒邪内侵,脾阳受困,症见脘腹冷痛,呕吐泻利。或肝经寒凝,少腹冷痛,头痛疝痛。或心肾阳衰,阴寒内盛的亡阳厥逆,脉微欲绝。此外,还能用于胸痹心痛、肺寒喘咳等。

使用温里药尚需注意,本类药物性多辛热燥烈,易耗阴助火,凡属实热证、阴虚火旺、津血亏虚者忌用,孕妇慎用。

or body fluid or blood deficiency, and it is cautious to apply for pregnant women.

Aconiti Lateralis Radix Praeparata (fu zi)

It is the dried product from the daughter root of *Aconitum carmichaeli* Debx., family Ranunculaceae. The medicinal herb is mainly produced in Sichuan Province. It is collected from late June to early August by removing parent root, applied in prepared form.

Features Flavor: pungent and sweet. Property: extremely hot and poisonous. Meridian tropism: the Heart Meridian, the Kidney Meridian and the Spleen Meridian.

Actions Bring back yang, rescue from the collapse, reinforce fire, assist yang, eliminate cold and stop pain.

Application

(1) Yang collapse pattern. The medicinal herb is extremely hot and dry in property, as the major herb to bring back yang and rescue from the collapse. In the treatment of yang collapse pattern, it is combined with *Zingiberis Rhizoma* (gan jiang) and *Glycyrrhizae Radix et Rhizoma* (gan cao), to form up Counterflow Cold Decoction (Si Ni Tang). In the treatment of loss of qi along with bleeding, it is combined with *Ginseng Radix et Raizoma* (ren shen), to form up Ginseng and Aconite Decoction (Shen Fu Tang).

(2) Yang deficiency pattern. The medicinal herb acts to reinforce fire and assist yang, so as to assist heart yang, warm spleen yang and reinforce kidney yang, applied to treat various types of yang deficiency pattern. In the treatment of kidney yang

附子

为毛茛科植物乌头的子根的加工品。主产于四川等地。6月下旬至8月上旬采收,除去母根。制用。

性味归经 辛、甘,大热;有毒。归心、肾、脾经。

功效 回阳救逆,补火助阳,散寒止痛。

应用

(1)亡阳证。本品辛甘大热,纯阳燥烈,为回阳救逆之要药。治亡阳证,常与干姜、甘草等同用,即四逆汤。若治气随血脱者,可与人参同用,即参附汤。

(2)阳虚证。本品有补火助阳之功,能助心阳、温脾阳、补肾阳,善治各脏阳虚证。治肾阳衰弱,阳痿宫冷,可与肉桂、熟地黄等同用,如

deficiency pattern manifested by impotence and frigidity, it is combined with *Cinnamomi Cortex* (rou gui) and *Rehmanniae Radix Praeparata* (shu di huang), to form up Cinnamon Bark and Aconite Eight Ingredients Pills (Gui Fu Ba Wei Wan). In the treatment of spleen yang deficiency pattern manifested by vomiting, diarrhea and cold pain at epigastria and abdomen, it is combined with *Codonopsis Radix* (dang shen), *Atractylodis Macrocephalae Rhizoma* (bai zhu) and *Zingiberis Rhizoma* (gan jiang), to form up Aconite Center-Rectifying Pills (Fu Zi Li Zhong Wan). In the treatment of spleen and kidney yang deficiency pattern manifested by edema, it is combined with *Poria* (fu ling), *Atractylodis Macrocephalae Rhizoma* (bai zhu) and *Zingiberis Rhizoma Recens* (sheng jiang), to form up True Warrior Decoction (Zhen Wu Tang). In the treatment of heart yang deficiency leading to heart yang obstruction manifested by chest pain, cardiac pain, palpitation and shortness of breath, it is combined with *Ginseng Radix et Raizoma* (ren shen), *Cinnamomi Ramulus* (gui zhi) and gan cao. In the treatment of yang deficiency pattern complicated with exogenous pathogen attack, it is combined with *Asari Radix et Rhizoma* (xi xin) and *Ephedrae Herba* (ma huang), to form up Ephedra, Monkshood and Asarum Decoction (Ma Huang Fu Zi Xi Xin Tang).

桂附八味丸。治脾阳亏虚，虚寒吐泻、脘腹冷痛，可与党参、白术、干姜等同用，如附子理中丸。治脾肾阳虚之水肿，可与茯苓、白术、生姜等同用，如真武汤。治心阳衰弱，胸阳痹阻的胸痹心痛、心悸气短，可与人参、桂枝、甘草等同用。治阳虚外感，可与细辛、麻黄同用，即麻黄附子细辛汤。

(3) Bi (Obturation) Pattern due to cold. The medicinal herb is pungent, dispersing, warm and opening in property and acts to eliminate cold and stop pain. In the treatment of Bi (Obturation) Pattern due to wind, cold and damp manifested by general joint pain, it is combined with gui zhi, bai zhu

(3) 寒痹证。本品辛散温通，散寒止痛。治风寒湿痹，周身骨节疼痛，可与桂枝、白术、甘草等同用。

and gan cao.

Usage and dosage Apply 3～15 g in decoction by decocting first and for long time. It is advisable to prepare the medicinal herb for oral administration.

用法用量 煎服，3～15克。宜先煎，久煎。内服须炮制后用。

Precautions for use It is prohibited to apply for those with yin deficiency and yang hyperactivity and pregnant women. The medicinal herb is incompatible with *Pinelliae Rhizoma* (ban xia), *Trichosanthis Fructus* (gua lou), *Fritillariae Cirrhosae Bulbus* (chuan bei mu), *Bulbus Fritillariae Thunbergii* (zhe bei mu), *Bletillae Rhizoma* (bai ji) and *Radix Ampelopsis* (bai lian).

使用注意 阴虚阳亢者及孕妇忌用。反半夏、瓜蒌、贝母、白及、白蔹。

Remarks *Aconiti Radix* (chuan wu) and *Aconiti Lateralis Radix Praeparata* (fu zi)

Both the medicinal herbs are the products from the *Aconitum carmichaeli* Debx., family Ranunculaceae, pungent, hot and poisonous in property, and act to eliminate cold and stop pain. Chuan wu is the product from the parent root and acts to eliminate wind and cold and stop pain, applied to treat Bi (Obturation) Pattern due to cold-damp and pain. Fu zi is the product from the daughter root and acts to bring back yang and rescue from the collapse, reinforce fire and assist yang, applied to treat yang collapse pattern and yang deficiency pattern.

按语 川乌与附子

二药均来源于毛茛科植物乌头，均为辛热、有毒之品。均具散寒止痛功效。不同的是川乌药用母根，功能祛风散寒，尤善止痛，多用于寒湿痹痛及疼痛证。附子药用子根，功能回阳救逆、补火助阳，尤善回阳，多用于亡阳证及阳虚诸证。

Cinnamomi Cortex (rou gui)

It is the dried product from the bark of *Cinnamomum cassia* Presl, family Lauraceae. The medicinal herb is collected in autumn by barking and drying, applied in crude form.

Features Flavor: pungent and sweet. Property: extremely hot. Meridian tropism: the Kidney

肉桂

为樟科植物肉桂的干燥树皮。秋季剥取，刮去粗皮。生用。

性味归经 辛、甘，大热。归肾、脾、心、肝经。

Meridian, the Spleen Meridian, the Heart Meridian and the Liver Meridian.

Actions Reinforce fire, assist yang, guide fire back to its source, eliminate cold, stop pain, warm meridians and dredge collaterals.

功效 补火助阳，引火归元，散寒止痛，温经通脉。

Application

(1) Kidney yang deficiency pattern. The medicinal herb is pungent, sweet and extremely hot in property, and acts to reinforce fire and assist yang, as the major herb to treat kidney yang deficiency pattern. In the treatment of kidney yang deficiency pattern manifested by fear of cold, chills in limbs, weakness at low back and knees, impotence and frigidity, it is combined with *Aconiti Lateralis Radix Praeparata* (fu zi), *Rehmanniae Radix Praeparata* (shu di huang) and *Corni Fructus* (shan zhu yu). In the treatment of cold in the lower and false yang floating upward, it acts to guide fire back to its source.

(2) Cold pain at chest and abdomen, vomiting and diarrhea due to deficiency and cold, and abdominal pain due to cold-type hernia. The medicinal herb is extremely hot and acts to eliminate cold and stop pain. In the treatment of cold blocking heart yang manifested by chest pain and cardiac pain, it is combined with *Trichosanthis Fructus* (gua lou) and *Cinnamomi Ramulus* (gui zhi). In the treatment of deficiency and cold pattern manifested by cold pain at epigastria and abdomen, vomiting and diarrhea, it is applied singly by grinding into powder for oral administration, or combined with fu zi and *Zingiberis Rhizoma* (gan jiang). In the treatment of abdominal pain due to cold-type hernia, it is combined with *Foeniculi Fructus* (xiao hui xiang) and *Euodiae Fructus* (wu zhu yu).

应用

（1）肾阳虚证。本品辛甘大热，善补火助阳，为治肾阳虚证常用药。治肾阳不足，畏寒肢冷、腰膝软弱、阳痿宫冷，常与附子、熟地黄、山茱萸同用。治下元虚冷，虚阳上浮证，有引火归元之效。

（2）心腹冷痛，虚寒吐泻，寒疝腹痛。本品大热，散寒止痛力强。治寒遏胸阳，胸痹心痛，可与瓜蒌、桂枝等同用。治虚寒所致的脘腹冷痛或吐泻，单味研末吞服，或与附子、干姜等同用。治寒疝腹痛，可配伍小茴香、吴茱萸等同用。

(3) Dysmenorrhea and amenorrhea. The medicinal herb acts to warm meridians and dredge collaterals. In the treatment of cold congealing and blood stasis manifested by dysmenorrhea and amenorrhea, it is combined with *Angelicae Sinensis Radix* (dang gui) and *Chuanxiong Rhizoma* (chuan xiong).

(3) 痛经,经闭。本品能温经通脉。治寒凝血滞的痛经、经闭,常与当归、川芎等同用。

(4) Yin-type furuncle. In the treatment of yin-type furuncle or non-ruptured furuncle with purulence due to deficiency and cold in qi and blood, it is combined with *Rehmanniae Radix Praeparata* (shu di huang), *Colla Cornus Cervi* (lu jiao jiao) and *Ephedrae Herba* (ma huang), to form up Yang-Harmonizing Decoction (Yang He Tang).

(4) 阴疽。治阴疽或气血虚寒,痈肿脓成不溃,可与熟地黄、鹿角胶、麻黄等同用,如阳和汤。

Furthermore, it is advisable to add small dose of the medicinal herb to the qi-reinforcing and blood-nourishing formula, so as to inspire the growth of qi and blood.

此外,在补益气血方中少量配以本品,能鼓舞气血生长。

Usage and dosage Apply 1～5 g in decoction and decoct it later. Apply 1～2 g of grinded powder.

用法用量 煎服,1～5克。宜后下。研末冲服,每次1～2克。

Precautions for use It is cautious to apply for pregnant women or those with tendency of bleeding. It is not advisable to apply it with *Halloysitum Rubrum* (chi shi zhi).

使用注意 孕妇及有出血倾向者慎用。不宜与赤石脂同用。

Remarks *Cinnamomi Ramulus* (gui zhi) and *Cinnamomi Cortex* (rou gui)

按语 桂枝与肉桂

Both the medicinal herbs are the products from the plant of *Cinnamomum cassia* Presl, family Lauraceae, and act to warm and dredge meridians, eliminate cold and stop pain. Gui zhi is the product from the tender twig, warm in property, and acts to make sweating and relieve exterior pattern, as the major herb to treat exterior pattern of wind-cold

二药均来源于樟科植物肉桂,均能温通经脉,散寒止痛。不同的是桂枝药用嫩枝,性温发散,功善发汗解肌,为风寒表证表实无汗或表虚有汗之常用,还能助阳化气。肉桂药用树皮,性热

without sweating or exterior deficiency pattern with sweating, and also acts to assist yang to transform into qi. Rou gui is the product from the bark, hot in property, and acts to warm the interior, reinforce fire, assist yang and guide fire back to its source, as the major herb to treat kidney yang deficiency pattern.

温里，功善补火助阳、引火归元，为肾阳不足之常用。

Zingiberis Rhizoma (gan jiang)

It is the dried product from the rhizome of the perennial herb, *Zingibor officinale* Rosc, family Zingiberaceae. The medicinal herb is collected in winter, applied in crude form.

Features Flavor: pungent. Property: hot. Meridian tropism: the Spleen Meridian, the Stomach Meridian, the Kidney Meridian, the Heart Meridian and the Lung Meridian.

Actions Warm middle energizer, eliminate cold, bring back yang, dredge vessels, warm lung and dissolve rheum.

Application

(1) Spleen-stomach cold pattern. The medicinal herb is pungent, hot and dry, and attributive to the spleen and stomach, and acts to warm middle energizer and eliminate cold. It is applied to treat the spleen-stomach cold pattern of excess type or deficiency type. In the treatment of spleen-stomach cold pattern of deficiency type manifested by cold pain at epigastria and abdomen, vomiting and diarrhea, it is combined with *Codonopsis Radix* (dang shen), *Glycyrrhizae Radix et Rhizoma* (gan cao) and *Atractylodis Macrocephalae Rhizoma* (bai zhu), to form up Center-Rectifying Pills (Li Zhong Wan). In the treatment of spleen-stomach cold pat-

干姜

为姜科植物姜的干燥根茎。冬季采挖。生用。

性味归经 辛，热。归脾、胃、肾、心、肺经。

功效 温中散寒，回阳通脉，温肺化饮。

应用

（1）脾胃寒证。本品辛热燥烈，主入脾胃，擅长温中散寒。治脾胃寒证，无论是实寒或虚寒证均可应用。治脾胃虚寒的脘腹冷痛，呕吐泄泻，常与党参、甘草、白术等同用，如理中丸。治脾胃有寒的吐泻腹痛，单用研末服，或配伍温中散寒药同用。

tern of excess type manifested by vomiting, diarrhea and abdominal pain, it is applied singly by grinding into powder or combined with the center-warming and cold-eliminating herbs.

(2) Yang collapse pattern. The medicinal herb is pungent and hot in property, and attributive to the Heart and Kidney Meridians, and acts to bring back yang and rescue from the collapse. In the treatment of yang collapse pattern, it is combined with *Aconiti Lateralis Radix Praeparata* (fu zi) in mutual reinforcement.

（2）亡阳证。本品辛、热，入心肾经，能回阳通脉。治亡阳证，可与附子相须为用。

(3) Panting and cough due to cold and rheum. The medicinal herb acts to warm lung and dissolve rheum. In the treatment of panting and cough due to cold and rheum, it is combined with *Ephedrae Herba* (ma huang), *Asari Radix et Rhizoma* (xi xin) and *Schisandrae Chinensis Fructus* (wu wei zi), to form up Minor Green Dragon Decoction (Xiao Qing Long Tang).

（3）寒饮喘咳。本品能温肺化饮。治寒饮咳喘，常与麻黄、细辛、五味子等同用，如小青龙汤。

Usage and dosage Apply 3～10 g in decoction.

用法用量 煎服，3～10克。

Euodiae Fructus (wu zhu yu)

吴茱萸

It is the dried product from the nearly ripe fruit of *Evodia rutaecarpa* (Juss) Benth. *Evodia rutaecarpa* (Juss.) Benth. var. officinalis (Dode) Huang, *Evodia rutaecarpa* (Juss) Benth. var. *bodinieri* (Dode) Huang, family Rutaceae. The medicinal herb is collected from August to November when the fruits are not split open, applied in crude form or prepared form.

为芸香科植物吴茱萸、石虎或疏毛吴茱萸的干燥近成熟果实。8～11月果尚未开裂时采收。生用或制用。

Features Flavor: pungent and bitter. Property: hot and slightly poisonous. Meridian tropism: the Liver Meridian, the Spleen Meridian, the Stom-

性味归经 辛、苦，热；有小毒。归肝、脾、胃、肾经。

ach Meridian and the Kidney Meridian.

Actions Eliminate cold, stop pain, subdue up-reverse flowing qi, stop vomiting, assist yang and stop diarrhea.

功效 散寒止痛,降逆止呕,助阳止泻。

Application

(1) Jueyin headache, abdominal pain due to cold-type hernia, beriberi due to cold-damp, abdominal pain in menstruation, and diarrhea due to deficiency and cold. The medicinal herb is pungent and hot in property, and acts to eliminate cold, promote liver qi flow and stop pain. In the treatment of Jueyin headache, it is combined with *Ginseng Radix et Raizoma* (ren shen), *Zingiberis Rhizoma Recens* (sheng jiang) and *Fructus Ziziphi Jujubae* (da zao), to form up Evodia Decoction (Wu Zhu Yu Tang). In the treatment of abdominal pain due to cold-type hernia, it is combined with *Foeniculi Fructus* (xiao hui xiang) and *Linderae Radix* (wu yao). In the treatment of beriberi due to cold-damp, it is combined with *Chaenomelis Fructus* (mu gua). In the treatment of abdominal pain in menstruation, it is combined with *Angelicae Sinensis Radix* (dang gui) and *Carthami Flos* (hong hua).

应用

(1) 厥阴头痛,寒疝腹痛,寒湿脚气,经行腹痛,虚寒泄泻。本品辛热,既散寒凝,又疏肝气,且能止痛。治厥阴头痛,常与人参、生姜、大枣等同用,如吴茱萸汤。治寒疝腹痛,可与小茴香、乌药等配伍。治寒湿脚气,可与木瓜等同用。治经行腹痛,可配伍当归、红花等同用。

(2) Vomiting and acid regurgitation. The medicinal herb acts to soothe liver, subdue up-reverse flowing qi and stop vomiting. In the treatment of vomiting and acid regurgitation caused by disharmony between liver and stomach, it is combined with *Coptidis Rhizoma* (huang lian), to form up Coptis and Evodia Pills (Zuo Jin Wan). In the treatment of vomiting due to cold in stomach, it is combined with *Pinelliae Rhizoma* (ban xia) and *Zingiberis Rhizoma Recens* (sheng jiang).

(2) 呕吐吞酸。本品具疏肝降逆、止呕作用。治肝胃不和的呕吐吞酸,可与黄连同用,即左金丸。治胃寒呕吐,常与半夏、生姜等同用。

(3) Diarrhea due to deficiency and cold. The

(3) 虚寒泄泻。本品辛

medicinal herb is pungent and hot in property and attributive to the Spleen and Kidney Meridians, and acts to warm spleen and kidney, assist yang and stop diarrhea. In the treatment of chronic diarrhea or dawn diarrhea due to deficiency and cold in spleen and kidney, it is combined with *Psoraleae Fructus* (bu gu zhi), *Schisandrae Chinensis Fructus* (wu wei zi) and *Myristicae Semen* (rou dou kou), to form up Four Divinities Pills (Si Shen Wan).

热,入脾肾经,能温暖脾肾,助阳止泻。治脾肾虚寒的久泻、五更泻,可与补骨脂、五味子、肉豆蔻同用,即四神丸。

Usage and dosage Apply 2～5 g in decoction. Apply a proper amount for external use. The medicinal herb is dry in crude form. After preparation with *Glycyrrhizae Radix et Rhizoma* (gan cao), its poison is decreased and its dry property is modified. It is applied in prepared form for oral administration.

用法用量 煎服,2～5克。外用适量。生用性燥,用甘草制后既减毒,又缓和燥性,内服多制用。

Precautions for use It is prohibited to apply for those with yin deficiency and heat.

使用注意 阴虚有热者忌用。

Caryophylli Flos (ding xiang)

丁香

It is the dried product from the flower bud of *Eugenia caryophyllata* Thunb., family Myrtaceae. The medicinal herb, also called "gong ding xiang", is collected when the flower bud is changing from green to red, applied in crude form.

为桃金娘科植物丁香的干燥花蕾。又名公丁香。花蕾由绿转红时采收。生用。

Features Flavor: pungent. Property: warm. Meridian tropism: the Spleen Meridian, the Stomach Meridian and the Kidney Meridian.

性味归经 辛,温。归脾、胃、肾经。

Actions Warm middle energizer, subdue up-reverse flowing qi, reinforce kidney and assist yang.

功效 温中降逆,补肾助阳。

Application

应用

(1) Hiccup due to cold in stomach, and diarrhea due to deficiency and cold. The medicinal herb is warm and fragrant in property, and acts to warm

(1) 胃寒呕逆,虚寒泄泻。本品性温气香,能温中散寒,尤善降逆。治胃寒呕

middle energizer, eliminate cold and subdue up-reverse flowing qi. In the treatment of vomiting and hiccup due to cold in stomach, it is combined with *Ginseng Radix et Raizoma* (ren shen), *Zingiberis Rhizoma Recens* (sheng jiang) and *Kaki Calyx* (shi di), to form up Cloves and Kaki Calyx Decoction (Ding Xiang Shi Di Tang). In the treatment of diarrhea due to deficiency and cold in spleen and stomach, it is combined with *Atractylodis Macrocephalae Rhizoma* (bai zhu) and *Codonopsis Radix* (dang shen).

吐、呃逆,可与人参、生姜、柿蒂等同用,如丁香柿蒂汤。治脾胃虚寒的泄泻,可与白术、党参等同用。

(2) Kidney yang deficiency pattern manifested by impotence. The medicinal herb acts to reinforce kidney and assist yang. In the treatment of kidney yang deficiency pattern manifested by impotence, aching and pain at low back and knees, it is combined with *Aconiti Lateralis Radix Praeparata* (fu zi), *Cinnamomi Cortex* (rou gui) and *Epimedii Folium* (yin yang huo).

(2) 肾虚阳痿。本品具补肾助阳之功。治肾虚阳痿、腰膝酸痛,可与附子、肉桂、淫羊藿等同用。

Usage and dosage Apply 1～3 g in decoction.

用法用量 煎服,1～3克。

Precautions for use It is not advisable to apply with *Curcumae Radix* (yu jin).

使用注意 不宜与郁金同用。

Appendix *Caryopaylli Fructus* (mu ding xiang)

附药 母丁香

It is the dried product from the nearly ripe fruit of *Eugenia caryophyllata* Thunb., family Myrtaceae, also called "ji she xiang". The medicinal herb is pungent in flavor, warm in property and attributive to the Spleen Meridian, the Stomach Meridian, the Lung Meridian and the Kidney Meridian. It acts to warm middle energizer, subdue up-reverse flowing qi, reinforce kidney and assist yang, applied to treat spleen-stomach deficiency and cold pattern manifested

为丁香的干燥近成熟果实,又名鸡舌香。性味辛、温,归脾、胃、肺、肾经。功能温中降逆、补肾助阳,适用于脾胃虚寒、食少吐泻、呃逆呕吐,以及肾虚阳痿,心腹冷痛。煎服,1～3克。不宜与郁金同用。

by poor appetite, hiccup and vomiting, and to treat kidney deficiency pattern manifested by impotence, cold pain at chest and abdomen. Apply 1～3 g in decoction. It is not advisable to apply with yu jin.

Foeniculi Fructus (xiao hui xiang)

It is the dried product from the ripe fruit of *Foeniculum vulgare* Mill., family Umbelliferae. The medicinal herb is collected in autumn when the fruits are ripe, applied in crude form or prepared form by frying with salty solution.

Features Flavor: pungent. Property: warm. Meridian tropism: the Liver Meridian, the Kidney Meridian, the Spleen Meridian and the Stomach Meridian.

Actions Eliminate cold, stop pain, regulate qi flow and harmonize middle energizer.

Application

(1) Abdominal pain due to cold-type hernia, drop-weighty sensation at scrotum, cold pain at lower abdomen and dysmenorrhea. The medicinal herb is attributive to the Liver Meridian and acts to warm liver, eliminate cold and stop pain. In the treatment of abdominal pain due to cold-type hernia, it is combined with *Cinnamomi Cortex* (rou gui) and *Linderae Radix* (wu yao). In the treatment of drop-weighty sensation and pain at scrotum, it is combined with the qi-moving and pain-relieving herbs. In the treatment of cold congealing in the Liver Meridian manifested by cold pain at lower abdomen or dysmenorrhea, it is combined with *Cyperi Rhizoma* (xiang fu) and *Angelicae Sinensis Radix* (dang gui), or applied singly by frying to hot and wrapping in a cloth bag for application at lower abdomen.

小茴香

为伞形科植物茴香的干燥成熟果实。秋季果实成熟时采收。生用或盐水炒用。

性味归经 辛，温。归肝、肾、脾、胃经。

功效 散寒止痛，理气和中。

应用

（1）寒疝腹痛，睾丸偏坠，少腹冷痛，痛经。本品入肝经，善暖肝散寒凝，且能止痛。治寒疝腹痛，可与肉桂、乌药等同用。治睾丸偏坠胀痛，可与行气止痛药同用。治肝经寒凝的少腹冷痛或痛经，可与香附、当归等同用；亦可单味炒热，布包温熨下腹部。

(2) Cold and qi stagnation in middle energizer. The medicinal herb acts to eliminate cold and stop pain, and also to regulate qi flow and harmonize middle energizer. In the treatment of cold and qi stagnation in stomach manifested by distending pain at epigastria and abdomen, vomiting and poor appetite, it is combined with *Zingiberis Rhizoma* (gan jiang) and *Aucklandiae Radix* (mu xiang).

（2）中寒气滞证。本品既散寒止痛，又理气和中。治胃寒气滞的脘腹胀痛，呕吐食少，可与干姜、木香等同用。

Usage and dosage Apply 3～6 g in decoction. Apply a proper amount for external use. The medicinal herb acts to eliminate cold, regulate qi flow and harmonize middle energizer in crude form, while acts to warm kidney, eliminate cold and stop pain in prepared form by frying with salt.

用法用量 煎服，3～6克。外用适量。生用散寒理气和中，盐炒暖肾散寒止痛。

Zanthoxyli Pericarpium (hua jiao)

花椒

It is the dried product from the ripe peel of *Zanthoxylum schinifolium* Sieb. et Zucc. or *Zanthoxylum bungeanum* Maxim., family Rutaceae. The medicinal herb produced in Sichuan Province is in a high quality, so it is also called "chuan jiao" or "shu jiao". It is collected in autumn, applied in crude form or prepared form by frying.

为芸香科植物青椒或花椒的干燥成熟果皮。以四川产者为佳，故名川椒、蜀椒。秋季采收。生用或炒用。

Features Flavor: pungent. Property: warm. Meridian tropism: the Spleen Meridian, the Stomach Meridian and the Kidney Meridian.

性味归经 辛，温。归脾、胃、肾经。

Actions Warm middle energizer, stop pain, kill worms and relieve itching.

功效 温中止痛，杀虫止痒。

Application

应用

(1) Spleen-stomach deficiency and cold pattern. The medicinal herb is attributive to the Spleen and Stomach Meridians, and acts to warm middle energizer, eliminate cold and stop pain. In the treatment of spleen-stomach deficiency and cold pattern

（1）脾胃虚寒证。本品入脾、胃经，能温中散寒、止痛。治脾胃虚寒，脘腹冷痛，呕吐，常与人参、干姜等同用，或将本品炒热布包温熨

manifested by cold pain at epigastria and abdomen and vomiting, it is combined with *Ginseng Radix et Raizoma* (ren shen) and *Zingiberis Rhizoma* (gan jiang). Or fry the medicinal herb to hot and wrap it in a cloth bag for application at painful area.

痛处。

(2) Abdominal pain due to parasites, eczema and pruritus vulvae. The medicinal herb acts to kill worms and relieve itching. In the treatment of abdominal pain due to parasites, it is applied singly or combined with *Mume Fructus* (wu mei), *Zingiberis Rhizoma* (gan jiang) and *Coptidis Rhizoma* (huang lian), to form up Black Plum Pills (Wu Mei Wan). It is applied to treat eczema and pruritus vulvae for external use, applied singly or combined with *Sophorae Flavescentis Radix* (ku shen), *Kochiae Fructus* (di fu zi) and *Cnidii Fructus* (she chuang zi) by decocting for external wash.

（2）虫积腹痛，湿疹，阴痒。本品具杀虫、止痒之功。治虫积腹痛，可单用，或配伍乌梅、干姜、黄连等同用，如乌梅丸。外用治湿疹、阴痒，可单用或配伍苦参、地肤子、蛇床子等煎汤外洗。

Usage and dosage　Apply 3～6 g in decoction. Apply a proper amount for external use.

用法用量　煎服，3～6克。外用适量。

Brief summary

小　结

Both *Aconiti Lateralis Radix Praeparata* (fu zi) and *Zingiberis Rhizoma* (gan jiang) are pungent and hot in property and act to bring back yang, rescue from the collapse, warm middle energizer and eliminate cold, applied to treat yang collapse pattern and spleen-stomach cold pattern manifested by cold pain at epigastria and abdomen, vomiting and diarrhea. Fu zi is extremely hot and poisonous, as the major herb to bring back yang and rescue from the collapse, and acts to reinforce primary yang, benefit fire and diminish yin, applied to treat kidney yang deficiency pattern, fire decline at Vital Gate

附子、干姜，均性味辛热，具回阳救逆、温中散寒之功，治亡阳证及脾胃寒证之脘腹冷痛、呕吐泄泻。其中，附子大热有毒，为回阳救逆之要药；又善峻补元阳，益火消阴，善治肾阳不足、命门火衰之证，以及诸脏阳虚证；其散寒止痛力佳，为治寒凝诸痛之常用。干姜功能回阳通脉，回阳救逆力虽弱，但与附子同用，既增附子回阳之力，

pattern and various types of yang deficiency pattern. It also acts to eliminate cold and stop pain, applied to treat various types of pain due to cold congealing. Gan jiang acts to bring back yang and rescue from the collapse. It is weaker than fu zi in bringing back yang rescuing from the collapse, but it strengthens action of fu zi in bringing back yang rescuing from the collapse and reduce the toxicity of fu zi when it is applied with fu zi. The medicinal herb is attributive to spleen and stomach, and acts to warm middle energizer and eliminate cold, applied to treat spleen-stomach cold pattern of deficiency type or excess type, as the major herb to warm middle energizer and eliminate cold. It also warm lung and dissolve rheum, applied to treat cough and panting due to cold and rheum.

又减附子之毒；主入脾胃，功偏温中散寒，善治脾胃寒证，无论虚实，故为温中散寒之要药；且能温肺化饮，治寒饮咳喘。

Both *Cinnamomi Cortex* (rou gui) and *Euodiae Fructus* (wu zhu yu) are pungent and hot in property and act to eliminate cold and stop pain. Rou gui is extremely hot and attributive to the Kidney Meridian, and acts to reinforce fire, assist yang and guide fire back to its source, as the major herb to treat kidney yang deficiency pattern, deficiency and cold in the lower and false yang floating upwards. It also acts to warm and dredge meridians, applied to treat dysmenorrhea and amenorrhea due to cold congealing and blood stasis. Wu zhu yu is attributive to the Liver Meridian, and acts to eliminate cold, promote liver qi flow and stop pain, as the major herb to treat Jueyin headache. It acts to soothe liver, subdue up-reverse flowing qi and stop vomiting, applied to treat vomiting and acid regurgitation due to disharmony between liver and stomach. It also acts to assist yang and stop diarrhea, applied to

肉桂、吴茱萸，均性味辛热，具散寒止痛作用。其中肉桂性大热，主入肾经，功善补火助阳、引火归元，为肾阳虚证，以及下元虚冷、虚阳上浮之证的常用药；且能温通经脉，亦治寒凝血滞之痛经经闭等证。吴茱萸主入肝经，既散寒凝、疏肝气，且能止痛，为治厥阴头痛之要药；还能疏肝、降逆止呕，治肝胃不和之呕吐吞酸；又能助阳止泻，治脾肾阳虚的泄泻。

treat diarrhea due to spleen-kidney yang deficiency.

Both Flos Caryophylli (ding xiang) and *Zanthoxyli Pericarpium* (hua jiao) act to warm middle energizer, applied to treat spleen-stomach deficiency and cold pattern. Ding xiang is attributive to the Spleen, Stomach and Kidney Meridians, acts to warm middle energizer, eliminate cold, warm kidney, assist yang and subdue up-reverse flowing qi, as the major herb to treat vomiting, hiccup, and impotence due to kidney deficiency. Hua jiao acts to warm middle energizer and eliminate cold, applied to treat spleen-stomach deficiency and cold, for both oral administration and external use. It also acts to kill worms and relieve itching, applied to treat abdominal pain due to parasites.

丁香、花椒,均能温中,善治脾胃虚寒证。其中丁香入脾、胃、肾经,既温中散寒,又温肾助阳,尤善降逆,为治呕吐、呃逆之要药,且治肾虚阳痿。花椒功善温中散寒,治脾胃虚寒,内服外用均可;且能杀虫止痒,尤善治虫积腹痛。

Foeniculi Fructus (xiao hui xiang) is pungent and warm in property and attributive to the Liver and Stomach Meridians, and acts to eliminate cold in the Liver Meridian, applied to treat abdominal pain due to cold-type hernia and drop-weighty sensation of scrotum. It also acts to regulate qi flow and harmonize stomach, applied to treat cold and qi stagnation pattern of middle energizer.

小茴香,性味辛温,主入肝、胃经,既散肝经寒凝,治寒疝腹痛、睾丸偏坠,又理气和胃,治中寒气滞证。

Chapter 8 Qi-Regulating Herbs

第8章 理气药

The medicinal herbs acting to regulate and manage qi activities, relieve qi stagnation or treat up-reverse flowing qi pattern are called qi-regulating herbs, also called qi-moving herbs. Those with strong action to regulate qi flow are also called qi-breaking herbs.

以疏理气机，消除气滞或气逆证为主要作用的药物，称理气药，又谓行气药。其中理气力强者，又称破气药。

The qi-regulating herbs are mostly pungent and bitter in flavor and warm in property, so they are moving, dispersing, reducing, warming and dredging. They act to regulate qi flow to strengthen spleen, soothe liver to relieve depression, regulate qi flow to dilate chest, and move qi to stop pain. Some of medicinal herbs also act to desiccate damp, dissolve phlegm, break qi clump, dissipate stasis, subdue up-reverse flowing qi and stop vomiting. They are applied to treat spleen-stomach qi stagnation pattern manifested by distending pain at epigastria and abdomen, vomiting, nausea, acid regurgitation, constipation or diarrhea. They are applied to treat liver qi stagnation pattern manifested by stuffiness and pain at chest and hypochondria, distending pain at breasts, pain due to hernia, or irregular menstruation. They are also applied to treat lung failing to disperse and descend pattern or lung qi accumulation and stagnation pattern manifested by stuffy chest, cough and panting.

理气药多味辛苦性温，其辛香行散、苦泄温通。功能理气健脾、疏肝解郁、理气宽胸和行气止痛。部分药物还有燥湿化痰、破气散结、降逆止呕等作用。主要用于脾胃气滞证，症见脘腹胀痛、呕恶泛酸、便秘或腹泻。肝郁气滞证，症见胸胁闷痛、乳房胀痛、疝气疼痛，或月经不调。肺失宣肃、肺气壅滞证，症见胸闷不畅、咳嗽气喘。

The medicinal herbs are mostly pungent, fragrant, warm and dry, so they are easy to consume qi and exhaust yin, therefore it is cautious to apply for those with yin deficiency or qi deficiency. It is cautious to apply qi-breaking herbs which have strong action for pregnant women. It is not advisable to decoct the medicinal herbs for long time.

本类药物大多辛香温燥，易耗气伤阴，故阴亏气虚者慎用。作用峻猛的破气药，孕妇慎用。入汤剂一般不宜久煎。

Citri Reticulatae Pericarpium (chen pi)

陈皮

It is the dried product from the ripe pericarp of *Citrus reticulate* Blanco, and similar varietal species by cultivation, family Rutaceae. The medicinal herb is collected when the fruit is ripe, applied in crude form.

为芸香科植物橘及其栽培变种的干燥成熟果皮。采摘成熟果实，剥取果皮。生用。

Features Flavor: bitter and pungent. Property: warm. Meridian tropism: the Spleen Meridian and the Lung Meridian.

性味归经 苦、辛，温。归脾、肺经。

Actions Regulate qi flow, strengthen spleen, desiccate damp and dissolve phlegm.

功效 理气健脾，燥湿化痰。

Application

应用

(1) Spleen-stomach qi stagnation pattern. The medicinal herb acts to regulate qi flow and strengthen spleen. In the treatment of spleen-stomach qi stagnation pattern manifested by distension and fullness at epigastria and abdomen, it is combined with *Aurantii Fructus* (zhi qiao) and *Aucklandiae Radix* (mu xiang). It acts to regulate qi flow and desiccate damp. In the treatment of damp and qi stagnation of middle energizer manifested by distension and fullness at epigastria and abdomen, poor appetite, vomiting and diarrhea, it is combined with *Atractylodis Rhizoma* (cang zhu) and *Magnoliae Officinalis Cortex* (hou po), to form up Stomach-Calming Powder (Ping Wei San). In the treatment of spleen

（1）脾胃气滞证。本品功善理气健脾。治脾胃气滞，脘腹胀满，可与枳壳、木香等同用。其能理气燥湿，若湿阻气滞的脘腹胀满，食少吐泻，常与苍术、厚朴等同用，如平胃散。治脾虚气滞，脘腹胀满，纳呆便溏，可与党参、白术、茯苓等同用，如异功散。

deficiency and qi stagnation pattern manifested by distension and fullness at epigastria and abdomen, poor appetite and loose feces, it is combined with *Codonopsis Radix* (dang shen), *Atractylodis Macrocephalae Rhizoma* (bai zhu) and *Poria* (fu ling), to form up Fantastic Efficacy Powder (Yi Gong San).

(2) Cough with excessive sputum. The medicinal herb acts to regulate lung qi flow, strengthen spleen and desiccate damp-phlegm. In the treatment of cough with excessive sputum due to phlegm-damp, it is combined with *Pinelliae Rhizoma* (ban xia) and fu ling, to form up Double Vintage Decoction (Er Chen Tang).

（2）咳嗽痰多。本品能理肺气、健脾运、燥湿痰。治痰湿所致的咳嗽、痰多，可与半夏、茯苓等同用，如二陈汤。

Usage and dosage Apply 3～10 g in decoction.

用法用量 煎服，3～10克。

Citri Reticulatae Pericarpium Viride (qing pi)

青皮

It is the dried product from the unripe fruit or its pericarp of *Citrus reticuta* Blanco, and similar varietal species by cultivation, family Rutaceae. The medicinal herb is collected in May and June for young fruit, or in July and August for unripe fruit, applied in crude form or prepared for by stir-frying with vinegar.

为芸香科植物橘及其栽培变种的干燥幼果或未成熟果实的干燥果皮。5～6月间收集自落的幼果，或7～8月间采收未成熟果实。生用或醋炙用。

Features Flavor: bitter and pungent. Property: warm. Meridian tropism: the Liver Meridian, the Gallbladder Meridian and the Stomach Meridian.

性味归经 苦、辛，温。归肝、胆、胃经。

Actions Soothe liver, break qi clump, digest food and dissolve stasis.

功效 疏肝破气，消积化滞。

Application

应用

(1) Liver qi stagnation pattern. The medicinal herb acts to soothe liver and break qi clump. In the treatment of liver qi stagnation manifested by dis-

（1）肝郁气滞证。本品善疏肝破气。治肝郁气滞的胸胁胀痛，常与柴胡、郁金等

tending pain at chest and hypochondria, it is combined with *Bupleuri Radix* (chai hu) and *Curcumae Radix* (yu jin). In the treatment of distending pain at breasts, it is combined with chai hu, *Paeoniae Radix Alba* (bai shao). In the treatment of early stage of acute mastitis, it is combined with *Trichosanthis Fructus* (gua lou), *Lonicerae Japonicae Flos* (jin yin hua) and *Taraxaci Herba* (pu gong ying).

同用。治乳房胀痛,可与柴胡、白芍等同用。治乳痈初起,多与瓜蒌、金银花、蒲公英等同用。

(2) Food retention due to qi stagnation. The medicinal herb acts to digest food and dissolve stasis. In the treatment of indigestion, distension and fullness at epigastria and abdomen, it is combined with *Crataegi Fructus* (shan zha), *Hordei Fructus Germinatus* (mai ya) and *Massa Medicata Fermentata* (shen qu), to form up Green Tangerine Peel Pills (Qing Pi Wan).

(2) 食积气滞证。本品善消积化滞且力强。治食积不化,脘腹胀满,可与山楂、麦芽、神曲等同用,如青皮丸。

Usage and dosage　Apply 3～10 g in decoction. It acts to break qi clump and dissolve stasis in crude form, while it is attributive to liver and acts to soothe liver and stop pain in prepared form with vinegar.

用法用量　煎服,3～10克。生用破气、消积。醋制入肝,疏肝止痛力强。

Precautions for use　It is cautious to apply for those with qi deficiency.

使用注意　气虚者慎用。

Remarks　*Citri Reticulatae Pericarpium* (chen pi) and *Citri Reticulatae Pericarpium Viride* (qing pi)

按语　陈皮与青皮

Both the medicinal herbs are the products from *Citrus reticuta* Blanco, family Rutaceae. *Pericarpium Citri Tangerinae* (chen pi) is the product from the ripe pericarp, while *Pericarpium Citri Reticulatae Viride* (qing pi) is the product from the unripe fruit or its pericarp. Chen pi is attributive to the Lung and Spleen Meridians, and acts to regulate qi

二药均来源于芸香科橘。不同的是陈皮药用成熟果实果皮,青皮药用未成熟幼果或未成熟果实果皮。陈皮入肺脾经,药性和缓,能理气健脾、燥湿化痰;青皮入肝胆经,药性峻急,能破气疏

flow, strengthen spleen, desiccate damp and dissolve phlegm. Qing pi is attributive to the Liver and Gallbladder Meridians, and acts to break qi clump, soothe liver, digest food and dissolve stasis.

肝、消积化滞。

Aurantii Fructus Immaturus (zhi shi)

枳实

It is the dried product from the young fruit of *Citrus aurantium* L., or *Citrus wilsonii* Tana ka, and similar varietal species by cultivation, family Rutaceae. The medicinal herb is collected in May and June, cut into slices applied in crude form or prepared form by frying with wheat bran.

为芸香科植物酸橙及其栽培变种或甜橙的干燥幼果。5～6月采收。切片，生用或麸炒用。

Features Flavor: bitter and pungent. Property: slightly cold. Meridian tropism: the Spleen Meridian and the Stomach Meridian.

性味归经 苦、辛，微寒。归脾、胃经。

Actions Break qi clump, digest food, dissolve phlegm and dissipate masses.

功效 破气消积，化痰除痞。

Application

应用

(1) Food retention due to qi stagnation manifested by distension and fullness at epigastria and abdomen. The medicinal herb acts to break qi clump, digest food, relieve distension and dissolve stasis. In the treatment of food retention due to indigestion manifested by distension and fullness at epigastria and abdomen, it is combined with *Crataegi Fructus* (shan zha) and *Hordei Fructus Germinatus* (mai ya). In the treatment of constipation due to heat accumulation manifested by pain, distension and fullness at abdomen, it is combined with *Magnoliae Officinalis Cortex* (hou po) and *Rhei Radix et Rhizoma* (da huang), to form up Minor Purgative Decoction (Xiao Cheng Qi Tang). In the treatment of dysentery and tenesmus due to damp-heat, it is combined with *Scutellariae Radix* (huang

（1）食积气滞，脘腹胀满。本品长于破气消积、除胀导滞。治食积不化，脘腹胀满，可与山楂、麦芽等同用。治热结便秘的腹痛胀满，可与厚朴、大黄等同用，如小承气汤。治湿热泻痢后重，可与黄芩、黄连、茯苓等同用，如枳实导滞丸。

qin), *Coptidis Rhizoma* (huang lian) and *Poria* (fu ling), to form up Immature Citrus Stagnation-Abducing Pills (Zhi Shi Dao Zhi Wan).

(2) Phlegm blockage and qi stagnation pattern. The medicinal herb acts to break qi clump, dissolve phlegm and dissipate masses, applied to treat phlegm blockage and qi stagnation pattern. In the treatment of phlegm blocking chest yang manifested by chest pain and cardiac pain, it is combined with *Alli Macrostemi Bulbus* (xie bai), *Cinnamomi Ramulus* (gui zhi) and *Trichosanthis Fructus* (gua lou), to form up Immature Citrus, Longstaner Onion Bulb and Cinnamon Decoction (Zhi Shi Xie Bai Gui Zhi Tang). In the treatment of phlegm-heat accumulating in chest, it is combined with huang lian, gua lou and *Pinelliae Rhizoma* (ban xia), to form up Minor Chest-Bind with Immature Citrus Added Decoction (Xiao Xian Xiong Jia Zhi Shi Tang).

(2) 痰阻气滞证。本品能破气化痰、以除痞满，善治痰阻气滞证。治痰阻胸阳的胸痹心痛，常与薤白、桂枝、瓜蒌等同用，如枳实薤白桂枝汤。治痰热结胸，可与黄连、瓜蒌、半夏同用，即小陷胸加枳实汤。

Furthermore, the medicinal herb is applied to treat prolapse of internal organs.

此外，本品还可用于治疗脏器下垂。

Usage and dosage Apply 3～10 g in decoction. It is strong to break qi clump in crude form, while its action is moderate after frying with wheat bran.

用法用量 煎服，3～10克。生用破气力强，麸炒后药性较缓。

Appendix *Aurantii Fructus* (zhi qiao)

It is the dried product from the unripe fruit of *Citrus aurantium* L. and similar varietal species by cultivation, family Rutaceae. The medicinal herb is bitter, pungent and sour in flavor, slightly cold in property, and attributive to the Spleen Meridian and the Stomach Meridian. It acts to regulate qi flow, dilate middle energizer, move qi and relieve distension, applied to treat qi stagnation in chest

附药 枳壳

为酸橙或其栽培变种的未成熟果实。味苦、辛、酸，性微寒，归脾、胃经，功能理气宽中、行气消胀，适用于胸胁气滞、胀满疼痛、食积不化、痰饮内停、内脏下垂等。煎服。3～10克。孕妇慎用。

and hypochondria, distension, fullness and pain, food retention due to indigestion, internal accumulation of phlegm-rheum and prolapse of internal organs. Apply 3～10 g in decoction. It is cautious to apply for pregnant women.

Remarks *Aurantii Fructus Immaturus* (zhi shi) and *Aurantii Fructus* (zhi qiao)

Both *Aurantii Fructus Immaturus* (zhi shi) and *Aurantii Fructus* (zhi qiao) are from the same source with similar actions. Zhi shi is stronger in moving qi with drastic action, as the herb to break qi clump. Zhi qiao is weaker in moving qi with moderate action, as the herb to move qi and relieve distension.

按语 枳实与枳壳

二药来源相同，功效相似。枳实行气力强，药性峻急，为破气之品。枳壳行气力弱，药性和缓，为行气除胀之品。

Aucklandiae Radix (mu xiang)

木香

It is the dried product from the root of *Aucklandia lappa* Decne., family Compositae. The medicinal herb is mainly produced in Yunnan Province, and collected in autumn and winter. It is applied in crude form or prepared form by roasting.

为菊科植物木香的干燥根。主产于云南。秋、冬季采挖。生用或煨用。

Features Flavor: pungent and bitter. Property: warm. Meridian tropism: the Spleen Meridian, the Stomach Meridian, the Large Intestine Meridian, the Triple Energizer Meridian and the Gallbladder Meridian.

性味归经 辛、苦，温。归脾、胃、大肠、三焦、胆经。

Actions Move qi, stop pain, strengthen spleen and digest food.

功效 行气止痛，健脾消食。

Application

(1) Spleen-stomach qi stagnation pattern. The medicinal herb is pungent, dispersing, warm and dredging, and acts to move qi and relieve pain, in the treatment of spleen-stomach qi stagnation pattern manifested by distension and fullness at epi-

应用

（1）脾胃气滞证。本品辛散温通，能行气止痛，尤善治脾胃气滞，症见脘腹胀满、食欲不振，可与枳壳、川楝子等同用。治脾虚气滞、脘腹

gastria and abdomen, and poor appetite, it is combined with *Aurantii Fructus* (zhi qiao) and *Toosendan Fructus* (chuan lian zi). In the treatment of spleen deficiency with qi stagnation pattern manifested by distension and fullness at epigastria and abdomen, poor appetite and loose feces, it is combined with *Codonopsis Radix* (dang shen), *Atractylodis Macrocephalae Rhizoma* (bai zhu) and *Amomi Fructus* (sha ren), to form up Costus Root and Amomum with Six Nobles Decoction (Xiang Sha Liu Jun Zi Tang).

胀满、食少便溏,可与党参、白术、砂仁等同用,如香砂六君子汤。

(2) Diarrhea, dysentery and tenesmus. The medicinal herb is attributive to the Large Intestine Meridian and acts to relieve qi stagnation in large intestine. In the treatment of diarrhea and dysentery due to damp-heat, it is combined with *Coptidis Rhizoma* (huang lian), to form up Aucklandia and Coptis Pills (Xiang Lian Wan), or combined with *Arecae Semen* (bing lang) and *Aurantii Fructus Immaturus* (zhi shi), to form up Aucklandia and Areca Nut Pills (Mu Xiang Bing Lang Wan).

(2) 泻痢后重。本品入大肠经,能行大肠滞气。治湿热泻痢,可与黄连同用,如香连丸。或与槟榔、枳实等同用,如木香槟榔丸。

(3) Food retention pattern. The medicinal herb acts to move qi, harmonize middle energizer, strengthen spleen and digest food. In the treatment of food retention due to indigestion manifested by poor appetite, it is combined with *Crataegi Fructus* (shan zha) and *Massa Medicata Fermentata* (shen qu).

(3) 食积证。本品能行气调中、健脾消食。治食积不消,不思饮食,可与山楂、神曲等配伍同用。

Furthermore, the medicinal herb is applied to treat hypochondriac pain due to liver qi stagnation or jaundice due to damp-heat.

此外,本品亦能治肝郁胁痛或湿热黄疸。

Usage and dosage Apply 3～10 g in decoction. The medicinal herb acts to move qi in crude form, while acts to stop diarrhea in prepared form

用法用量 煎服,3～10克。生用行气,煨用止泻。

by roasting.

Cyperi Rhizoma (xiang fu)

香附

It is the dried product from the rhizome of *Cyperus rotundus* L., family Cyperaceae. The medicinal herb is collected in autumn, applied in crude form or prepared form by stir-frying with vinegar.

为莎草科植物莎草的干燥根茎。秋季采挖。生用或醋炙用。

Features Flavor: pungent, slightly bitter and slightly sweet. Property: neutral. Meridian tropism: the Liver Meridian, the Spleen Meridian and the Triple Energizer Meridian.

性味归经 辛、微苦、微甘,平。归肝、脾、三焦经。

Actions Soothe liver, relieve stagnation, regulate qi flow, dilate middle energizer, regulate menstruation and stop pain.

功效 疏肝解郁,理气宽中,调经止痛。

Application

应用

(1) Liver qi stagnation pattern. The medicinal herb is attributive to the Liver Meridian and acts to soothe liver, relieve stagnation and stop pain. In the treatment of liver qi stagnation pattern manifested by hypochondriac pain, it is combined with *Bupleuri Radix* (chai hu) and *Paeoniae Radix Alba* (bai shao) to form up Bupleurum Liver-Soothing Powder (Chai Hu Shu Gan San). In the treatment of distending pain at breasts, it is combined with *Folium Citri Reticulatae* (ju ye) and *Curcumae Radix* (yu jin). In the treatment of lower abdomen pain due to hernia, it is combined with *Linderae Radix* (wu yao) and *Foeniculi Fructus* (xiao hui xiang).

(1) 肝郁气滞证。本品性平入肝,擅长疏肝解郁、止痛。治肝郁胁痛,可与柴胡、白芍等同用,如柴胡疏肝散。治乳房胀痛,可与橘叶、郁金等同用。治疝气疼痛,可与乌药、小茴香等同用。

(2) Spleen-stomach qi stagnation pattern. The medicinal herb acts to regulate qi flow and dilate middle energizer. In the treatment of spleen-stomach qi stagnation pattern manifested by distension

(2) 脾胃气滞证。本品亦能理气宽中。治脾胃气滞,脘腹胀满,可与陈皮、枳壳等同用。

and fullness at epigastria and abdomen, it is combined with *Citri Reticulatae Pericarpium* (chen pi) and *Aurantii Fructus* (zhi qiao).

(3) Irregular menstruation, amenorrhea and dysmenorrhea. The medicinal herb, termed as "the major herb for gynecology", acts to soothe liver, promote qi flow, regulate menstruation and stop pain. In the treatment of liver qi stagnation pattern manifested by irregular menstruation, abdominal pain in menstruation, or amenorrhea, it is combined with *Angelicae Sinensis Radix* (dang gui), chai hu and *Chuanxiong Rhizoma* (chuan xiong).

（3）月经不调，经闭痛经。本品为"女科之主帅"，既疏肝行气，又调经止痛，为调经常用。治肝郁月经不调、经行腹痛或经闭等证，常与当归、柴胡、川芎同用。

Usage and dosage　Apply 6～10 g in decoction.

用法用量　煎服，6～10克。

Linderae Radix (wu yao)

乌药

It is the dried product from the tuber of *Lindera aggregata* (Sims) Kosterm., family Lauraceae. The medicinal herb is collected all over the year, applied in crude form.

为樟科植物乌药的干燥块根。全年均可采挖。生用。

Features　Flavor: pungent. Property: warm. Meridian tropism: the Lung Meridian, the Spleen Meridian, the Kidney Meridian and the Bladder Meridian.

性味归经　辛，温。归肺、脾、肾、膀胱经。

Actions　Move qi, stop pain, warm kidney and eliminate cold.

功效　行气止痛，温肾散寒。

Application

应用

(1) Cold congealing and qi stagnation pattern. The medicinal herb is warm in property and acts to move qi, eliminate cold and stop pain. In the treatment of cold congealing and qi stagnation pattern manifested by stuffy chest and hypochondriac pain, it is combined with *Alli Macrostemi Bulbus* (xie bai), *Pericarpium Trichosanthis* (gua lou pi) and

（1）寒凝气滞证。本品性温，善行气散寒止痛。治寒凝气滞的胸闷、胁痛，可与薤白、瓜蒌皮、延胡索等同用。治脘腹胀痛，可与木香、枳壳等同用。治寒疝腹痛，配伍小茴香、青皮等同用，如天台乌

Corydalis Rhizoma (yan hu suo). In the treatment of distending pain at epigastria and abdomen, it is combined with *Aucklandiae Radix* (mu xiang) and *Aurantii Fructus* (zhi qiao). In the treatment of abdominal pain due to cold-type hernia, it is combined with *Foeniculi Fructus* (xiao hui xiang) and *Citri Reticulatae Pericarpium Viride* (qing pi), to form up Tian Tai Lindera Powder (Tian Tai Wu Yao San). In the treatment of abdominal pain in menstruation, it is combined with *Cyperi Rhizoma* (xiang fu), *Angelicae Sinensis Radix* (dang gui) and *Chuanxiong Rhizoma* (chuan xiong).

药散。治经行腹痛,可与香附、当归、川芎等同用。

(2) Enuresis and frequency of urination. The medicinal herb acts to warm kidney, eliminate cold, astringe urine and stop enuresis. In the treatment of deficiency and cold in bladder manifested by frequency of urination and enuresis, it is combined with *Alpiniae Oxyphyllae Fructus* (yi zhi) and *Dioscoreae Rhizoma* (shan yao), to form up Spring-Reducing Pills (Suo Quan Wan).

（2）遗尿尿频。本品能温肾散寒、缩尿止遗。治膀胱虚寒所致的尿频、遗尿,常与益智仁、山药等同用,如缩泉丸。

Usage and dosage Apply 6～10 g in decoction.

用法用量 煎服,6～10克。

Aquilariae Lignum Resinatum (chen xiang)

沉香

It is dried product from the dark brown resinous wood of *Aquilaria sinensis* (Lour) Gilg, family Thymelaeaceae. The medicinal herb is collected all over the year and applied to cut the resinous part from the wood, remove the non-resinous part and dry in shade. It is cut into small pieces and smashed or ground into powder, applied in crude form.

为瑞香科植物白木香含有树脂的木材。全年均可采收。割取含树脂的木材,除去不含树脂的部分,阴干。劈成小块,捣碎或锉末。生用。

Features Flavor: pungent and bitter. Property: slightly warm. Meridian tropism: the Spleen Meridian, the Stomach Meridian and the Kidney

性味归经 辛、苦,微温。归脾、胃、肾经。

Meridian.

Actions Move qi, stop pain, warm middle energizer, stop vomiting, accept qi and soothe panting.

功效 行气止痛，温中止呕，纳气平喘。

Application

应用

(1) Cold congealing and qi stagnation pattern. The medicinal herb is pungent, fragrant, warm and dredging, and acts to eliminate yin-cold in chest and abdomen. In the treatment of cold congealing and qi stagnation pattern manifested by distending pain at chest and abdomen, it is combined with *Linderae Radix* (wu yao), *Aucklandiae Radix* (mu xiang) and *Arecae Semen* (bing lang), to form up Chinese Eaglewood Four Smalls Decoction (Chen Xiang Si Mo Tang).

(1) 寒凝气滞证。本品辛香温通，能祛除胸腹阴寒。治寒凝气滞的胸腹胀痛，常与乌药、木香、槟榔等同用，如沉香四磨汤。

(2) Cold in stomach manifested by vomiting and hiccup. The medicinal herb acts to warm middle energizer, eliminate cold, subdue up-reverse flowing qi and stop vomiting. In the treatment of cold in stomach manifested by vomiting and hiccup, it is combined with *Citri Reticulatae Pericarpium* (chen pi), *Semen Amomi Fructus Rotundus* (bai dou kou) and *Kaki Calyx* (shi di).

(2) 胃寒呕吐呃逆。本品能温中散寒、降逆止呕。治胃寒呕吐、呃逆，可与陈皮、白豆蔻、柿蒂等同用。

(3) Panting pattern of deficiency type. The medicinal herb acts to warm kidney, eliminate cold, accept qi and soothe panting. In the treatment of kidney deficiency manifested by panting, it is combined with *Cinnamomi Cortex* (rou gui), *Aconiti Lateralis Radix Praeparata* (fu zi) and *Psoraleae Fructus* (bu gu zhi). In the treatment of upper excess and lower deficiency pattern manifested by cough and panting due to phlegm-rheum, it is combined with *Perillae Folium* (zi su zi), *Pinelliae Rhizoma* (ban xia) and chen pi.

(3) 虚喘证。本品能温肾散寒、纳气平喘。治肾虚气喘，可与肉桂、附子、补骨脂等同用。治上盛下虚的痰饮咳喘，常与紫苏子、半夏、陈皮等同用。

Usage and dosage Apply 1～5 g in decoction

用法用量 煎服，1～5

and decoct it later.

克。宜后下。

Precautions for use It is prohibited to apply for those with qi deficiency and sinking or those with yin deficiency with fire hyperactivity.

使用注意 气虚下陷，阴虚火旺者忌用。

***Toosendan Fructus* (chuan lian zi)**

川楝子

It is the dried product from the ripe fruit of *Melia toosendan* Sieb. et Zucc., family Meliaceae. The medicinal herb is mainly produced in Sichuan Province and collected in winter. It is applied in crude form or prepared form by frying.

为楝科植物川楝的干燥成熟果实。主产于四川。冬季采收。生用或炒用。

Features Flavor: bitter. Property: cold and slightly poisonous. Meridian tropism: the Liver Meridian, the Small Intestine Meridian and the Bladder Meridian.

性味归经 苦，寒；有小毒。归肝、小肠、膀胱经。

Actions Move qi, stop pain, soothe liver, reduce heat and kill worms.

功效 行气止痛，疏肝泄热，杀虫。

Application

应用

(1) Liver stagnation transforming to fire pattern. The medicinal herb is bitter and cold in property and acts to move qi, stop pain, soothe liver and reduce heat. In the treatment of liver stagnation transforming to fire pattern or disharmony between liver and stomach manifested by distending pain at chest, hypochondria, epigastria or abdomen, it is combined with *Corydalis Rhizoma* (yan hu suo), to form up Melia Toosendan Powder (Jin Ling Zi San).

(1) 肝郁化火证。本品苦寒，能行气止痛、疏肝泄热。治肝郁化火或肝胃不和所致的胸胁、脘腹胀痛，常与延胡索同用，如金铃子散。

(2) Abdominal pain due to parasites. The medicinal herb acts to kill worms and stop pain. In the treatment of abdominal pain due to parasites, it is combined with *Arecae Semen* (bing lang).

(2) 虫积腹痛。本品能杀虫、止痛，治虫积腹痛常与槟榔等同用。

Furthermore, the medicinal herb is baked and ground into powder, then made into soft ointment to treat tinea capitis for external use.

此外，本品焙黄研末，制为软膏涂敷，治头癣。

Usage and dosage Apply 5～10 g in decoction. Apply a proper amount for external use. The medicinal herb acts to move qi, soothe liver and reduce heat in crude form, while it is to modify its bitter and cold property after stir-frying.

用法用量 煎服，5～10克。外用适量。生用行气、疏肝泄热，炒用苦寒之性得减。

Precautions for use It is cautious to apply for those with deficiency and cold in spleen and stomach. It is not advisable to apply it in overdose or in continuity.

使用注意 脾胃虚寒者慎用。不宜过量或持续服用。

Citri Saroodactylis Fructus (fo shou)

佛手

It is the dried product from the fruit of the *Citrus medica* L. var. *sarcodactuy* Swingle, family Rutaceae. The medicinal herb is collected in autumn when the fruits are not turning yellow or just turning yellow, applied in crude form.

为芸香科植物佛手的干燥果实。秋季果实尚未变黄或刚变黄时采收。生用。

Features Flavor: pungent, bitter and sour. Property: warm. Meridian tropism: the Liver Meridian, the Spleen Meridian, the Stomach Meridian and the Lung Meridian.

性味归经 辛、苦、酸，温。归肝、脾、胃、肺经。

Actions Soothe liver, relieve depression, regulate qi flow, harmonize middle energizer, desiccate damp and dissolve phlegm.

功效 疏肝解郁，理气和中，燥湿化痰。

Application

应用

(1) Liver qi stagnation pattern. The medicinal herb is pungent and dispersing, bitter and draining, and acts to soothe liver, relieve depression, promote qi flow and stop pain. In the treatment of liver qi stagnation pattern manifested by hypochondriac pain and stuffy chest, it is combined with *Bupleuri Radix* (chai hu) and *Curcumae Radix* (yu jin).

(1) 肝郁气滞证。本品辛散苦泄，善疏肝解郁、行气止痛。治肝气郁结的胁痛胸闷，常与柴胡、郁金等同用。

(2) Spleen and stomach qi stagnation pattern. The medicinal herb is fragrant and acts to promote qi flow, harmonize stomach, soothe liver and regu-

(2) 脾胃气滞证。本品气味清香，具行气和胃、疏肝理气之功，尤善治肝胃不和、

late qi flow. In the treatment of liver and stomach disharmony pattern or spleen and stomach qi stagnation pattern manifested by distending pain at epigastria and abdomen, nausea and poor appetite, it is combined with *Aucklandiae Radix* (mu xiang), *Amomi Fructus* (sha ren) and *Citri Reticulatae Pericarpium* (chen pi).

脾胃气滞的脘腹胀痛、呕恶纳呆等证,常与木香、砂仁、陈皮等同用。

(3) Cough with excessive sputum. The medicinal herb is bitter and warm to desiccate damp and pungent and fragrant to promote qi flow, and acts to desiccate damp and dissolve phlegm. In the treatment of cough with excessive sputum, stuffy chest pain and hypochondriac pain, it is combined with *Pinelliae Rhizoma* (ban xia) and *Pericarpium Trichosanthis* (gua lou pi).

(3) 咳嗽痰多。本品苦温燥湿,辛香行气,具燥湿化痰之功。治咳嗽痰多,胸闷胁痛,可与半夏、瓜蒌皮等同用。

Usage and dosage Apply 3～10 g in decoction.

用量用法 煎服,3～10克。

Alli Macrostemi Bulbus (xie bai)

薤白

It is the dried product from the bulb of *Allium maerostemon* Bunge, or *Allium chinene* G. Don, family Liliaceae. The medicinal herb is collected in summer and autumn, applied in crude form.

为百合科植物小根蒜或薤的干燥鳞茎。夏、秋季采挖。生用。

Features Flavor: pungent and bitter. Property: warm. Meridian tropism: the Heart Meridian, the Lung Meridian, the Stomach Meridian and the Large Intestine Meridian.

性味归经 辛、苦,温。归心、肺、胃、大肠经。

Actions Activate yang, disperse accumulation, promote qi flow and relieve stagnation.

功效 通阳散结,行气导滞。

Application

应用

(1) Chest pain and cardiac pain. The medicinal herb acts to warm and activate the chest yang and disperse the accumulation due to yin cold and phlegm, the key herb to treat chest Bi (Obturation) Pattern with cardiac pain. In the treatment of chest

(1) 胸痹心痛。本品功善温通胸阳、散阴寒痰凝之结,为治胸痹心痛之要药。常与瓜蒌、半夏、枳实、桂枝等配伍同用。如瓜蒌薤白白

pain and cardiac pain, it is combined with *Trichosanthis Fructus* (gua lou), *Pinelliae Rhizoma* (ban xia), *Aurantii Fructus Immaturus* (zhi shi) and *Cinnamomi Ramulus* (gui zhi), to form up Snakegourd, Longstaner Onion Bulb and Liquor (Gua Lou Xie Bai Bai Jiu Tang), Snakegourd, Longstaner Onion Bulb and Pinellia Decoction (Gua Lou Xie Bai Ban Xia Tang) or Immature Citrus, Longstaner Onion Bulb and Cinnamon Decoction (Zhi Shi Xie Bai Gui Zhi Tang).

酒汤、瓜蒌薤白半夏汤、枳实薤白桂枝汤等。

(2) Stomach and intestine qi stagnation, diarrhea, dysentery and tenesmus. The medicinal herb acts to promote qi flow and relieve stagnation. In the treatment of masses, fullness, distension and pain at epigastria and abdomen, or diarrhea, dysentery and tenesmus, it is combined with the qi-moving and middle energizer-dilating herbs as zhi shi and *Aucklandiae Radix* (mu xiang), or with the heat-clearing and dysentery-stopping herbs as *Coptidis Rhizoma* (huang lian) and *Fraxini Cortex* (qin pi).

（2）胃肠气滞，泻痢后重。本品能行气导滞。治脘腹痞满胀痛或泻痢后重，可与行气宽中的枳实、木香或清热止痢的黄连、秦皮等同用。

Usage and dosage Apply 5～10 g in decoction.

用量用法 煎服，5～10克。

Precautions for use It is cautious to apply for those with qi deficiency but without stagnation, or stomach weakness manifested by poor appetite and garlic odor intolerance.

使用注意 气虚无滞者及胃弱纳呆、不耐蒜味者慎用。

Arecae Semen (bing lang)

槟榔

It is the dried product from the ripe seed of *Areca catechu* L., family Palmae. The medicinal herb is collected from late spring to early autumn when the seeds are ripe, by peeling and taking out seeds, applied in crude form or carbonized form.

为棕榈科植物槟榔的成熟种子。春末至秋初采集成熟果实，剥去果皮，取出种子。生用或炒焦。

Features Flavor: bitter and pungent. Proper-

性味归经 苦、辛，温。

ty: warm. Meridian tropism: the Stomach Meridian and the Large Intestine Meridian.

归胃、大肠经。

Actions Promote qi flow, promote water, dissolve accumulation, kill worms and treat malaria.

功效 行气利水，消积，杀虫，截疟。

Application

应用

(1) Edema and beriberi. The medicinal herb acts to promote qi flow and promote water flow. In the treatment of edema, panting and stuffy chest, it is combined with *Alismatis Rhizoma* (ze xie) and *Akebiae Caulis* (mu tong), to form up Dredging and Excavating Drink (Shu Zao Yin Zi). In the treatment of beriberi due to cold-damp, it is combined with *Chaenomelis Fructus* (mu gua) and *Euodiae Fructus* (wu zhu yu).

（1）水肿，脚气。本品有行气利水之功。治水肿喘满，可与泽泻、木通等同用，如疏凿饮子。治寒湿脚气，常与木瓜、吴茱萸等同用。

(2) Food retention due to indigestion, diarrhea, dysentery and tenesmus. The medicinal herb is attributive to the stomach and intestines and acts to subdue qi, dissolve accumulation, relieve stagnation and eliminate fullness. In the treatment of food retention due to indigestion, diarrhea, dysentery and tenesmus, it is combined with *Aucklandiae Radix* (mu xiang), *Citri Reticulatae Pericarpium Viride* (qing pi) and *Rhei Radix et Rhizoma* (da huang), to form up Aucklandia and Areca Nut Pills (Mu Xiang Bing Lang Wan).

（2）食积不消，泻痢后重。本品善入胃肠，能下气消积，导滞除满。治食积不消、积滞泻痢、里急后重等，常与木香、青皮、大黄等同用，如木香槟榔丸。

(3) Abdominal pain due to parasites. The medicinal herb acts to eliminate and kill various types of intestinal parasites, such as tapeworm, roundworm, Fasciolopsis buski, etc., it is applied singly or combined with other worm-killing herbs.

（3）虫积腹痛。本品对多种肠寄生虫如绦虫、蛔虫、姜片虫等有驱杀作用，可单用，或与其他杀虫药同用。

(4) Malaria. In the treatment of malaria, it is combined with *Artemisiae Annuae Herba* (qing hao) and *Magnoliae Officinalis Cortex* (hou po).

（4）疟疾。本品治疟疾，可与青蒿、厚朴等同用。

Usage and dosage Apply 3～10 g in decoc-

用法用量 煎服，3～10

tion, and apply 30～60 g to eliminate tapeworm and Fasciolopsis buski. The medicinal herb is applied to promote water flow, kill worms and treat malaria in crude form, while applied to dissolve accumulation and relieve stagnation (after being stir-baked to brown).

克。驱绦虫、姜片虫，30～60克。生用利水、杀虫、截疟，炒焦用消积导滞。

Precautions for use It is prohibited to apply for those with spleen deficiency manifested by loose feces, or those with qi deficiency and sinking.

使用注意 脾虚便溏或气虚下陷者忌用。

Appendix *Arecae Pericarpium* (da fu pi)

It is the dried product from the pericarp of Betelnutpalm, *Areca catechu* L., family Palmae. The medicinal herb is pungent in flavor, slightly warm in property, and attributive to the Spleen Meridian, the Stomach Meridian, the Large Intestine Meridian and the Small Intestine. It acts to promote qi flow, dilate middle energizer, move water and dissipate swell, applied to treat damp blockage and qi stagnation manifested by distension and fullness at epigastria and abdomen, edema, beriberi and difficult urination. Apply 5～10 g in decoction.

附药 大腹皮

为棕榈科植物槟榔的干燥果皮。味辛性微温。归脾、胃、大肠、小肠经。功能行气宽中、行水消肿；适用于湿阻气滞、脘腹胀满、水肿、脚气、小便不利。煎服。5～10克。

Kaki Calyx (shi di)

柿蒂

It is the dried product from the persistent calyx of *Diospyros Kaki* Thunb., family Ebenaceae. The medicinal herb is collected in winter when the fruits are ripe, applied in crude form.

为柿树科植物柿干燥宿萼。冬季果实成熟时采摘。生用。

Features Flavor: bitter and astringent. Property: neutral. Meridian tropism: the Stomach Meridian.

性味归经 苦、涩，平。归胃经。

Actions Subdue qi and stop hiccup.

功效 降气止呃。

Application

应用

Hiccup. The medicinal herb is bitter, dispersing and descending, and acts to subdue stomach qi and stop hiccup. In the treatment of hiccup, it is

呃逆证。本品苦泄性降，善降胃气、止呃逆，为治呃逆的要药。可单用，或与

applied singly or combined with *Haematitum* (zhe shi) and *Inulae Flos* (xuan fu hua).

赭石、旋覆花等同用。

Usage and dosage Apply 5～10 g in decoction.

用法用量 煎服，5～10克。

Brief summary

小　结

Both *Citri Reticulatae Pericarpium* (chen pi) and *Aurantii Fructus Immaturus* (zhi shi) act to promote qi flow. Chen pi is bitter and pungent in flavor, warm in property, and attributive to the Spleen and Lung Meridians, and acts to regulate qi flow, strengthen spleen, desiccate damp and dissolve phlegm, applied to treat spleen and stomach qi stagnation, distension and fullness at epigastria and abdomen, and cough with excessive sputum. Zhi shi is bitter and pungent in flavor, slightly cold in property, and attributive to the Spleen and Stomach Meridians, and acts to promote qi flow and break qi clump, to dissolve accumulation, relieve distension and dissolve phlegm, applied to treat food retention with distension and fullness, and phlegm blockage and qi stagnation with painful chest and stuffy chest.

陈皮、枳实，均功能行气。其中陈皮苦辛性温，入脾肺经，长于理气健脾兼以燥湿化痰，凡脾胃气滞、脘腹胀满、咳嗽痰多皆可应用。枳实苦辛微寒，入脾胃经，行气力强，为破气之品，善破气消积除胀、破气消痰，善治食积停滞之胀满，以及痰阻气滞的胸痹、结胸。

All *Citri Reticulatae Pericarpium Viride* (qing pi), *Cyperi Rhizoma* (xiang fu) and *Citri Saroodactylis Fructus* (fo shou) act to soothe liver and promote qi flow, applied to treat liver qi stagnation pattern. Qing pi is warm and acts to soothe liver, break qi clump, dissolve accumulation and relieve stagnation, applied to treat food retention and qi stagnation manifested by distension and fullness at epigastria and abdomen. Xiang fu is neutral in property, and acts to soothe liver, promote qi flow,

青皮、香附、佛手，均能疏肝行气，治肝气郁滞之证。其中青皮性温，为疏肝破气之品，且能消积化滞，治食积气滞，脘腹胀满。香附性平，善疏肝行气、止痛；亦能理气宽中，治脾胃气滞证；还能调经止痛，为调经所常用。佛手性温，既疏肝解郁，又理气和胃，尤善治肝胃不和之证；且

stop pain, regulate qi flow and dilate middle energizer, applied to treat spleen and stomach qi stagnation pattern. It also acts to regulate menstruation and stop pain, applied to treat irregular menstruation and dysmenorrhea. Fo shou is warm in property, and acts to soothe liver, relieve depression, regulate qi flow and harmonize stomach, applied to treat liver and stomach disharmony pattern. It is bitter in flavor and acts to desiccate damp and dissolve phlegm, applied to treat sputum with excessive sputum.

味苦燥湿化痰,治咳嗽痰多。

All *Aucklandiae Radix* (mu xiang), *Linderae Radix* (wu yao) and *Aquilariae Lignum Resinatum* (chen xiang) are warm in property and act to promote qi flow and stop pain. Mu xiang acts to relieve qi stagnation of stomach and intestines, applied to treat spleen and stomach qi stagnation pattern manifested by distension and fullness at epigastria and abdomen, and applied to treat large intestine qi stagnation pattern manifested by diarrhea, dysentery and tenesmus. It also acts to strengthen spleen and digest food. Wu yao acts to promote qi flow, eliminate cold and stop pain, applied to treat cold congealing and qi stagnation pattern. It is attributive to lower energizer and acts to disperse cold congealing in lower energizer, warm kidney, eliminate cold, astringe urine and stop enuresis. Chen xiang acts to disperse cold congealing in chest and abdomen, applied to treat cold congealing and qi stagnation pattern manifested by distending pain at chest and abdomen. It also acts to warm middle energizer, eliminate cold, subdue up-reverse flowing qi and stop vomiting, applied to treat stomach cold pattern. It also acts to warm kidney, eliminate

木香、乌药、沉香,均性温,均具行气止痛之功。其中木香善调肠胃气滞,既治脾胃气滞、脘腹胀满,又疗大肠气滞、泻痢后重;还能健脾消食。乌药功善行气散寒止痛,常用治寒凝气滞证;且入下焦,理下焦寒凝,温肾散寒、缩尿止遗。沉香善除胸腹寒凝,治寒凝气滞的胸腹胀痛;又温中散寒、降逆止呕,治胃寒之证;且能温肾散寒、纳气平喘,治肾不纳气之虚喘。

cold, accept qi and soothe panting, applied to treat deficiency-type asthma due to kidney failing to accept qi.

Both *Toosendan Fructus* (chuan lian zi) and *Arecae Semen* (bing lang) act to promote qi flow. Chuan lian zi is bitter in flavor and cold in property, and acts to promote qi flow, stop pain, soothe liver and reduce heat, applied to treat liver stagnation transforming to fire. It also acts to kill worms, applied to treat abdominal pain due to parasites. Bing lang is bitter and pungent in flavor and warm in property, and acts to promote qi flow and water flow, dissolve accumulation, kill worms and treat malaria, applied to treat food retention due to indigestion, diarrhea, dysentery, tenesmus, abdominal pain due to parasites and malaria.

川楝子、槟榔，均能行气。其中川楝子味苦性寒，既行气止痛，又疏肝泄热，常用于肝郁化火证；且能杀虫，治虫积腹痛。槟榔味苦辛性温，既行气又利水，且能消积、杀虫、截疟，治食积不消、泻痢后重，以及虫积腹痛、疟疾等证。

Alli Macrostemi Bulbus (xie bai) is pungent and bitter in flavor and warm in property, and acts to activate yang at chest and dissolve accumulation due to yin-cold, applied to treat chest pain. It also acts to promote qi flow and relieve stagnation, applied to treat stomach-intestine qi stagnation pattern, diarrhea, dysentery and tenesmus.

薤白，味辛苦性温，善通胸中之阳，散阴寒之结，为治胸痹要药；且能行气导滞，治胃肠气滞、泻痢后重。

Kaki Calyx (shi di) is attributive to the Stomach Meridian and acts to subdue stomach qi and stop hiccup. It is neutral in property, applied to treat hiccup caused by various factors.

柿蒂，专入胃经，善降胃气、止呃逆，其性平和，可用治多种病因所致的呃逆证。

Chapter 9 Food-Digesting Herbs

第9章 消食药

The medicinal herbs acting to dissolve accumulation, relieve stagnation and promote digestion are called the food-digesting herbs.

The medicinal herbs are mostly sweet in flavor and neutral in property, and act to digest food, relieve stagnation and strengthen transporting and transforming function of spleen and stomach, applied to treat food retention manifested by distension and fullness at epigastria and abdomen, belching, acid regurgitation, nausea, vomiting, poor appetite and abnormal defecation, and also applied to treat indigestion due to spleen and stomach deficiency.

The causative factors vary in food retention pattern. The medicinal herb are only applied to treat the superficial symptoms, therefore it is advisable to combine the medicinal herbs with other different herbs according to different causes and symptoms. For food retention and qi stagnation pattern, it is advisable to combine with the qi-regulating herbs. For spleen and stomach deficiency and failing to transport and transform, it is advisable to combine with the qi-reinforcing and spleen-strengthening herbs and the middle energizer-harmonizing herbs. For deficiency and cold in middle energizer, it is advisable to combine with the middle energizer-warming and cold-eliminating herbs. For

以消积导滞、促进消化为主要作用的药物,称为消食药。

本类药物大多味甘性平,功能消食导滞、健运脾胃。主要用于饮食积滞所引起的脘腹胀闷、嗳腐吞酸、恶心呕吐、不思饮食、大便失常,以及脾胃虚弱之消化不良等证。

食积停滞证的病因各异,本类药仅为治标之品,故使用本类药物应根据不同的病因或症状作相应的配伍。若食积气滞明显者,配理气药同用。若脾胃虚弱,运化无力者,当配伍补气健脾、和中药同用。若中焦虚寒者,当与温中散寒药同用。湿浊中阻者,可配伍芳香化湿药等。

damp-turbidity blocking middle energizer, it is advisable to combine with the fragrant-flavor and damp-dissolving herbs.

The food-digesting herbs are moderate in actions, but some herbs can consume qi. Therefore, it is not advisable to apply them for too long time, so as to prevent consuming the Zheng (Anti-Pathogenic) Qi.

消食药虽作用缓和，但部分药也有耗气之弊，故不宜过用久服，以免耗伤正气。

Crataegi Fructus (shan zha)

山楂

It is the dried product from the fruit of *Crataegus* Pinnatifida Bge. var. major N. E. Br., or *Crataegus pinnatifida* Bge, family Rosaceae. The meclicinal herb is collected in autumn when the fruits are ripe, anplied in crude form or prepared form by frying.

为蔷薇科植物山里红或山楂的干燥成熟果实。秋季果实成熟时采收。生用或炒用。

Features Flavor: sour and sweet. Property: slightly warm. Meridian tropism: the Spleen Meridian, the Stomach Meridian and the Liver Meridian.

性味归经 酸、甘，微温。归脾、胃、肝经。

Actions Digest food, strengthen spleen, promote qi flow, dissipate stagnation, dissolve turbidity and reduce lipid.

功效 消食健脾，行气散瘀，化浊降脂。

Application

(1) Meat-type food retention. The medicinal herb acts to relieve accumulation and stagnation and strengthen spleen and stomach. In the treatment of meat-type food retention, it is applied singly and combined with other food-digesting herbs. In the treatment of food retention with distension and fullness at epigastria and abdomen, it is combined with the qi-regulating herbs as *Aurantii Fructus* (zhi qiao) and *Aucklandiae Radix* (mu xiang). In the treatment of food retention with abdominal pain and diarrhea, it is applied singly by frying and grinding into powder.

应用

（1）肉食积滞证。本品善消积滞、健脾胃，尤其善消肉食积滞。可单用煎服，或与其他消食积药同用。若食积见脘腹胀满明显者，可与枳壳、木香等行气药同用。若食积见腹痛泄泻者，可单味炒后研末冲服。

(2) Blood stasis pattern. The medicinal herb is attributive to the Xue (Blood) Phase, and acts to promote qi flow, dissolve stasis and stop pain. In the treatment of amenorrhea due to blood stasis, it is combined with *Angelicae Sinensis Radix* (dang gui) and *Carthami Flos* (hong hua). In the treatment of abdominal pain and lochia retention due to blood stasis after delivery, it is combined with *Leonuri Herba* (yi mu cao) and *Chuanxiong Rhizoma* (chuan xiong). In the treatment of chest pain and cardiac pain, it is combined with *Salviae Miltiorrhizae Radix et Rhizoma* (dan shen) and *Cinnamomi Ramulus* (gui zhi). In the treatment of abdominal pain due to hernia, it is combined with the qi-regulating and accumulation-dissolving herbs.

(2) 瘀血证。本品入血分，能行气散瘀、止痛。治瘀滞经闭，可与当归、红花等同用。治产后瘀滞腹痛、恶露不尽，可与益母草、川芎等同用。治胸痹心痛，可与丹参、桂枝等同用。治疝气疼痛，常与行气散结之品同用。

(3) Hyperlipemia. The medicinal herb acts to reduce lipid and dissolve turbidity. In the treatment of hyperlipemia, it is combined with *Alismatis Rhizoma* (ze xie) and *Polygonati Odorati Rhizoma* (yu zhu).

(3) 高脂血症。本品降脂化浊，治高脂血症，可与泽泻、玉竹等同用。

Usage and dosage Apply 9～12 g in decoction. The medicinal herb is applied to digest food, promote qi flow, dissipate stasis, reduce lipid and dissolve turbidity in crude form, while to digest food, dissolve accumulation and stop diarrhea and dysentery after being stir-baked to brown.

用法用量 煎服，9～12克。生用消食行气散瘀、降脂化浊，炒焦消食化积、止泻止痢。

Massa Medicata Fermentata (shen qu)

神曲

It is the product from the mixture of fermented powders of wheat flour, *Armeniacae Amarum Semen*, sprout of *Semen Phaseoli*, *Herba Artmisiae Annuae*, *Fructus Xanthii*, and *Herba Polygoni Hydropiperis*, etc. The mixed product is covered by hemp fimble leaf to keep warm for fermentation for

为面粉和其他药物混合后经发酵而成的加工品，全国各地均产。其制法是以面粉或麸皮与杏仁泥、赤小豆粉，以及鲜青蒿、鲜苍耳、鲜辣蓼自然汁混合搅匀，做成

one week. It is done when the yellow mycelia grows up, then it is dried in the sun, applied in crude form or fried form.

小块，复以麻叶或楮叶，保温发酵一周，长出黄菌丝时取出，晒干即成。生用或炒用。

Features Flavor: sweet and pungent. Property: warm. Meridian tropism: the Spleen Meridian and the Stomach Meridian.

性味归经 甘、辛，温。归脾、胃经。

Actions Digest food and harmonize stomach.

功效 消食和胃。

Application

应用

Food retention. The medicinal herb acts to digest food, strengthen stomach and harmonize middle energizer, often combined with fried *Hordei Fructus Germinatus* (mai ya) and fried *Crataegi Fructus* (shan zha), as "the three carbonized immortals". In the treatment of food retention due to indigestion manifested by distension and fullness at epigastria and abdomen, abdominal pain, diarrhea and dysentery, it is combined with mai ya, shan zha and *Raphani Semen* (lai fu zi), to form up Harmony-Preserving Pills (Bao He Wan). In the treatment of food retention due to spleen deficiency, it is combined with *Codonopsis Radix* (dang shen), *Atractylodis Macrocephalae Rhizoma* (bai zhu) and *Citri Reticulatae Pericarpium* (chen pi).

食积证。本品能消食健胃和中。常与炒麦芽、炒山楂三者习称"焦三仙"。治食积不化、脘腹胀满或腹痛泻痢，常配伍麦芽、山楂、莱菔子等同用，如保和丸。治脾虚食滞，可与党参、白术、陈皮等配伍同用。

Besides, the pills made of minerals and shells are often prepared with shen qu paste, for the purpose to protect spleen and stomach and assist digestion.

此外，含有金石贝壳类的丸药，常以神曲糊丸，以护脾胃、助消化。

Usage and dosage Apply 6～15 g in decoction.

用法用量 煎服，6～15克。

Hordei Fructus Germinatus (mai ya)

麦芽

It is the dried product from the germinant fruit of *Hordeum vulgare* L., family Gramineae. The wheat grains are soaked in water in proper tempera-

为禾本科植物大麦的成熟果实经发芽干燥的炮制加工品。将麦粒用水浸泡后，

ture and humidity. When the germinal sprouts are 5 mm long, they are dried in the sun or in low temperature. The medicinal herb is applied in crude form or fried form.

保持适宜温、湿度，待幼芽长至约 5 毫米时，晒干或低温干燥。生用或炒用。

Features Flavor: sweet. Property: neutral. Meridian tropism: the Spleen Meridian and the Stomach Meridian.

性味归经 甘，平。归脾、胃经。

Actions Promote qi flow, digest food, strengthen spleen, promote appetite, withdraw lactation and relieve distension.

功效 行气消食，健脾开胃，回乳消胀。

Application

应用

(1) Food retention due to indigestion manifested by distending pain at epigastria and abdomen. The medicinal herb acts to promote qi flow, digest food, strengthen spleen and promote appetite. In the treatment of food retention due to indigestion manifested by distension and fullness at epigastria and abdomen and poor appetite, it is applied singly or combined with other food-digesting herbs. In the treatment of food retention due to spleen deficiency manifested by distension and fullness at epigastria and abdomen, it is combined with *Codonopsis Radix* (dang shen), *Atractylodis Macrocephalae Rhizoma* (bai zhu) and *Citri Reticulatae Pericarpium* (chen pi).

（1）食积不化，脘腹胀痛。本品既行气消食，又健脾开胃，常用于食积不化，脘腹胀满、纳呆等证。可单用煎服，亦可与其他消食药同用。若脾虚食积、脘腹胀满者，可与党参、白术、陈皮等同用。

(2) Withdrawal of lactation. The medicinal herb acts to withdraw lactation, applied singly in large dose.

（2）妇女断乳。本品具回乳之功。可用于哺乳期妇女的断乳，单味大剂量煎服即可。

Furthermore, the medicinal herb acts to soothe liver, applied to treat liver qi stagnation pattern manifested by hypochondriac pain or liver-stomach disharmony pattern.

此外，本品具疏肝作用，可治肝郁胁痛及肝胃不和证。

Usage and dosage Apply 10～15 g in decoc-

用法用量 煎服，10～

tion. Apply 60 g to withdraw lactation in fried form. The medicinal herb acts to strengthen spleen, harmonize stomach, soothe liver and promote qi flow in crude form, applied to promote qi flow, digest food and withdraw lactation in fried form, and applied to digest food and dissolve stasis after being stir-baked to brown.

15克。回乳炒用60克。生用健脾和胃、疏肝行气；炒用行气消食回乳；炒焦消食化滞。

Precautions for use It is not advisable to apply for those women in lactation period.

使用注意 哺乳妇女不宜使用。

Raphani Semen (lai fu zi)

莱菔子

It is the dried product from the ripe seed of Garden Radish, *Raphanus sativus* L., family Cruciferae. The medicinal herb is collected in summer, applied in crude form or fried form.

为十字花科植物萝卜的干燥成熟种子。夏季采收。生用或炒用。

Features Flavor: pungent and sweet. Property: neutral. Meridian tropism: the Lung Meridian, the Spleen Meridian and the Stomach Meridian.

性味归经 辛、甘，平。归肺、脾、胃经。

Actions Digest food, relieve distension, subdue qi and dissolve phlegm.

功效 消食除胀，降气化痰。

Application

应用

(1) Food retention and qi stagnation pattern. The medicinal herb acts to digest food, dissolve stasis, promote qi flow and relieve distension. In the treatment of food retention and qi stagnation pattern manifested by distension and fullness at epigastria and abdomen, abdominal pain and diarrhea, it is combined with *Citri Reticulatae Pericarpium* (chen pi), *Crataegi Fructus* (shan zha) and *Massa Medicata Fermentata* (shen qu).

（1）食积气滞证。本品功善消食化积，行气除胀。治食积气滞所致的脘腹胀满、腹痛泄泻等，常与陈皮、山楂、神曲等同用。

(2) Constipation, diarrhea and dysentery due to accumulation and stagnation. The medicinal herb acts to promote qi flow and dissolve accumulation. In the treatment of constipation, it is applied singly

（2）大便秘结，积滞泻痢。本品行气消积力强。治大便秘结，可单味服用，或与通便药同用。治积滞泻痢，

or combined with the defecation-promoting herbs. In the treatment of diarrhea and dysentery due to accumulation and stagnation, it is combined with *Aucklandiae Radix* (mu xiang) and *Coptidis Rhizoma* (huang lian).

可与木香、黄连等同用。

(3) Cough and panting due to phlegm accumulation. The medicinal herb acts to subdue qi and dissolve phlegm. In the treatment of cough and panting due to phlegm accumulation, it is combined with *Sinapis Semen Albae* (bai jie zi) and *Perillae Folium* (zi su zi), to form up Three Seed Filial Devotion Decoction (San Zi Yang Qin Tang).

(3) 痰壅咳喘。本品长于降气化痰。治痰壅咳喘上气，常与白芥子、紫苏子等同用，如三子养亲汤。

Usage and dosage Appy 5～12 g in decoction. The medicinal herb is applied to subdue qi and dissolve phlegm in crude form, while applied to digest food and relieve distension in fried form.

用法用量 煎服，5～12克。生用降气化痰。炒用消食除胀。

Precautions for use It is not advisable to apply for those with weak body and those with spleen deficiency without food retention. It is not advisable to apply together with *Ginseng Radix et Raizoma* (ren shen).

使用注意 体虚者及脾虚无食积者不宜。不可与人参等同用。

Galli Gigerii Endothelium Corneum (ji nei jin)

鸡内金

It is the dried product from the lining membrane of the gizzard of *Gallus gallus domesticus* Brisson, family Phasianidae. The gizzard of fowl is taken out immediately after the fowl is killed. The lining membrane is peeled off, cleaned and dried. The medicinal herb is applied in crude form or fried form.

为雉科动物家鸡的干燥砂囊内壁。杀鸡后，取出鸡肫，立即剥下内壁，洗净，干燥。生用或炒用。

Features Flavor: sweet. Property: neutral. Meridian tropism: the Spleen Meridian, the Stomach Meridian, the Small Intestine Meridian and the Bladder Meridian.

性味归经 甘，平。归脾、胃、小肠、膀胱经。

Actions Digest food, strengthen stomach, astringe essence to stop emission, treat stranguria and dissolve stones.

功效 消食健胃，涩精止遗，通淋化石。

Application

应用

(1) Food retention due to indigestion, infantile malnutrition. The medicinal herb acts to strengthen spleen and stomach, digest food and dissolve accumulation. In the treatment of food retention of mild condition, it is applied singly by grinding into powder. In the treatment of food retention due to indigestion manifested by distension and fullness at epigastria and abdominal, it is combined with *Crataegi Fructus* (shan zha) and *Citri Reticulatae Pericarpium* (chen pi). In the treatment of infantile malnutrition due to spleen deficiency, it is combined with the spleen-strengthening and qi-benefiting herbs and accumulating-dissolving and retention-relieving herbs.

（1）食积不化，小儿疳积。本品能运脾健胃、消食化积，且作用较强。食积轻者，单味研末。食积不化，脘腹胀满者，可与山楂、陈皮等同用。治小儿脾虚疳积，常配伍健脾益气、消积除疳药同用。

(2) Enuresis and seminal emission. The medicinal herb acts to astringe essence to stop emission. In the treatment of seminal emission due to kidney deficiency, it is applied singly by grinding into powder or combined with kidney-reinforcing and essence-astringing herbs. In the treatment of enuresis, it is combined with *Nelumbinis Semen* (lian zi) and *Cuscutae Semen* (tu si zi).

（2）遗精遗尿。本品能涩精止遗。本品焙干研末，或与补肾涩精药同用，治精关不固之遗精。亦治遗尿，可与莲子、菟丝子等同用。

(3) Stones. The medicinal herb acts to treat stranguria and dissolve stones. In the treatment of stranguria due to stones manifested by difficult and painful urination, it is combined with *Lysimachiae Herba* (jin qian cao) and *Lygodii Spora* (hai jin sha). In the treatment of gallstones, it is combined with jin qian cao, *Curcumae Radix* (yu jin) and *Artemisiae Scopariae Herba* (yin chen).

（3）结石证。本品能通淋化石。治石淋涩痛，常与金钱草、海金沙等同用。治胆结石，常与金钱草、郁金、茵陈等同用。

Usage and dosage Apply 3～10 g in decoction, or grind into powder and apply 1.5～3 g each time. The medicinal herb is applied to astringe essence and to dissolve stones in crude form, while applied to digest food and strengthen spleen in fried form which is easier to grind to powder.

用法用量 煎服，3～10克。研末服，每次1.5～3克。生用涩精、化石；炒用消食健脾，且易于研末。

Brief summary

小　结

All *Crataegi Fructus* (shan zha), *Massa Medicata Fermentata* (shen qu), *Hordei Fructus Germinatus* (mai ya), *Raphani Semen* (lai fu zi) and *Galli Gigerii Endothelium Corneum* (ji nei jin) act to digest food, applied to treat all types of food retention.

山楂、神曲、麦芽、莱菔子、鸡内金，均能消食，治食积诸证。

Shan zha acts to treat meat-type food retention, promote qi flow and strengthen spleen. It is also attributive to the Xue (Blood) Phase and acts to promote qi flow, to dissolve stasis and stop pain, applied to treat abdominal pain after delivery due to blood stasis.

其中山楂善消肉食积滞，且能行气健脾；入血分能行气散瘀、止痛，治产后瘀滞腹痛。

Shen qu acts to digest food and harmonize stomach, applied to treat food retention due to indigestion. Its paste is applied in preparation of pills for the purpose to protect spleen and stomach and assist digestion.

神曲善消食和胃，为食积不化证之常用；以此糊丸，有护脾胃、助消化之功。

Mai ya acts to soothe liver, promote qi flow, strengthen spleen and promote appetite, applied to treat food retention due to disharmony between liver and stomach and hypochondriac pain due to liver qi stagnation. It is also applied to withdraw lactation.

麦芽消食兼能疏肝行气、健脾开胃，尤善治肝胃不和之食积不化，亦治肝郁胁痛；还能回乳。

Lai fu zi acts to dissolve accumulation, promote qi flow and relieve distension, applied to treat food

莱菔子善消积行气，尤以行气除胀之功见长，故为

retention and qi stagnation, diarrhea and dysentery due to accumulation and stagnation. It also acts to subdue qi and dissolve phlegm, applied to treat cough and panting due to phlegm accumulation.

治食积气滞、积滞泻痢所常用;还长于降气化痰,治痰壅咳喘。

Ji nei jin acts to strengthen spleen and stomach, digest food and dissolve accumulation, applied to treat food retention due to indigestion and infantile malnutrition. It also acts to astringe essence to stop emission, treat stranguria and dissolve stones, applied to treat seminal emission, enuresis and stones.

鸡内金善运脾健胃、消食化积,既治食积不化,亦治小儿疳积;且能涩精止遗、通淋化石,常用治遗精遗尿,以及结石证。

Chapter 10 Blood-Stanching Herbs

第 10 章 止血药

The medicinal herbs acting to stanch internal and external hemorrhage and applying to treat bleeding patterns are called the blood-stanching herbs.

以制止体内外出血，治疗出血证为主要作用的药物，称为止血药。

The medicinal herbs are attributive to the Xue (Blood) Phase, applied to treat hematemesis, epistaxis, hemoptysis, hematochezia, hematuria, metrorrhagia and metrostaxis, and hemorrhage due to traumatic injury. According to their properties and actions, the medicinal herbs are divided into four types of blood-cooling and blood-stanching herbs, stasis-dissolving and blood-stanching herbs, astringing and blood-stanching herbs and meridian-warming and blood-stanching herbs.

本类药物入血分，可用于吐血、衄血、咳血、便血、尿血、崩漏，以及外伤出血等。根据其药性及功效的不同，可分为凉血止血、化瘀止血、收敛止血、温经止血四类。

The blood-cooling and blood-stanching herbs are mostly cold and cool in property, and act to cool blood, clear heat and stop bleeding, applied to treat bleeding pattern due to heat in blood, manifested by fresh red-colored blood, restlessness, thirst and red tongue body, such as *Cirsii Japonici Radix* (da ji), *Cirsii Herba* (xiao ji), *Sanguisorbae Radix* (di yu), *Sophorae Flos* (huai hua), *Platyclaoi Cacumen* (ce bai ye) and *Imperatae Rhizoma* (bai mao gen).

凉血止血类药性多寒凉，功能凉血分之热、制止出血，主要用于血热妄行的出血证，症见血色鲜红，或伴有烦躁、口渴舌红。如大蓟、小蓟、地榆、槐花、侧柏叶、白茅根。

The stasis-dissolving and blood-stanching herbs are mostly warm or neutral in property, and act to stop bleeding and dissolve stasis, applied to treat

化瘀止血类药性温或平，既止血，又化瘀，功能消散瘀血、制止出血，主要用于

bleeding pattern due to blood stasis, manifested by purple-colored or dark-colored blood, or blood clots, or local pain, such as *Notoginseng Radix et Rhizoma* (san qi), *Rubiae Radix Et Rhizoma* (qian cao) and *Typhae Pollen* (pu huang).

瘀血内阻，以致血不循经的出血证，症见血色紫暗，或有瘀块，或伴有局部疼痛。如三七、茜草、蒲黄。

The astringing and blood-stanching herbs are mostly astringent in flavor and neutral or cool in property, and act to astringe blood and stop bleeding, applied to treat various types of bleeding pattern, such as *Bletillae Rhizoma* (bai ji) and *Agrimoniae Herba* (xian he cao).

收敛止血类药大多味涩，其性多平或凉而不寒，功能收敛止血，可用于各种出血。如白及、仙鹤草。

The meridian-warming and blood-stanching herbs are mostly warm or hot in property, and act to warm meridians, eliminate cold and stop bleeding, applied to treat deficiency-type and cold-type bleeding pattern caused by spleen failing to control blood or debility of Thoroughfare Vessel, manifested by dark-colored or light-colored blood, such as *Artemisiae Argyi Folium* (ai ye) and *Zingiberis Rhizoma Praeparatum* (pao jiang).

温经止血类药性多温热，功能温经散寒、制止出血。主要用于脾不统血，冲脉不固之虚寒性出血，出血色暗且淡。如艾叶、炮姜。

In the application of the blood-cooling and blood-stanching herbs and the astringing and blood-stanching herbs, it is necessary to notice if any stasis exists, so as to avoid production of stasis. In severe bleeding pattern with qi deficiency, it is necessary to reinforce the Yuan (Primary) Qi with the qi-reinforcing herbs.

使用凉血止血和收敛止血药时，应注意有无瘀滞，以免产生留瘀之弊。若出血过多致气虚欲脱，当急固元气，配大补元气之品同用。

Cirsii Japonici Radix (da ji)

It is the dried product from the root and aerial herb of *Cirsium japonicum* Fisch. ex DC., family Compositae. The aerial part of the medicinal herb is collected in summer and autumn when it is flowering, while its root is dug in late autumn, applied in

大蓟

为菊科植物蓟的干燥地上部分或根。夏、秋二季花开时割取地上部分，或秋末挖根。生用或炒炭用。

crude form or carbonized form.

Features Flavor: sweet and bitter. Property: cool. Meridian tropism: the Heart Meridian and the Liver Meridian.

性味归经 甘、苦，凉。归心、肝经。

Actions Cool blood, stanch blood, dissolve stasis, relieve toxin and dissipate carbuncles.

功效 凉血止血，散瘀解毒消痈。

Application

应用

(1) Bleeding pattern due to heat in blood. The medicinal herb is attributive to the Xue (Blood) Phase and acts to cool blood and stanch blood. In the treatment of hematemesis, epistaxis, hemoptysis, hematuria, metrorrhagia and metrostaxis due to heat in blood, it is applied singly in decoction or by smashing its fresh product to take out the juice, or combined with *Cirsii Herba* (xiao ji) and *Platyclaoi Cacumen* (ce bai ye), to form up Ten Ashes Powder (Shi Hui San).

(1) 血热出血证。本品性凉入血分，有凉血止血之效。可用于血热妄行引起的吐衄、咯血、尿血、崩漏等，单用浓煎或鲜品捣汁，或与小蓟、侧柏叶等同用，如十灰散。

(2) Carbuncle and furuncle due to heat-toxin. The medicinal herb acts to dissolve stasis, relieve toxin and dissipate carbuncle. In the treatment of carbuncle, ulcer and furuncle due to heat-toxin, it is applied by smashing its fresh product to take out the juice or by smashing its fresh product for topical application, or combined with other heat-clearing and toxin-relieving herbs.

(2) 热毒疮痈。本品能散瘀解毒消痈。治痈疽疮毒，鲜品捣汁服或外用捣敷，亦可与其他清热解毒药同用。

Usage and dosage Apply 9～15 g in decoction. Apply a proper amount for external use. The medicinal herb acts to cool blood, dissolve stasis and relieve toxin in crude form, while acts to stanch blood in carbonized form.

用法用量 煎服，9～15克。外用适量。生用凉血、散瘀解毒，炒炭止血。

***Cirsii Herba* (xiao ji)**

小蓟

It is the dried product from the whole plant of the perennial herbage, *Cirsium setosum* (Willd.)

为菊科植物刺儿菜的干燥地上部分。夏、秋季花开

MB, family Compositae. The medicinal herb is collected in summer and autumn when it is flowering, applied in crude form or carbonized form.

时采收。生用或炒炭用。

Features Flavor: sweet and bitter. Property: cool. Meridian tropism: the Heart Meridian and the Liver Meridian.

性味归经 甘、苦，凉。归心、肝经。

Actions Cool blood, stanch blood, dissolve stasis, relieve toxin and subside swell.

功效 凉血止血，散瘀解毒消肿。

Application

应用

(1) Bleeding pattern due to heat in blood. Similar to *Cirsii Japonici Radix* (da ji) in cooling blood and stanching blood, it is weaker but acts to promote urination. In the treatment of hematuria and stranguria with bleeding, it is combined with *Platyclaoi Cacumen* (ce bai ye), da ji and *Imperatae Rhizoma* (bai mao gen), *Talcm* (hua shi), to form up Cephalanoplos Drink (Xiao Ji Yin Zi) or Ten Ashes Powder (Shi Hui San).

（1）血热出血证。本品凉血止血功似大蓟而力弱，兼能利尿，尤宜于尿血、血淋，常与侧柏叶、大蓟、白茅根、滑石等同用，如小蓟饮子、十灰散等。

(2) Carbuncle and furuncle due to heat-toxin. The medicinal herb acts to clear heat and to subside swell. It is applied singly in decoction, or by smashing the fresh product for topical application.

（2）热毒疮痈。本品能清热消肿。可单用内服，亦可用鲜品捣烂敷于患处。

Usage and dosage Apply 9～15 g in decoction. Apply a proper amount for external use. The medicinal herb acts to cool blood, dissolve stasis and relieve toxin in crude form, while acts to stanch blood in carbonized form.

用法用量 煎服，9～15克。外用适量。生用凉血、散瘀解毒，炒炭止血。

Sanguisorbae Radix (di yu)

地榆

It is the dried product from the root of the perennial herbage, *Sanguisorba officinalis* L., or *Sanguisorba officinalis* L. var. *Longifolia* (Bert.) Yü et Li, family Rosaceae. The medicinal herb is collected in spring when it is sprouting or in autumn when

为蔷薇科植物地榆或长叶地榆的干燥根。春季将发芽时或秋季植株枯萎时采挖。生用或炒炭用。

it is withered, applied in crude form or carbonized form.

Features Flavor: bitter, sour and astringent. Property: slightly cold. Meridian tropism: the Liver Meridian and the Large Intestine Meridian.

性味归经 苦、酸、涩,微寒。归肝、大肠经。

Actions Cool blood, stanch blood, relieve toxin and astringe carbuncle.

功效 凉血止血,解毒敛疮。

Application

应用

(1) Bleeding pattern due to heat in blood. The medicinal herb is bitter, sour and cold in property and acts to cool blood stanch blood and astringing, often applied to treat bleeding pattern with heat in blood in lower energizer, such as hematochezia, anal bleeding due to hemorrhoids, bloody dysentery, hematuria, metrorrhagia and metrostaxis. In the treatment of hematochezia and anal bleeding due to hemorrhoids, it is combined with *Sophorae Flos* (huai hua) and *Gardeniae Fructus* (zhi zi). In the treatment of dysentery with purulent and bloody feces and tenesmus, it is combined with *Coptidis Rhizoma* (huang lian) and *Aucklandiae Radix* (mu xiang). In the treatment of metrorrhagia and metrostaxis, it is combined with *Rehmanniae Radix* (sheng di huang) and *Scutellariae Radix* (huang qin).

(1) 血热出血证。本品苦酸而寒,有凉血止血、收敛之功,尤多用于便血、痔血、血痢、尿血及崩漏等下焦血热出血之证。治便血、痔血,多配伍槐花、栀子等同用。治下痢脓血、里急后重,可配伍黄连、木香等。治崩漏,常与生地黄、黄芩等同用。

(2) Carbuncle and furuncle due to heat-toxin. The medicinal herb acts to reduce fire and relieve toxin. In the treatment of carbuncle and furuncle in early stage when purulence is not formed, it is applied singly by smashing the fresh product for topical application, or combined with the heat-clearing and toxin-relieving herbs.

(2) 痈疽肿毒。本品具泻火解毒之功。痈疽初起未成脓者,可单用捣敷,或配清热解毒药同用。

(3) Scalding by water, burning by fire, eczema and skin ulcer. The medicinal herb acts to relieve

(3) 水火烫伤,湿疹,皮肤溃烂。本品能解毒敛疮,

toxin and astringe carbuncle, the bey herb to treat scalding by water and burning by fine. In the treatment of scalding by water and burning by fire, it is applied singly by grinding into powder, or combined with *Rhei Radix et Rhizoma* (da huang). In the treatment of eczema and skin ulcer, it is combined with *Sophorae Flavescentis Radix* (ku shen) and da huang in decoction or by taking out the juice for topical application, or combined with calcined *Gypsum Fibrosum* (shi gao) and *Alumen* (bai fan) by grinding into powder and mixing with Vaseline for external use.

尤为治水火烫伤之要药。可单用研末，或配伍大黄同用。治湿疹及皮肤溃烂，可与苦参、大黄同煎，取汁湿敷，或配煅石膏、枯矾研末，加凡士林调涂。

Usage and dosage Apply 9～15 g in decoction. Apply a proper amount for external use. The medicinal herb acts to relicve toxin and astringe carbuncle in crude form, while acts to stanch blood in carbonized form.

用法用量 煎服，9～15克。外用适量。生用解毒敛疮，炒炭止血。

Precautions for use It is not advisable to apply topically in large area burn, so as to prevent massive absorption of tannin so as to cause toxic hepatitis.

使用注意 大面积烧伤，不宜外涂，以防鞣质被大量吸收而引起中毒性肝炎。

Sophorae Flos (huai hua)

槐花

It is the dried product from the flower or bud of *Sophora japonica* L., family Leguminosae. The flower is customarily called "huai hua", while the bud is called "huai mi". The medicinal herb is collected in summer, applied in crude form, fried form or carbonized form.

为豆科植物槐的干燥花及花蕾。前者习称"槐花"，后者称"槐米"。夏季采收。生用或炒用、炒炭用。

Features Flavor: bitter. Property: slightly cold. Meridian tropism: the Liver Meridian and the Large Intestine Meridian.

性味归经 苦，微寒。归肝、大肠经。

Actions Cool blood, stanch blood, purify liver and reduce fire.

功效 凉血止血，清肝泻火。

Application

(1) Bleeding pattern due to heat in blood. The medicinal herb is cool, bitter and descending in property and acts to clear heat in Xue (Blood) Phase, cool blood and stanch blood, more applied to treat bleeding caused by blood heat in lower part. In the treatment of hematemesis and epistaxis, it is combined with *Agrimoniae Herba* (xian he cao) and *Imperatae Rhizoma* (bai mao gen). In the treatment of hematochezia and anal bleeding due to hemorrhoids, it is combined with *Sanguisorbae Radix* (di yu) in mutual reinforcement.

(2) Redness of eyes and headache due to liver fire. The medicinal herb acts to purify liver and reduce fire. It is combined with the heat-clearing herbs, such as *Prunellae Spica* (xia ku cao), *Scutellariae Radix* (huang qin), *Gardeniae Fructus* (zhi zi) and *Chrysanthemi Flos* (ju hua).

Usage and dosage　Apply 5～10 g in decoction. The medicinal herb acts to purify liver and reduce fire in crude form, while acts to stanch blood in fried form or carbonized form.

应用

（1）血热出血证。本品性凉苦降，善清血分之热而凉血止血，尤宜于下部血热出血。治吐血、衄血，常配仙鹤草、白茅根等同用。治便血、痔血，常与地榆相须为用。

（2）肝火目赤、头痛。本品能清肝泻火。常与夏枯草、黄芩、栀子、菊花等清热药同用。

用法用量　煎服，5～10克。生用清肝泻火，炒制或炒炭止血。

Platyclaoi Cacumen (ce bai ye)

It is the dried product from the tender branch and leaf of *Platycladus orientalis*(L.) Franco, family Cupressaceae. The medicinal herb is collected in summer and autumn, applied in crude form and carbonized form.

Features　Flavor: bitter and astringent. Property: cold. Meridian tropism: the Lung Meridian, the Liver Meridian and the Spleen Meridian.

Actions　Cool blood, stanch blood, dissolve phlegm and stop cough.

侧柏叶

为柏科植物侧柏的干燥枝梢及叶。夏、秋季采收。生用或炒炭用。

性味归经　苦、涩，寒。归肺、肝、脾经。

功效　凉血止血，化痰止咳。

Application

(1) Various types of bleeding pattern. The medicinal herb is astringent in property and acts to cool blood and stanch blood. In the treatment of hematemesis and epistaxis due to heat in blood, it is combined with fresh *Rehmanniae Radix* (sheng di huang) and fresh *Artemisiae Argyi Folium* (ai ye), to form up Four Crude Ingredients Pills (Si Sheng Wan). In the treatment of hematochezia, metrorrhagia and metrostaxis, it is combined with *Sophorae Flos* (huai hua) and *Sanguisorbae Radix* (di yu), or with ai ye and *Zingiberis Rhizoma Praeparatum* (pao jiang).

(2) Cough and panting with excessive sputum. The medicinal herb acts to clear heat in lung, dissolve phlegm and stop cough. In the treatment of cough with yellow, sticky and thick sputum due to heat in lung, it is applied singly or combined with *Scutellariae Radix* (huang qin) and *Trichosanthis Fructus* (gua lou).

Furthermore, the medicinal herb is prepared into tincture for external use for the treatment of hair loss and premature grey hair.

Usage and dosage Apply 6～12 g in decoction. Apply a proper amount for external use. The medicinal herb acts to dissolve phlegm and stop cough in crude form, while acts to stanch blood in carbonized form.

应用

（1）各种出血证。本品具有凉血止血之功，味涩兼能收敛。治血热吐血、衄血，常与鲜生地黄、鲜艾叶等同用，如四生丸。治便血或崩漏，可与槐花、地榆或艾叶、炮姜等同用。

（2）咳喘痰多。本品能清泄肺热，化痰止咳。治肺热咳嗽，痰黄黏稠，可单用或配黄芩、瓜蒌等同用。

此外，本品制成酊剂外涂，还可治脱发及须发早白。

用法用量 煎服，6～12克；外用适量。生用化痰止咳，炒炭止血。

Imperatae Rhizoma (bai mao gen)

It is the dried product from the rhizome of *Imperata cylindrica* Beauv. var. *major* (Nees) C. E. Hubb., family Gramineae. The medicinal herb is collected in spring and autumn, applied in crude

白茅根

为禾本科植物白茅的干燥根茎。春、秋季采挖。生用或炒炭用。

form or carbonized form.

Features Flavor: sweet. Property: cold. Meridian tropism: the Lung Meridian, the Stomach Meridian and the Bladder Meridian.

性味归经 甘，寒。归肺、胃、膀胱经。

Actions Cool blood, stanch blood, clear heat and promote urination.

功效 凉血止血，清热利尿。

Application

应用

(1) Bleeding pattern due to heat in blood. The medicinal herb acts to cool blood and stanch blood. In the treatment of hematemesis, epistaxis and hematuria, it is applied singly in decoction or combined with *Cirsii Japonici Radix* (da ji), *Cirsii Herba* (xiao ji) and *Rubiae Radix Et Rhizoma* (qian cao), to form up Ten Ashes Powder (Shi Hui San).

（1）血热出血证。本品具凉血止血之功。可用于血热妄行所致吐衄、尿血诸证，尤多用于尿血，可单用大量煎服，或配大蓟、小蓟、茜草根等同用，如十灰散。

(2) Stranguria due to heat with difficult and painful urination, edema with scanty urine, and jaundice due to damp-heat. The medicinal herb acts to clear heat and promote urination. In the treatment of stranguria due to heat or stranguira with bleeding, it is combined with *Plantaginis Semen* (che qian zi), *Akebiae Caulis* (mu tong) and *Lysimachiae Herba* (jin qian cao). In the treatment of edema with scanty urine, it is combined with *Poriae Cutis* (fu ling pi) and *Arecae Pericarpium* (da fu pi). In the treatment of jaundice due to damp-heat, scanty and dark urine, it is combined with *Artemisiae Scopariae Herba* (yin chen) and *Gardeniae Fructus* (zhi zi).

（2）热淋涩痛，水肿尿少，湿热黄疸。本品能清热利尿。治热淋或血淋，可与车前子、木通、金钱草等同用。治水肿尿少，可与茯苓皮、大腹皮等同用。治湿热黄疸，小便短赤，可与茵陈、栀子等同用。

Furthermore, the medicinal herb is applied to treat febrile disease manifested by restlessness and thirst, vomiting and hiccup due to heat in stomach, and panting and cough due to heat in lung.

此外，本品还可治热病烦渴，胃热呕逆及肺热喘咳等证。

Usage and dosage Apply 9～30 g in decoction. The medicinal herb acts to cool blood, clear

用法用量 煎服，9～30克。生用凉血、清热利尿，炒

heat and promote urination in crude form, while acts to stanch blood in carbonized form.

炭止血。

Notoginseng Radix et Rhizoma (san qi)

三七

It is the dried product from the root and rhizome of *Panax notoginseng* (Burk.) F. H. Chen, family Araliaceae. The medicinal herb is mainly produced in Yunnan Province, collected in autumn before it is flowering. It is applied in crude form or in powdered form.

为五加科植物三七的干燥根和根茎。主产云南。秋季花开前采挖。生用或研细粉。

Features Flavor: sweet and slightly bitter. Property: warm. Meridian tropism: the Liver Meridian and the Stomach Meridian.

性味归经 甘、微苦,温。归肝、胃经。

Actions Dissolve stasis, stanch blood, subside swell and stop pain.

功效 散瘀止血,消肿定痛。

Application

应用

(1) Various types of bleeding pattern. The medicinal herb acts to stanch blood and dissolve stasis, applied to treat bleeding pattern with blood stasis. In the treatment of various types of external and internal bleeding pattern, it is applied singly for oral administration or external application, or combined with other blood-stanching herbs.

(1) 各种出血证。本品止血作用广泛,又能散瘀,故出血兼瘀者尤为适宜。对体内外各种出血,可单用本品内服或外敷,或配伍其他止血药同用。

(2) Swelling and pain due to traumatic injury, sharp-stabbing pain at chest and abdomen. The medicinal herb acts to activate, dissolve stasis, subside swell and stop pain, as the major herb for traumatic diseases. In the treatment of swelling and pain due to traumatic injury, it is applied singly for oral administration or external application, for oral administration or external application, or combined with other blood-activating herbs. In the treatment of sharp-stabbing pain at chest and abdomen due to blood stasis, it is combined with *Salviae Miltiorrhizae Radix et Rhizoma* (dan shen), *Corydalis*

(2) 跌仆肿痛,胸腹刺痛。本品既活血散瘀,又消肿定痛,尤为伤科要药。治跌仆伤痛,可单用内服或外敷,亦可活血药同用。治瘀滞胸腹刺痛,常与丹参、延胡索、川芎等同用。

Rhizoma (yan hu suo) and *Chuanxiong Rhizoma* (chuan xiong).

Usage and dosage Apply 3～10 g in decoction. Apply 1～3 g of ground powder. Apply a proper amount for external use.

用法用量 煎服，3～10克。研末吞服，每次1～3克。外用适量。

Rubiae Radix Et Rhizoma (qian cao)

茜草

It is the dried product from the root of *Rubia cordifolia* L., family Rubiaceae. The medicinal herb is collected in spring and autumn, applied in crude form or carbonized form.

为茜草科植物茜草的干燥根及根茎。春、秋季采挖。生用或炒炭用。

Features Flavor: bitter. Property: cold. Meridian tropism: the Liver Meridian.

性味归经 苦，寒。归肝经。

Actions Cool blood, stanch blood, dissolve stasis and dredge meridians.

功效 凉血止血，祛瘀通经。

Application

(1) Bleeding pattern due to heat in blood. The medicinal herb acts to cool blood and stanch blood. In the treatment of various types of bleeding pattern due to heat in blood, it is combined with *Platyclaoi Cacumen* (ce bai ye) and *Cirsii Japonici Radix* (da ji).

(2) Amenorrhea due to blood stasis, traumatic injury, and Bi (Obturation) Pattern due to wind-damp. The medicinal herb acts to activate blood and dredge meridians, applied to treat blood stasis pattern in gynecology. In the treatment of amenorrhea due to blood stasis, it is combined with *Carthami Flos* (hong hua), *Angelicae Sinensis Radix* (dang gui) and *Cyperi Rhizoma* (xiang fu). In the treatment of traumatic injury and Bi (Obturation) pattern due to wind-damp, it is applied singly by making into medicinal liquor, or combined with other herbs.

应用

（1）血热出血证。本品能凉血止血。治血热出血诸证，可与侧柏叶、大蓟等同用。

（2）血瘀经闭，跌打损伤，风湿痹痛。本品有活血通经作用，尤宜于妇科血瘀证。治血瘀经闭，常与红花、当归、香附等同用。治跌打损伤、风湿痹痛，可单用泡酒服，或入复方服用。

Usage and dosage Apply 6～10 g in decoction. The medicinal herb acts to activate blood in crude form, while acts to stanch blood in carbonized form.

用法用量 煎服，6～10克。生用活血，炒炭止血。

Typhae Pollen (pu huang)

蒲黄

It is the dried product from the pollen of *Typha angustifolia* L., *Typha orientalis* Presl or other species of the same genus, family Typhaceae. The medicinal herb is collected in summer when it is flowering by collecting and drying the yellow male tassels. It is applied in crude form or carbonized form.

为香蒲科植物水烛香蒲、东方香蒲或同属植物的干燥花粉。夏季采收蒲棒上部的黄色雄花穗，晒干后碾轧筛取花粉。生用或炒炭用。

Features Flavor: sweet. Property: neutral. Meridian tropism: the Liver Meridian and the Heart Meridian.

性味归经 甘，平。归肝、心经。

Actions Stanch blood, dissolve stasis and treat stranguria.

功效 止血，化瘀，通淋。

Application

应用

(1) Various types of bleeding pattern. The medicinal herb acts to dissolve stasis and stanch blood, applied to treat bleeding pattern with blood stasis due to its neutral property. It is applied singly or combined with other herbs according to the causes of bleeding. It is applied to treat bleeding due to wound for external use.

（1）各种出血证。本品能化瘀止血，且性平，应用范围广，尤以出血属夹瘀者为宜。可单用，亦可根据出血原因随证配伍。外敷可治创伤出血。

(2) Amenorrhea, dysmenorrhea, sharp-stabbing pain at chest and abdomen, and swelling and pain due to traumatic injury. The medicinal herb acts to dissolve stasis and stop pain. In the treatment of various types of pain due to blood stasis, it is combined with *Faeces Trogopterorum* (wu ling zhi) for mutual reinforcement, to form up Great Guffaw Powder (Shi Xiao San).

（2）经闭痛经，心腹刺痛，跌打伤痛。本品有良好的化瘀止痛之功。治各种瘀滞作痛，常与五灵脂相须为用，即失笑散。

(3) Stranguria with bleeding. The medicinal

（3）血淋。本品有化瘀、

herb acts to dissolve stasis, promote urination and treat stranguria. In the treatment of stranguria with bleeding manifested by difficult and painful urination, it is combined with *Plantaginis Semen* (che qian zi) and *Akebiae Caulis* (mu tong), to form up Cattail Pollen Powder (Pu Huang San).

利尿通淋之功。对血淋涩痛,可与车前子、木通等同用,如蒲黄散。

Usage and dosage Apply 5～10 g in decoction by wrapping. Apply a proper amount for external use. The medicinal herb acts to dissolve stasis in crude form, and acts to stanch blood in carbonized form.

用法用量 煎服,5～10克。宜布包煎。外用适量。生用化瘀,炒炭止血。

Precautions for use It is cautious to apply for pregnant women.

使用注意 孕妇慎服。

Bletillae Rhizoma (bai ji)

白及

It is the dried product from the tuber of *Bletilla striata* (Thunb.) Reichb. f., family Orchidaceae. The medicinal herb is collected in summer and autumn, applied in crude form.

为兰科植物白及的干燥块茎。夏、秋季采挖。生用。

Features Flavor: bitter, sweet and astringent. Property: slightly cold. Meridian tropism: the Lung Meridian, the Liver Meridian and the Stomach Meridian.

性味归经 苦、甘、涩,微寒。归肺、肝、胃经。

Actions Astringe and stanch blood, subside swell and engender flesh.

功效 收敛止血,消肿生肌。

Application

应用

(1) Various types of bleeding pattern. The medicinal herb is sticky and astringent in property and acts to stanch blood. In the treatment of bleeding of lung and stomach, it is applied singly by grinding into powder and taking with glutinous rice congee, the so-called Solo Sage Powder (Du Sheng San), or combined with other herbs according to the causes of bleeding of lung and stomach. In the treatment

(1) 各种出血证。本品质地黏涩、收敛止血,多用于肺、胃出血,可单味研末,糯米汤调服,即独圣散。或依据肺、胃出血之病因,随证加减。治外伤出血,可单用或配伍煅石膏研末外敷。

of bleeding due to traumatic injury, it is applied singly or combined with calcined *Gypsum Fibrosum* (shi gao) by grinding into powder for external use.

(2) Carbuncle and furuncle due to heat-toxin, scalding by water, burning by fire, anal fissure, and chapped skin at hands and feet. The medicinal herb acts to subside swell, engender flesh and astringe carbuncle. In the treatment of carbuncle and furuncle in early stage, it is applied singly for external use, or combined with *Lonicerae Japonicae Flos* (jin yin hua), *Olibanum* (ru xiang). In the treatment of ulcerated carbuncle and furuncle without healing, it is applied by grinding into powder for external use. In the treatment of scalding by water, burning by fire, anal fissure and chapped skin at hands and feet, it is applied singly by grinding into powder and mixing with sesame oil for external use.

（2）疮疡肿毒，水火烫伤，肛裂、手足皲裂。本品有消肿生肌、敛疮收口之功。治痈肿初起，可单用外敷，或与金银花、乳香等同用。若痈肿已溃，久不收口，可研粉外敷。治水火烫伤、肛裂、手足皲裂，可用白及粉麻油调敷。

Usage and dosage Apply 6～15 g in decoction. Apply 3～6 g powder. Apply a proper amount for external use.

用法用量 煎服，6～15克。研末吞服，3～6 克。外用适量。

Precautions for use It is cautious to apply for those with hemoptysis due to exogenous factors, pulmonary abscess in early stage or heat of excess type in lung and stomach. It is incompatible with *Aconiti Radix* (wu tou) and *Aconiti Lateralis Radix Praeparata* (fu zi).

使用注意 外感咯血、肺痈初起及肺胃实热者慎服。反乌头、附子。

Agrimoniae Herba (xian he cao)

仙鹤草

It is the dried product from the aerial herb of *Agrimonia pilosa* ledeb., family Rosaceae. The medicinal herb is collected in summer and autumn when the stems and leaves are flourishing, applied in crude form.

为蔷薇科植物龙芽草的干燥地上部分。夏、秋季茎叶茂盛时采收。生用。

Features Flavor: bitter and astringent. Prop-

性味归经 苦、涩，平。

erty: neutral. Meridian tropism: the Heart Meridian and the Liver Meridian.

归心、肝经。

Actions Astringe and stanch blood, stop dysentery, reinforce body, treat malaria and relieve toxin.

功效 收敛止血，止痢，补虚，截疟，解毒。

Application

应用

(1) Various types of bleeding pattern. The medicinal herb is astringent and neutral in property and acts to astringe and stanch blood. In the treatment of various types of bleeding pattern, it is applied singly or combined with other herbs according to the causes of bleeding. In the treatment of bleeding pattern due to heat in blood, it is combined with fresh *Rehmanniae Radix* (sheng di huang), *Scrophulariae Radix* (xuan shen) and *Moutan Cortex* (mu dan pi). In the treatment of bleeding pattern due to false cold, it is combined with *Folium Artemisiae Aygyi* (ai ye) and *Zingiberis Rhizoma Praeparatum* (pao jiang).

（1）多种出血证。本品味涩、性平，有收敛止血之功，可用于各种出血证。单味应用，或根据出血病因随证配伍。治血热出血，常与鲜生地黄、玄参、牡丹皮等同用。虚寒出血者，则与艾叶、炮姜等同用。

(2) Chronic dysentery. The medicinal herb is astringent in property and acts to stop dysentery. In the treatment of chronic diarrhea or dysentery, it is applied singly.

（2）泻痢日久。本品能收涩止痢。尤宜于久泻久痢，单用即效。

(3) Loss of energy and strains. The medicinal herb acts to strengthen the body. In the treatment of loss of energy and strains manifested by low spirit and lassitude, it is combined with *Fructus Ziziphi Jujubae* (da zao).

（3）脱力劳伤。本品具补虚强壮之功。治脱力劳伤，神疲乏力，可与大枣同用。

(4) Malaria. The medicinal herb acts to treat malaria and kill worms. In the treatment of malaria, it is applied singly.

（4）疟疾。本品能截疟、杀虫。治疟疾可单用。

(5) Carbuncle and furuncle due to heat-toxin, and pruritus vulvae. The medicinal herb acts to relieve toxin and kill worms. In the treatment of carbuncle and furuncle due to heat-toxin, it is applied

（5）痈肿疮毒，外阴瘙痒。本品能解毒、杀虫。治疮疖痈肿，可外用，亦可内服。治外阴瘙痒，煎汤外洗，

for external use or oral administration. In the treatment of pruritus vulvae, it is applied by decocting and washing for the purpose to kill worms and stop itching.

能杀虫止痒。

Usage and dosage Apply 6～12 g in decoction. Apply a proper amount for external use.

用法用量 煎服，6～12克。外用适量。

Artemisiae Argyi Folium (ai ye)

艾叶

It is the dried product from the leaf of *Artemisia argyi* levl. et Vant., family Compositae. The medicinal herb is collected in early summer before it is flowering, applied in crude form or carbonized form.

为菊科植物艾的干燥叶。夏初花未开采摘。生用或炒炭用。

Features Flavor: pungent and bitter. Property: warm and slightly poisonous. Meridian tropism: the Liver Meridian, the Spleen Meridian and the Kidney Meridian.

性味归经 辛、苦，温；有小毒。归肝、脾、肾经。

Actions Warm meridians, stanch blood, eliminate cold and stop pain, and dissolve damp and stop itching for external use.

功效 温经止血，散寒止痛，外用祛湿止痒。

Application

应用

(1) Bleeding pattern due to false cold. The medicinal herb is warm in property and acts to warm meridians and stanch blood, applied to treat bleeding pattern due to false cold. In the treatment of metrorrhagia and metrostaxis, threatened miscarriage, it is combined with *Rehmanniae Radix Praeparata* (shu di huang) and *Asini Corii Colla* (e jiao), to form up Donkey-Hide Gelatin and Mugwort Leaf Decoction (Jiao Ai Tang).

（1）虚寒性出血证。本品性温，能温经止血，尤宜于虚寒性出血。治崩漏下血、妊娠胎漏，常与熟地黄、阿胶等同用，如胶艾汤。

(2) Abdominal pain due to false cold. The medicinal herb acts to warm meridians, eliminate damp and stop pain. In the treatment of false cold pattern manifested by irregular menstruation and abdominal

（2）虚寒性腹痛。本品能温经脉、逐散湿、止疼痛。治虚寒所致的月经不调、经行腹痛，可与当归、肉桂等同

pain during menstruation, it is combined with *Angelicae Sinensis Radix* (dang gui) and *Cinnamomi Cortex* (rou gui). In the treatment of false cold in spleen and stomach manifested by cold pain at abdomen, it is combined with *Zingiberis Rhizoma* (gan jiang) and *Citri Reticulatae Pericarpium* (chen pi).

用。治脾胃虚寒引起的腹中冷痛,可与干姜、陈皮等同用。

(3) Skin itch. The medicinal herb acts to dissolve damp and stop itching for external use. In the treatment of skin itch, it is applied singly or combined with *Phellodendri Cortex Chiensis* (huang bo), *Zanthoxyli Pericarpium* (hua jiao) and *Saposhnikoviae Radix* (fang feng), or combined with *Alumen* (bai fan) by grinding into powder for external use.

(3) 皮肤瘙痒。本品外用祛湿止痒。治皮肤瘙痒,可单用或与黄柏、花椒、防风等煎水外洗,或配枯矾研末外敷。

Usage and dosage Apply 3～9 g in decoction. The medicinal herb acts to eliminate cold, stop pain, dissolve damp and stop itching in crude form, and acts to warm meridians and stanch blood in carbonized form stir-fried by vinegar. Apply a proper amount for external use.

用法用量 煎服,3～9克。生用散寒止痛、祛湿止痒,醋制炒炭温经止血。外用适量。

Zingiberis Rhizoma Praeparatum (pao jiang)

炮姜

It is the dried product from the prepared rhizome of *Zingiber officinale* Rosc., family Zingiberaceae.

为干姜的炮制加工品。

Features Flavor: pungent. Property: hot. Meridian tropism: the Spleen Meridian, the Stomach Meridian and the Kidney Meridian.

性味归经 辛,热。归脾、胃、肾经。

Actions Warm meridians, stanch blood, warm middle energizer and stop pain.

功效 温经止血,温中止痛。

Application

应用

(1) Bleeding pattern due to false cold. The medicinal herb acts to warm meridians and stanch blood. In the treatment of spleen yang deficiency or

(1) 虚寒性出血证。本品有温经止血作用,为治脾阳亏虚、脾不统血之吐血、便

spleen failing to control blood manifested by hematemesis and hematochezia, it is applied singly by grinding into powder, or combined with carbonized *Artemisiae Argyi Folium* (ai ye), carbonized *Platyclaoi Cacumen* (ce bai ye) and carbonized *Mume Fructus* (wu mei).

血的要药。可单用为末服之,亦可与艾叶炭、侧柏炭、乌梅炭等同用。

(2) Abdominal pain and diarrhea due to false cold. The medicinal herb acts to warm middle energizer and stop pain. In the treatment of false cold in middle energizer or disharmony between spleen and stomach manifested by abdominal pain, vomiting and diarrhea, it is applied singly or combined with *Ginseng Radix et Raizoma* (ren shen) and *Atractylodis Macrocephalae Rhizoma* (bai zhu).

(2) 虚寒腹痛腹泻。本品能温中止痛。治中焦虚寒,脾胃不和,腹痛吐泻,单用即效,或与人参、白术等同用。

Usage and dosage Apply 3～6 g in decoction. Apply a proper amount for external use.

用法用量 煎服,3～6克。外用适量。

Remarks *Zingiberis Rhizoma Recens* (sheng jiang), *Zingiberis Rhizoma* (gan jiang) and *Zingiberis Rhizoma Praeparatum* (pao jiang)

按语 生姜、干姜与炮姜

All the three medicinal herbs are the products from the rhizome of family Zingberaceae, and act to warm the middle energizer. Sheng jiang, the fresh product, is pungent, dispersing and slightly warm in property, and acts to make sweating and relieve exterior symptoms, applied to treat exterior pattern due to wind-cold, and also acts to relieve toxin in herb, fish and crab. Gan jiang, the dried product, is hot in property and acts to warm the interior, warm middle energizer, eliminate cold, bring back yang, dredge meridians, warm lung and dissolve rheum, as the major herb to treat interior cold pattern. Pao jiang, the prepared product, is pungent and hot in property and attributive to the Xue (Blood) Phase, and acts to warm meridians and

三者均来源于姜科植物姜,均能温中。不同的是生姜为姜的新鲜品,辛散微温,能发汗解表,治疗风寒表证,还能解药物、鱼蟹毒。干姜为姜的干燥品,性热温里,尤善温中散寒,还能回阳通脉、温肺化饮,为治里寒证之要药。炮姜为干姜的炮制品,辛热入血分,能温经止血,善治虚寒出血,且能温中止痛。

stanch blood, applied to treat bleeding pattern due to false cold, and also acts to warm middle energizer and stop pain.

Brief summary

小　结

Both *Cirsii Japonici Radix* (da ji) and *Cirsii Herba* (xiao ji) are sweet and bitter in flavor and cool in property, attributive to the Heart and Liver Meridians, and act to cool blood, stanch blood, dissolve stasis, relieve toxin and dissipate carbuncle, applied to treat bleeding pattern due to heat in blood, carbuncle and furuncle due to heat-toxin. Da ji acts to cool blood, stanch blood, dissolve stasis and dissipate carbuncle. Xiao ji acts to promote urination, applied to treat hematuria and stranguria with bleeding.

大蓟、小蓟，均甘苦性凉，入心、肝经，均有凉血止血、散瘀解毒消痈之功，治疗血热出血证及热毒疮疡。其中大蓟功专凉血止血，散瘀消痈。小蓟兼能利尿，可用治尿血、血淋等证。

Both *Sanguisorbae Radix* (di yu) and *Sophorae Flos* (huai hua) are cool in property and attributive to the Liver and Large Intestine Meridians, and act to cool blood and stanch blood, applied to treat bleeding pattern due to heat in blood. In the treatment of hematochezia and anal bleeding due to hemorrhoids, they are applied in mutual reinforcement. Di yu is astringent in property, applied to treat metrorrhagia, metrostaxis and heavy blood flow in menstruation. It also acts to relieve toxin and astringe carbuncle, as the major herb to treat scalding by water and burning by fire. Huai hua acts to reduce fire in liver, applied to treat headache and redness of eyes due to liver fire.

地榆、槐花，均性凉，入肝、大肠经，均能凉血止血，治血热出血证，尤宜于下部便血、痔血，常相须为用。其中地榆兼收敛之性，又治妇女血热崩漏、月经过多；且能解毒敛疮，为治水火烫伤要药。槐花还善清肝火，治肝火头痛目赤。

Both *Platyclaoi Cacumen* (ce bai ye) and *Imperatae Rhizoma* (bai mao gen) are cold in property and act to cool blood and stanch blood, applied to

侧柏叶、白茅根，均性寒，能凉血止血，治血热出血。其中侧柏叶味苦涩，兼

treat bleeding pattern due to heat in blood. Ce bai ye is bitter and astringent in flavor and astringent in property, and acts to purify lung, dissolve phlegm and stop cough, applied to treat cough with sputum due to heat in lung. Bai mao gen is sweet and cold in property, and acts to clear heat and promote urination, applied to treat stranguria due to heat manifested by difficult and painful urination.

能收敛，且能清肺化痰止咳，治肺热痰嗽。白茅根味甘性寒，兼能清热利尿，可治热淋涩痛。

All *Notoginseng Radix et Rhizoma* (san qi), *Typhae Pollen* (pu huang) and *Rubiae Radix Et Rhizoma* (qian cao) act to dissolve stasis and stanch blood and possess the advantage to stop bleeding without stasis. They are applied to treat bleeding pattern due to blood stasis, and also to treat blood stasis pattern manifested by amenorrhea, dysmenorrhea, placenta retention after delivery, sharp-stabbing pain at chest and abdomen, and swelling and pain due to traumatic injury. San qi is warm in property and acts to stanch blood, dissolve stasis and stop pain, applied to treat various types of external and internal bleeding pattern, and swelling and pain due to traumatic injury. Pu huang is neutral in property, applied to treat bleeding pattern due to blood stasis with cold or with heat. It acts to dissolve stasis and stop pain, applied to treat various types of pain due to blood stasis, and also acts to promote urination and treat stranguria, applied to treat hematuria and stranguria with bleeding. Qian cao is bitter and cold in property and attributive to the Liver Meridian, and acts to cool blood, dissolve stasis and stanch blood, applied to treat bleeding pattern due to blood stasis or due to heat in blood. It also acts to activate blood and dredge meridians, applied to treat amenorrhea due to blood stasis.

三七、蒲黄、茜草，均善化瘀止血，有止血不留瘀之优点，既善治瘀滞出血，又用于血瘀经闭痛经、产后瘀阻、心腹瘀痛及外伤肿痛。其中三七性温，为止血、化瘀、止痛之良药，善治体内外多种出血；又治跌打伤痛，为伤科要药。蒲黄性平，治瘀滞出血不论寒热均可用之；且善化瘀止痛，可治各种瘀滞作痛，兼能利尿通淋，善治尿血及血淋。茜草苦寒，专入肝经，功能凉血化瘀止血，瘀滞或血热出血皆宜，且能活血通经，善治瘀滞经闭。

Both *Bletillae Rhizoma* (bai ji) and *Agrimoniae Herba* (xian he cao) are astringent in property and act to stanch blood, applied to treat external and internal pattern without blood stasis. Bai ji is slightly cold and sticky in property and acts to astringe and stanch blood, applied to treat bleeding of lung and stomach. It also acts to subside swell, engender flesh and astringe carbuncle, applied to treat carbuncle and furuncle due to heat-toxin, chapped skin at hands and feet, scalding by water, burning by fire and anal fissure. Xian he cao is neutral in property, applied to treat various types of bleeding pattern due to cold, heat, deficiency or excess. It acts to astringe and stop dysentery, applied to treat chronic dysentery. It acts to reinforce body, applied to treat loss of energy and strains. It also acts to treat malaria and relieve toxin, applied to malaria and carbuncle due to toxin.

白及、仙鹤草，均收敛止血，善治内外出血而无瘀滞者。其中白及性微寒、质黏涩，为收敛止血药要药，善治肺胃出血；且能消肿生肌敛疮，治痈疮肿毒、手足皲裂、水火烫伤、肛裂等证。仙鹤草性平，出血证无论寒热虚实均宜；又能收涩止痢，治久痢不愈；能补虚，治脱力劳伤；还能截疟、解毒，治疟疾、疮肿等。

Both *Artemisiae Argyi Folium* (ai ye) and *Zingiberis Rhizoma Praeparatum* (pao jiang) are warm in property and act to warm meridians and stanch blood, applied to treat bleeding due to deficiency and cold. Ai ye is good at treating uterine bleeding due to deficiency and cold. It also acts to warm meridians, eliminate cold and damp and relieve pain, applied to treat irregular menstruation and dysmenorrheal due to deficiency and cold. It acts to stop itching in topical application. Pao jiang is good at treating hematemesis and hematochezia due to spleen failing to control blood. It also acts to warm the middle energizer and relieve pain, applied to treat abdominal pain and diarrhea due to deficiency and cold in middle energizer.

艾叶、炮姜，均性温，有温经止血之功，适用于虚寒性出血证。其中艾叶善治虚寒性崩漏下血；又能温经脉、散寒湿、止疼痛，虚寒所致的月经不调、经行腹痛，亦为常用之品；外用祛湿止痒。炮姜善治脾不统血之的吐血、便血；又温中止痛，治中焦虚寒之腹痛、腹泻。

Chapter 11 Blood-Activating and Stasis-Dissolving Herbs

第 11 章 活血化瘀药

The medicinal herbs acting to dredge meridians, promote blood flow and dissolve blood stasis are called the blood-activating and stasis-dissolving herbs, also called the blood-activating and stasis-eliminating herbs, or the blood-activating herbs or the stasis-dissolving herbs in short.

以通利血脉、促进血行、消散瘀血为主要作用的药物,称为活血化瘀药,又称活血祛瘀药,简称活血药或化瘀药。

The medicinal herbs are mostly pungent and bitter in flavor and warm in property, because the pungent-flavor herbs act to move and dissipate stasis, the bitter-flavor herbs act to dredge and descend, and the warm-property herbs act to dredge the blood vessels. They act to move blood, dissolve stasis, dredge meridians, treat wounds and dissipate masses. According to their strength of actions, they are divided into the blood-harmonizing and blood-circulating herbs, the blood-activating and stasis-dissolving herbs and the blood-breaking and stasis-eliminating herbs.

本类药物味多辛苦性温,辛能行散瘀滞,苦能泄利通降,温能通行血脉。功能行血、散瘀、通经、疗伤、消癥等。根据药物作用强弱,有和血行血、活血化瘀、破血逐瘀之分。

The medicinal herbs are applied to treat blood stasis pattern, manifested by local sharp-stabbing pain with fixed location, local bruise and swelling, masses and blotchy areas. The blood stasis pattern involves the diseases in clinical departments, such as chest pain, hypochondriac pain due to blood stasis, Bi (Obturation) Pattern due to wind-damp, pain

本类药主要用于瘀血证,表现为局部刺痛,痛处固定;或局部青紫瘀肿;或见肿块、瘀斑等。瘀血证涉及临床各科,如胸痹胸痛、血瘀胁痛、风湿痹痛、跌打伤痛、癥瘕积聚、痛经经闭、产后瘀滞

due to traumatic injury, abdominal masses, dysmenorrhea, amenorrhea, abdominal pain due to blood stasis after delivery, hemiplegia due to wind stroke, etc.

腹痛、中风半身不遂等。

In the application of the medicinal herbs, it is necessary to follow the theory that "when qi flow, the blood flows". The medicinal herbs are often combined with the qi-regulating herbs. The medicinal herbs may consume blood and cause bleeding, so it is prohibited to apply for those with heavy blood flow in menstruation, bleeding pattern, or blood deficiency pattern without stasis. It is cautious or prohibited to apply for pregnant women.

使用本类药物需注意，根据“气行则血行”的理论，本类药常与理气药同用。本类药物易耗血动血，月经过多及出血证，或血虚无瘀者忌用。孕妇慎用或忌用。

Chuanxiong Rhizoma (chuan xiong)

川芎

It is the dried product from the rhizome of *Ligusticum chuanxiong* Hort., family Umbelliferae. The medicinal herb is collected in summer when the tuber on rhizome becomes bulging and slightly purple, applied in crude form.

为伞形科植物川芎的干燥根茎。夏季当茎上的节盘显著突出，并略带紫色时采挖。生用。

Features Flavor: pungent. Property: warm. Meridian tropism: the Liver Meridian, the Gallbladder Meridian and the Pericardium Meridian.

性味归经 辛，温。归肝、胆、心包经。

Actions Activate blood, move qi, eliminate wind and stop pain.

功效 活血行气，祛风止痛。

Application

应用

(1) Blood stasis and qi stagnation pattern. The medicinal herb acts to activate blood and move qi as well, termed as "the qi herb in the category of blood herbs", applied to treat blood stasis and qi stagnation pattern. In the treatment of cardiac pain, it is applied singly by grinding into powder and taking with liquor. In the treatment of liver qi stagnation pattern manifested by hypochondriac pain, it is

（1）血瘀气滞证。本品既活血又行气，为“血中气药”，善治血瘀气滞诸证。治胸痹心痛者，可单用为末，以酒送服。治肝郁胁痛，常与柴胡、香附等同用，治血瘀经闭、痛经、月经不调，常与赤芍、桃仁、丹参等同用。治跌

combined with *Bupleuri Radix* (chai hu) and *Cyperi Rhizoma* (xiang fu). In the treatment of blood stasis pattern manifested by amenorrhea, dysmenorrhea and irregular menstruation, it is combined with *Paeoniae Radix Rubra* (chi shao), *Persicae Semen* (tao ren) and *Salviae Miltiorrhizae Radix et Rhizoma* (dan shen). In the treatment of pain due to traumatic injury, it is combined with *Notoginseng Radix et Rhizoma* (san qi), *Olibanum* (ru xiang) and *Myrrha* (mo yao). In the treatment of abdominal masses, it is combined with *Sparganii Rhizoma* (san leng) and *Curcumae Rhizoma* (e zhu).

仆伤痛，与三七、乳香、没药等同用。治癥瘕积聚，可与三棱、莪术等同用。

(2) Headache. The medicinal herb acts to ascend to reach the head and eyes and to activate blood, eliminate wind and stop pain. It is said in ancient times that" the treatment of headache relies on *Chuanxiong Rhizoma* (chuan xiong)". In the treatment of headache due to wind-cold, it is combined with *Angelicae Dahuricae Radix* (bai zhi) and *Asari Radix et Rhizoma* (xi xin), to form up Tea-Blended Ligusticum Powder (Chuan Xiong Cha Tiao San). In the treatment of headache due to wind-heat, it is combined with *Chrysanthemi Flos* (ju hua) and *Gypsum Fibrosum* (shi gao). In the treatment of headache due to wind-damp, it is combined with *Notopterygii Rhizoma et Radix* (qiang huo) and *Radix Saposhuikoviae* (fang feng). In the treatment of headache due to blood stasis, it is combined with *Persicae Semen* (tao ren) and *Carthami Flos* (hong hua). In the treatment of headache due to blood deficiency, it is combined with the qi-reinforcing herbs and blood-reinforcing herbs.

（2）头痛。本品能上行头目，善活血祛风止痛，古有“头痛不离川芎”之说。治风寒头痛，常与白芷、细辛等配伍，如川芎茶调散。治风热头痛，与菊花、石膏等配伍。治风湿头痛，与羌活、防风等同用。治血瘀头痛，与桃仁、红花等同用。与补气血药配伍，治血虚头痛。

(3) Bi (Obturation) Pattern due to wind-damp. The medicinal herb acts to eliminate wind, dispel

（3）风湿痹痛。本品能祛风散寒、活血通经。治风

cold, activate blood and dredge meridians. In the treatment of Bi (Obturation) Pattern due to wind-damp, it is combined with *Angelicae Pubescentis Radix* (du huo) and qiang huo.

湿痹痛，常与独活、羌活等同用。

Usage and dosage　Apply 3～10 g in decoction.

用法用量　煎服，3～10克。

Precautions for use　It is prohibited to apply for those with headache due to yin deficiency and yang hyperactivity. It is cautious to apply for those with profuse sweating or those with heavy blood flow in menstruation.

使用注意　阴虚阳亢头痛者忌用。多汗、月经过多者慎用。

Corydalis Rhizoma (yan hu suo)

延胡索

It is the dried product from the tuber of the perennial herbage *Corydalis yanhusuo* W. T. Wang, family Papaveraceae. The medicinal herb is collected in early summer when the stems and leaves are withered, applied in crude form or in stir-baked form by vinegar.

为罂粟科植物延胡索的干燥块茎。夏初茎叶枯萎时采挖。生用或醋炙用。

Features　Flavor: pungent and bitter. Property: warm. Meridian tropism: the Liver Meridian and the Spleen Meridian.

性味归经　辛、苦，温。归肝、脾经。

Actions　Activate blood, move qi and stop pain.

功效　活血，行气，止痛。

Application

应用

Blood stasis and qi stagnation pattern manifested by various types of pain. The medicinal herb acts to activate blood and move qi, as the major herb to stop pain, "specially applied to treat various pains in the upper and the lower of the body". In the treatment of chest pain and cardiac pain, it is combined with *Salviae Miltiorrhizae Radix et Rhizoma* (dan shen), *Chuanxiong Rhizoma* (chuan xiong) and *Trichosanthis Fructus* (gua lou). In the

血瘀气滞诸痛证。功能活血行气，尤为止痛佳品，“专治一身上下诸痛”。治胸痹心痛，可与丹参、川芎、瓜蒌等同用。治脘腹疼痛者，可与川楝子同用，即金铃子散。治肝郁胸胁胀痛，可与柴胡、郁金等同用。治痛经经闭、产后腹痛，可与当归、

treatment of epigastric pain and abdominal pain, it is combined with *Toosendan Fructus* (chuan lian zi), to form up Melia Toosendan Powder (Jin Ling Zi San). In the treatment of liver qi stagnation manifested by distending pain at chest and hypochondria, it is combined with *Bupleuri Radix* (chai hu) and *Curcumae Radix* (yu jin). In the treatment of dysmenorrhea, amenorrhea and abdominal pain after delivery, it is combined with *Angelicae Sinensis Radix* (dang gui) and *Carthami Flos* (hong hua). In the treatment of pain due to traumatic injury, it is combined with *Olibanum* (ru xiang) and *Myrrha* (mo yao).

红花等同用。治跌打伤痛，与乳香、没药等配伍。

Usage and dosage Apply 3～10 g in decoction. Apply 1.5～3 g of powder. The medicinal herb becomes stronger in stopping pain after stir-baking with vinegar.

用法用量 煎服，3～10克。研末服1.5～3克。醋制后可增止痛之力。

Curcumae Radix (yu jin)

郁金

It is the dried product from the tuberous root of the perennial herbage *Curcuma Wenyujin* Y. H. Chen et C. Ling., or *Curcuma Longa* L., or *Curcuma kwangsiensis* S. G. Lee et C. F. Liang., or *Curcuma phaeocaulis* Val., family Zingiberaceae. The medicinal herb is collected in winter, applied in crude form.

为姜科植物温郁金、姜黄、广西莪术或蓬莪术的干燥块根。冬季采挖。生用。

Features Flavor: pungent and bitter. Property: cold. Meridian tropism: the Liver Meridian, the Heart Meridian and the Gallbladder Meridian.

性味归经 辛、苦，寒。归肝、心、胆经。

Actions Activate blood, stop pain, move qi, relieve stagnation, purify heart, cool blood, benefit gallbladder and treat jaundice.

功效 活血止痛，行气解郁，清心凉血，利胆退黄。

Application

应用

(1) Blood stasis and qi stagnation pattern. The

(1) 血瘀气滞证。本品

medicinal herb acts to activate blood and stop pain, and also acts to move qi and relieve stagnation as well. In the treatment of distending pain or sharp-stabbing pain at chest and hypochondria, it is combined with *Bupleuri Radix* (chai hu), *Salviae Miltiorrhizae Radix et Rhizoma* (dan shen) and *Cyperi Rhizoma* (xiang fu). In the treatment of chest pain and cardiac pain, it is combined with *Chuanxiong Rhizoma* (chuan xiong), *Cinnamomi Ramulus* (gui zhi) and *Trichosanthis Fructus* (gua lou). In the treatment of amenorrhea and dysmenorrhea, it is combined with *Angelicae Sinensis Radix* (dang gui), chai hu and *Paeoniae Radix Alba* (bai shao).

既活血止痛，又行气解郁。治胸胁胀痛或刺痛，常与柴胡、丹参、香附等同用。治胸痹心痛，可与川芎、桂枝、瓜蒌等同用。治经闭痛经，可与当归、柴胡、白芍等同用。

(2) Loss of consciousness in febrile disease, epilepsy and mania. The medicinal herb acts to cool blood, purify heart, relieve stagnation and open aperture. In the treatment of loss of consciousness in febrile disease, it is combined with *Acori Tatarinowii Rhizoma* (shi chang pu) and *Gardeniae Fructus* (zhi zi). In the treatment of epilepsy and mania, it is combined with *Alumen* (bai fan), to form up White and Golden Pills (Bai Jin Wan).

（2）热病神昏，癫痫发狂。本品凉血清心，解郁开窍。治热病神昏，常与石菖蒲、栀子等同用。治癫痫发狂，可与白矾配伍，即白金丸。

(3) Hematemesis, epistaxis and retrograde menstruation. The medicinal herb is combined with *Achyranthis Bidentatae Radix* (niu xi), *Moutan Cortex* (mu dan pi) and zhi zi.

（3）吐血、衄血、倒经。常与牛膝、牡丹皮、栀子等同用。

(4) Jaundice due to damp-heat. The medicinal herb acts to eliminate damp-heat and treat jaundice. In the treatment of damp-heat pattern manifested by jaundice, bitter taste in mouth and dark urine, it is combined with *Artemisiae Scopariae Herba* (yin chen), zhi zi and *Rhei Radix et Rhizoma* (da huang).

（4）湿热黄疸。本品能清湿热、退黄疸。治湿热黄疸、口苦尿赤，常与茵陈、栀子、大黄等同用。

Usage and dosage Apply 3～10 g in decoc-

用法用量 煎服，3～10

tion.

克。

Precautions for use It is not advisable to apply with *Caryophylli Flos* (ding xiang).

使用注意 不宜与丁香同用。

Curcumae Longae Rhizoma (jiang huang)

姜黄

It is the dried product from the rhizome of the perennial herbage *Curcuma longa* L., family Zingiberaceae. The medicinal herb is collected in winter, applied in crude form.

为姜科植物姜黄的干燥根茎。冬季采挖。生用。

Features Flavor: pungent and bitter. Property: warm. Meridian tropism: the Spleen Meridian and the Liver Meridian.

性味归经 辛、苦，温。归脾、肝经。

Actions Break blood, move qi, dredge meridians and stop pain.

功效 破血行气，通经止痛。

Application

应用

(1) Blood stasis and qi stagnation pattern. The medicinal herb is pungent and bitter and acts to break blood and move qi. In the treatment of sharp-stabbing pain at chest and hypochondria, it is combined with *Bupleuri Radix* (chai hu) and *Cyperi Rhizoma* (xiang fu). In the treatment of chest pain and cardiac pain, it is combined with *Salviae Miltiorrhizae Radix et Rhizoma* (dan shen), *Chuanxiong Rhizoma* (chuan xiong) and *Carthami Flos* (hong hua). In the treatment of amenorrhea and dysmenorrhea, it is combined with chuan xiong and *Curcumae Rhizoma* (e zhu).

（1）血瘀气滞证。本品辛行苦泄，能破血行气。治胸胁刺痛，常与柴胡、香附等同用。治胸痹心痛，与丹参、川芎、红花等同用。治经闭、痛经，常与川芎、莪术等配伍。

(2) Arm pain due to wind-cold. The medicinal herb externally acts to eliminate wind-cold and internally acts to move qi and blood, and it moves to the four limbs. In the treatment of shoulder and arm pain due to wind-cold-damp, it is combined with *Notopterygii Rhizoma et Radix* (qiang huo) and *Saposhnikoviae Radix* (fang feng).

（2）风寒臂痛。本品外散风寒，内行气血，长于行肢臂而通利血脉，善治风寒湿痹肩臂疼痛，常与羌活、防风等同用。

Usage and dosage Apply 3～10 g in decoction. Apply a proper amount for external use.

用法用量 煎服，3～10克。外用适量。

Olibanum (ru xiang)

乳香

It is the product from the resin at the dark of *Boswellia carterii* Birdw and other species in the sam genus, family Burseraceae. In spring and summer, the bark is cut and the resin is made to ooze out of the cut. The medicinal herb is collected when the resin coagulates into solid mass, applied in prepared form by stir-baking with vinegar.

为橄榄科植物卡氏乳香树及同属植物皮部渗出的树脂。春、夏将树干的皮部切伤，树脂从伤口渗出，凝成硬块后收集即得。醋炙用。

Features Flavor: pungent and bitter. Property: warm. Meridian tropism: the Heart Meridian, the Liver Meridian and the Spleen Meridian.

性味归经 辛、苦，温。归心、肝、脾经。

Actions Activate blood, stop pain, subside swell and engender flesh.

功效 活血止痛，消肿生肌。

Application

应用

(1) Blood stasis and qi stagnation pattern manifested by various types of pain. The medicinal herb is pungent, bitter, warm and dredging in property, and acts to activate blood, move qi and stop pain. In the treatment of cardiac pain, abdominal pain and abdominal masses, it is combined with *Angelicae Sinensis Radix* (dang gui) and *Salviae Miltiorrhizae Radix et Rhizoma* (dan shen). In the treatment of blood stasis and qi stagnation pattern manifested by epigastric pain, it is combined with *Corydalis Rhizoma* (yan hu suo) and *Toosendan Fructus* (chuan lian zi). In the treatment of traumatic injury, it is combined with *Carthami Flos* (hong hua) and *Myrrha* (mo yao). In the treatment of Bi (Obturation) Pattern due to wind-damp, it is combined with *Gentianae Macrophyllae Radix* (qin jiao) and *Angelicae Pubescentis Radix* (du huo).

(1) 血瘀气滞诸痛证。本品辛散苦泄温通，能活血行气止痛。治心腹疼痛、癥瘕积聚，常与当归、丹参等同用。治血瘀气滞胃脘痛，常与延胡索、川楝子等同用。治跌打损伤，常与红花、没药等配伍。治风湿痹痛，可与秦艽、独活等同用。

(2) Carbuncle, furuncle and ulcer. The medicinal herb acts to activate blood, move qi and stop pain, and also acts to subside swell and engender flesh, as the major herb in external medicine. In the treatment of carbuncle and furuncle in early stage manifested by redness, swelling, hotness and pain, it is combined with *Lonicerae Japonicae Flos* (jin yin hua) and *Myrrha* (mo yao), to form up Fairy Formula Life-Saving Drink (Xian Fang Huo Ming Yin). In the treatment of carbuncle and furuncle with unhealed ulcer, it is combined with mo yao by grinding into powder for external use, to form up Floating on Sea Powder (Hai Fu San).

（2）疮疡痈肿。本品能活血行气止痛，消肿生肌，为外科要药。治疮痈初起，红肿热痛，常与金银花、没药等同用，如仙方活命饮。治疮疡溃破久不收口，与没药研末外用，即海浮散。

Usage and dosage Apply 3～5 g in decoction. Apply a proper amount for external use. The medicinal herb is prepared by stir-baking with vinegar for degreasing.

用法用量 煎服，3～5克。外用适量。多醋炙去油后用。

Precautions for use The medicinal herb often causes vomiting. It is cautious to apply for those with weakness of stomach. It is prohibited to apply for pregnant women or those without blood stasis.

使用注意 易致呕吐，胃弱者慎用。孕妇及无瘀滞者忌用。

Myrrha (mo yao)

没药

It is the dried product from the resin of the bark of *Commiphora myrrha* Engl. or *Commiphora molmol* Engl., family Burseraceae. The medicinal herb is applied in fried form.

为橄榄科植物地丁树或哈地丁树的干燥树脂。炒用。

Features Flavor: pungent and bitter. Property: neutral. Meridian tropism: the Heart Meridian, the Liver Meridian and the Spleen Meridian.

性味归经 辛、苦，平。归心、肝、脾经。

Actions Activate blood, stop pain, subside swell and engender flesh.

功效 活血止痛，消肿生肌。

Application

应用

Blood stasis pattern. The medicinal herb acts to

瘀血证。本品能活血止

activate blood, stop pain, subside swell and engender flesh, applied to treat various types of blood stasis pattern. In the treatment of cardiac pain, abdominal pain and traumatic injury, it is combined with *Salviae Miltiorrhizae Radix et Rhizoma* (dan shen), *Chuanxiong Rhizoma* (chuan xiong) and *Paeoniae Radix Rubra* (chi shao). In the treatment of carbuncle and furuncle with unhealed ulcer, it is combined with *Olibanum* (ru xiang) for mutual reinforcement.

痛、消肿生肌，可治瘀滞诸证。治心腹诸痛，跌打损伤，常与丹参、川芎、赤芍等同用。治疮疡不敛，常与乳香相须为用。

Usage and dosage Apply 3～5 g in decoction. Make it into pills or powder. Apply a proper amount for external use. The medicinal herb is prepared by stir-baking with vinegar for degreasing.

用法用量 煎汤，3～5克。或入丸散。外用适量。多醋炙去油用。

Precautions for use It is prohibited to apply for pregnant women or those with weakness of stomach.

使用注意 孕妇及胃弱者忌服。

Persicae Semen (tao ren)

桃仁

It is the dried product from the seed of *Prunus persica* (L.) Batsch or *Prunus davidiana* (Carr.) Franch., family Rosaceae. The medicinal herb is collected when the fruits are ripe, by taking out the seeds. It is applied in crude form or in fried form.

为蔷薇科植物桃或山桃的干燥成熟种子。果实成熟后采收，取出种子。生用或炒用。

Features Flavor: bitter and sweet. Property: neutral and slightly poisonous. Meridian tropism: the Heart Meridian, the Liver Meridian and the Large Intestine Meridian.

性味归经 苦、甘，平；有小毒。归心、肝、大肠经。

Actions Activate blood, dissolve stasis, moisturize intestines, promote defecation, stop cough and soothe panting.

功效 活血祛瘀，润肠通便，止咳平喘。

Application

(1) Blood stasis pattern. The medicinal herb is bitter and dispersing in property and has a strong

应用

(1) 血瘀证。本品苦泄，活血力强，有破血之功。治

action to activate blood and break blood. In the treatment of blood stasis pattern manifested by dysmenorrhea and amenorrhea, it is combined with *Carthami Flos* (hong hua) and *Angelicae Sinensis Radix* (dang gui), to form up Peach Pit, Safflower and Four Agents Decoction (Tao Hong Si Wu Tang). In the treatment of lochia retention after delivery, it is combined with *Chuanxiong Rhizoma* (chuan xiong) and *Zingiberis Rhizoma Praeparatum* (pao jiang), to form up Production and Transformation Decoction (Sheng Hua Tang). In the treatment of swelling and pain due to traumatic injury, it is combined with *Olibanum* (ru xiang) and hong hua. In the treatment of abdominal masses, it is combined with *Cinnamomi Ramulus* (gui zhi) and *Moutan Cortex* (mu dan pi).

血瘀痛经、闭经，常与红花、当归等同用，如桃红四物汤。治产后恶露不尽，常与川芎、炮姜等同用，如生化汤。治跌打损伤肿痛，可与乳香、红花等同用。治癥瘕积聚，常与桂枝、牡丹皮等同用。

(2) Pulmonary abscess and acute appendicitis. The medicinal herb acts to activate blood, relieve abscess and drain purulence. In the treatment of pulmonary abscess, it is combined with *Phragmitis Rhizoma* (lu gen) and *Houttuyniae Herba* (yu xing cao). In the treatment of acute appendicitis, it is combined with *Rhei Radix et Rhizoma* (da huang) and mu dan pi.

（2）肺痈，肠痈。本品能活血消痈排脓。治肺痈，与芦根、鱼腥草同用。治肠痈，与大黄、牡丹皮等同用。

(3) Constipation due to dryness in intestines. The medicinal herb is full of fats and acts to moisturize intestines and promote defecation. In the treatment of constipation due to dryness in intestines, it is combined with *Cannabis Fructus* (huo ma ren) and *Pruni Semen* (yu li ren).

（3）肠燥便秘。本品富含油脂，能润肠通便，常与火麻仁、郁李仁等同用，治肠燥便秘。

(4) Cough and panting. The medicinal herb acts to stop cough and soothe panting. In the treatment of cough and panting, it is combined with *Armeniacae Amarum Semen* (ku xing ren).

（4）咳嗽气喘。本品有止咳平喘之效，治咳嗽气喘，可与杏仁等同用。

Usage and dosage Apply 5～10 g in decoction.

Precautions for use It is prohibited to apply for pregnant women.

用法用量 煎服，5～10克。

使用注意 孕妇忌用。

Carthami Flos (hong hua)

红花

It is the dried product from the flower of *Carthamus tinctorius* L., family Compositae. The medicinal herb is collected in summer when its flower is changing from yellow to red, applied in crude form.

为菊科植物红花的干燥花。夏季花色由黄变红的时候采收。生用。

Features Flavor: pungent. Property: warm. Meridian tropism: the Heart Meridian and the Liver Meridian.

性味归经 辛，温。归心、肝经。

Actions Activate blood, dredge meridians, dissolve stasis and stop pain.

功效 活血通经，散瘀止痛。

Application

应用

(1) Dysmenorrhea, amenorrhea and abdominal pain after delivery. The medicinal herb acts to activate blood and dredge meridians. In the treatment of blood stasis pattern manifested by dysmenorrhea, amenorrhea and abdominal pain after delivery, it is combined with *Persicae Semen* (tao ren) and *Angelicae Sinensis Radix* (dang gui), to form up Peach Pit, Safflower and Four Agents Decoction (Tao Hong Si Wu Tang).

（1）痛经经闭，产后腹痛。本品功善活血通经，治血瘀所致的痛经经闭、产后腹痛，常与桃仁、当归等配伍，如桃红四物汤。

(2) Chest pain, cardiac pain, abdominal masses and traumatic injury. In the treatment of heart vessel obstruction pattern manifested by chest pain and cardiac pain, it is combined with *Cinnamomi Ramulus* (gui zhi), *Trichosanthis Fructus* (gua lou) and *Salviae Miltiorrhizae Radix et Rhizoma* (dan shen). In the treatment of abdominal masses, it is combined with *Sparganii Rhizoma* (san leng) and *Curcumae Rhizoma* (e zhu). In the treatment of trau-

（2）胸痹心痛，癥瘕积聚，跌打损伤。治心脉瘀阻，胸痹心痛，常与桂枝、瓜蒌、丹参等配伍。治癥瘕积聚，常配伍三棱、莪术等。治跌打损伤，可与川芎、乳香等同用。

matic injury, it is combined with *Chuanxiong Rhizoma* (chuan xiong) and *Olibanum* (ru xiang).

(3) Macula in purple and dark color. In the treatment of heat accumulation and blood stasis pattern manifested by macula in purple and dark color, it is combined with dang gui, *Isatidis Folium* (da qing ye) and *Arnebiae Radix* (zi cao).

(3) 斑疹紫暗。治热郁血滞的斑疹紫暗,本品常与当归、大青叶、紫草等同用。

Usage and dosage Apply 3～10 g in decoction.

用法用量 煎服,3～10克。

Precautions for use It is cautious to apply for pregnant women or those with heavy blood flow in menstruation.

使用注意 孕妇及月经过多者慎用。

Appendix *Croci Stigma* (xi hong hua)

It is the dried product from the stigma of *Crocus sativus* L., family Iridaceae. The medicinal herb, also called "zang hong hua", is sweet in flavor and neutral in property, and attributive to the Heart Meridian and the Liver Meridian. It acts to activate blood, dissolve stasis, cool blood, relieve toxin, dissolve stagnation and calm mind, applied to treat amenorrhea, abdominal masses, abdominal pain after delivery, febrile disease with macula, convulsion, mania, emotional depression and stuffy chest. Apply 1～3 g in decoction or in boiling water. It is cautious to apply for pregnant women.

附药 西红花

为鸢尾科植物番红花的干燥柱头。又名藏红花。味甘性平,归心、肝经。功能活血化瘀,凉血解毒,解郁安神。适用于经闭癥瘕,产后腹痛,热病发斑,惊悸发狂,忧郁痞闷。煎服或沸水泡服,1～3克。孕妇慎用。

Salviae Miltiorrhizae Radix et Rhizoma (dan shen)

It is the dried product from the root and rhizome of *Salvia miltiorrhiza* Bung, family Labiatae. The medicinal herb is collected in spring and autumn, applied in crude form or in liquor-fried form.

丹参

为唇形科植物丹参的干燥根及根茎。春、秋两季采挖。生用或酒炒用。

Features Flavor: bitter. Property: slightly cold. Meridian tropism: the Heart Meridian and the Liver Meridian.

性味归经 苦,微寒。归心、肝经。

Actions Activate blood, dredge meridians, cool blood, relive carbuncle, purify heart and eliminate restlessness.

功效 活血通经,凉血消痈,清心除烦。

Application

应用

(1) Dysmenorrhea, amenorrhea, irregular menstruation and abdominal pain after delivery. The medicinal herb acts to activate blood, dissolve stasis, dredge meridians and stop pain, as the major herb in gynecology. In the treatment of blood stasis pattern manifested by dysmenorrhea, amenorrhea and irregular menstruation, it is combined with *Leonuri Herba* (yi mu cao), *Carthami Flos* (hong hua) and *Persicae Semen* (tao ren), to form up Red Sage Powder (Dan Shen San). Or it is applied singly by grinding into powder and taken with rice liquor.

(1) 痛经经闭,月经不调,产后瘀滞腹痛。本品善活血祛瘀,通经止痛,为妇科调经要药。治疗瘀血所致的痛经、经闭、月经不调,常与益母草、红花、桃仁等配伍,或单用为末,陈酒送服,即丹参散。

(2) Chest pain, cardiac pain and abdominal masses. The medicinal herb acts to activate blood, dissolve stasis, dissipate masses and relieve stagnation, as the major herb to activate blood and dissolve stasis. In the treatment of chest pain and cardiac pain, it is combined with *Santalum Album* (tan xiang) and *Amomi Fructus* (sha ren), to form up Red Sage Drink (Dan Shen Yin). In the treatment of abdominal masses, it is combined with *Sparganii Rhizoma* (san leng) and *Curcumae Rhizoma* (e zhu).

(2) 胸痹心痛,癥瘕积聚。本品能活血祛瘀、消癥散结,为活血化瘀之要药。治胸痹心痛,可与檀香、砂仁配伍,即丹参饮。治癥瘕积聚,常与三棱、莪术等同用。

(3) Carbuncle, furuncle and ulcer. The medicinal herb acts to cool blood, activate blood, dissolve stasis and relieve carbuncle. In the treatment of carbuncle, furuncle and ulcer, it is combined with the heat-clearing and toxin-relieving herbs.

(3) 疮疡痈肿。本品具凉血活血、散瘀消痈之功。治疗疮痈肿痛,常与清热解毒药同用。

(4) Restlessness, palpitation and insomnia. The medicinal herb acts to purify heart, relieve restlessness and calm mind. In the treatment of fe-

(4) 心烦、心悸失眠。本品能清心除烦、安神。治疗热病心烦不眠,可与生地黄、

brile disease manifested by restlessness and poor sleep, it is combined with *Rehmanniae Radix* (sheng di huang) and *Lophatheri Herba* (dan zhu ye). In the treatment of heart blood deficiency pattern manifested by palpitation and insomnia, it is combined with *Ziziphi Spinosae Semen* (suan zao ren) and *Ginseng Radix et Raizoma* (ren shen).

淡竹叶等同用。亦治心血虚的心悸、失眠,常与酸枣仁、人参等配伍同用。

Usage and dosage Appy 10～15 g in decoction. The medicinal herb acts to activate blood, cool blood and purify heart in crude form, and strongly acts to activate blood in liquor-fried form.

用法用量 煎服,10～15克。生用活血、凉血、清心,酒炒可增强活血之功。

Precautions for use The medicinal herb is incompatible with *Radix et Rhizoma Veratri Nigri* (li lu).

使用注意 反藜芦。

Leonuri Herba (yi mu cao)

益母草

It is the fresh or dried product from the aerial parts of *Leonurus* japonicus Houtt. Sweet, family Labiatae. The medicinal herb is collected in summer, applied in crude form.

为唇形科植物益母草的新鲜或干燥的地上部分。夏季采割。生用。

Features Flavor: bitter and pungent. Property: slight cold. Meridian tropism: the Liver Meridian, the Pericardium Meridian and the Bladder Meridian.

性味归经 苦、辛,微寒。归肝、心包、膀胱经。

Actions Activate blood, regulate menstruation, promote water flow, subside swell, clear heat and relieve toxin.

功效 活血调经,利水消肿,清热解毒。

Application

应用

(1) Menstrual and obstetrical diseases due to blood stasis. The medicinal herb acts to activate blood, dredge meridians, dissolve stasis and engender the new, applied to treat women's menstrual and obstetrical diseases, so it is called "yi mu (benefit mother)". In the treatment of blood stasis pat-

(1) 血瘀经产诸证。本品有活血通经,祛瘀生新作用,善治妇人经产诸证,故有"益母"之称。治瘀滞痛经、经闭、产后恶露不尽,可单味熬膏内服,或配伍活血调经

tern manifested by dysmenorrhea, amenorrhea and lochia retention after delivery, it is applied singly by making into poultice for oral administration, or combined with other blood-activating and menstruation-regulating herbs.

药同用。

(2) Edema and difficult urination. The medicinal herb acts to promote water flow and subside swell, and also acts to activate blood and dissolve stasis as well. In the treatment of edema due to water retention and blood stasis, it is applied singly or combined with *Herba Lycopi* (ze lan) and *Imperatae Rhizoma* (bai mao gen).

(2) 水肿，小便不利。本品既利水消肿，又活血化瘀，尤宜于水瘀互结之水肿，可单用，或与泽兰、白茅根等同用。

(3) Carbuncle and furuncle due to heat-toxin, and skin itch. The medicinal herb is cool in property and acts to clear heat. In the treatment of carbuncle and furuncle or skin itch, it is applied singly by decocting for external wash or by smashing for topical application, or combined with *Sophorae Flavescentis Radix* (ku shen) and *Phellodendri Cortex Chiensis* (huang bo).

(3) 疮痈肿毒，皮肤痒疹。本品性凉清热，单味煎汤外洗或鲜品捣烂外敷，治疮痈或皮肤痒疹。亦可配伍苦参、黄柏等同用。

Usage and dosage Apply 9～30 g in decoction. Apply a proper amount for external use.

用法用量 煎服，9～30克。外用适量。

Precautions for use It is prohibited to apply for pregnant women.

使用注意 孕妇忌用。

Achyranthis Bidentatae Radix **(niu xi)**

牛膝

It is the dried product from the root of the perennial herbage *Achyrantes bidentata* Blume, family Amaranthaceae. The medicinal herb is mainly produced in Henan Province, also called "huai niu xi". It is collected in winter and dried in sun, applied in crude form or vinegar-baked form.

为苋科植物牛膝的干燥根。主产于河南，又称"怀牛膝"。冬季采挖。晒干。生用或酒炙用。

Features Flavor: bitter, sweet and sour. Property: neutral. Meridian tropism: the Liver Me-

性味归经 苦、甘、酸，平。归肝、肾经。

ridian and the Kidney Meridian.

Actions Activate blood, dredge meridians, reinforce liver and kidney, strengthen tendons and bones, promote urination, treat stranguria, and guide blood to flow downwards.

功效 活血通经，补肝肾，强筋骨，利尿通淋，引血下行。

Application

应用

(1) Dysmenorrhea and amenorrhea. The medicinal herb acts to activate blood and dredge meridians. In the treatment of blood stasis pattern manifested by dysmenorrhea and amenorrhea, it is combined with *Carthami Flos* (hong hua) and *Persicae Semen* (tao ren), or applied singly by steaming with liquor.

（1）痛经、经闭。本品能活血通经，治瘀滞痛经、经闭，常与红花、桃仁等配伍，或单味以酒蒸服。

(2) Aching and pain at low back and knees, and weakness at lower limbs. The medicinal herb acts to reinforce liver and kidney, strengthen tendons and bones, with action direction of going downwards. In the treatment of liver and kidney deficiency pattern manifested by aching and pain at low back and knees, it is combined with *Eucommiae Cortex* (du zhong) and *Dipsaci Radix* (xu duan). In the treatment of damp-heat downward-infusing manifested by flaccidity and weakness of lower limbs, it is combined with *Atractylodis Rhizoma* (cang zhu) and *Phellodendri Cortex Chiensis* (huang bo), to form up Three Wonderful Herbs Pills (San Miao Wan).

（2）腰膝酸痛，下肢无力。本品既补肝肾、强筋骨，尤善下行。治肝肾虚的腰膝酸痛，常与杜仲、续断等同用。若湿热下注，下肢痿弱，常与苍术、黄柏同用，即三妙丸。

(3) Stranguria and edema. The medicinal herb is sinking and descending in property and acts to promote urination and treat stranguria. In the treatment of stranguria with burning or bleeding, it is combined with *Plantaginis Semen* (che qian zi) and *Talcum* (hua shi). In the treatment of edema and difficult urination, it is combined with *Alismatis*

（3）淋证，水肿。本品沉降下行，能利尿通淋。治热淋、血淋，常与车前子、滑石等同用。治水肿、小便不利，常与泽泻、茯苓等同用。

Rhizoma (ze xie) and *Poria* (fu ling).

(4) Hematemesis, epistaxis and toothache. The medicinal herb is bitter, reducing and descending in property, and acts to guide fire or blood to go downwards. In the treatment of upward-reverse movement of qi and fire or heat in blood manifested by hematemesis and epistaxis, it is combined with *Gardeniae Fructus* (zhi zi) and *Imperatae Rhizoma* (bai mao gen). In the treatment of stomach fire pattern manifested by swelling and pain at gum, and ulcers at tongue and mouth ulcer, it is combined with *Gypsum Fibrosum* (shi gao) and *Anemarrhenae Rhizoma* (zhi mu).

（4）吐血、衄血，齿痛。本品苦泄下行，能引火或引血下行。常用于气火上逆，血热妄行之吐血、衄血，可与栀子、白茅根等同用。治疗胃火牙龈肿痛、口舌生疮，常与石膏、知母等同用。

Usage and dosage Apply 5～12 g in decoction. The medicinal herb acts to activate blood, dredge meridians, promote urination, treat stranguria and guide blood to flow downwards in crude form, and acts to reinforce liver and kidney, and strengthen tendons and bones in liquor-prepared form.

用法用量 煎服，5～12克。生用活血通经、利尿通淋、引血下行。酒制补肝肾、强筋骨。

Precautions for use It is cautious to apply for pregnant women or those with heavy flow of blood in menstruation.

使用注意 孕妇及月经过多者慎用。

Appendix *Cyathulae Radix* (chuan niu xi)

It is the dried product from the root of *Cyathulae officinalis* Kuan, family Amaranthaceae. The medicinal herb is mainly produced in Sichuan Province. It is sweet and bitter in flavor and neutral in property, acts to dissolve stasis, dredge meridians, lubricate joints, promote urination and treat stranguria, applied to treat amenorrhea, abdominal masses, placenta retention, traumatic injury, Bi (Obturation) Pattern due to wind-damp, hematuria and stranguria with bleeding. Apply 5～10 g in decoction.

附药 川牛膝

为苋科植物川牛膝的干燥根。主产于四川。味甘、苦，性平。功能逐瘀通经，通利关节，利尿通淋。适用于经闭癥瘕，胞衣不下，跌仆损伤，风湿痹痛，尿血血淋等。煎服，5～10克。孕妇慎用。

It is cautious to apply for pregnant women.

Remarks *Cyathulae Radix* (chuan niu xi) and *Achyranthis Bidentatae Radix* (niu xi)

Both chuan niu xi and niu xi are the same species of family Amaranthaceae. Chuan niu xi is mainly produced in Sichuan Province, and acts to activate blood, dredge meridians and dissolve stasis, applied to treat various types of stasis and stagnation patterns. Niu xi is mainly produced in Henan Province, also called "huai niu xi", and acts to reinforce liver and kidney and strengthen tendons and bones, applied to treat liver and kidney deficiency pattern manifested by aching and weakness of feet and knees.

按语 川牛膝与牛膝

川牛膝与牛膝均为苋科植物。川牛膝主产于四川，功偏活血通经，祛瘀力强，为治瘀滞诸证多用。牛膝主产于河南，又称"怀牛膝"。功偏补肝、强筋骨，常用于肝肾虚亏、足膝酸软无力等证。

Spatholobi Caulis (ji xue teng)

It is the dried product from the vine and stem of *Spatholobus suberectus* Dunn, family Leguminosae. The medicinal herb is collected in autumn and winter, applied in crude form.

Features Flavor: bitter and sweet. Property: warm. Meridian tropism: the Liver Meridian and the Kidney Meridian.

Actions Activate blood, reinforce blood, regulate menstruation, stop pain, relax tendons and dredge collaterals.

Application

(1) Irregular menstruation, dysmenorrhea and amenorrhea. The medicinal herb acts to activate blood, reinforce blood, regulate menstruation and stop pain. In the treatment of blood stasis pattern or blood deficiency pattern manifested by irregular menstruation, dysmenorrhea and amenorrhea, it is combined with *Angelicae Sinensis Radix* (dang gui),

鸡血藤

为豆科植物密花豆的干燥藤茎。秋、冬二季采收。生用。

性味归经 苦、甘，温。归肝、肾经。

功效 活血补血，调经止痛，舒筋活络。

应用

（1）月经不调，痛经、经闭。本品具活血、补血，调经止痛之功。治血瘀或血虚的月经不调，痛经、经闭，常与当归、川芎、香附或熟地黄、白芍等同用。

Chuanxiong Rhizoma (chuan xiong) and *Cyperi Rhizoma* (xiang fu) or combined with *Rehmanniae Radix Praeparata* (shu di huang) and *Paeoniae Radix Alba* (bai shao).

(2) Bi (Obturation) Pattern due to wind-damp, numbness at body and limbs, and hemiplegia. The medicinal herb acts to nourish blood, activate blood, relax tendons and dredge collaterals. In the treatment of Bi (Obturation) Pattern due to wind-damp, and numbness at body and limbs, it is combined with *Achyranthis Bidentatae Radix* (niu xi) and *Eucommiae Cortex* (du zhong). In the treatment of hemiplegia due to wind stroke, it is combined with *Astragali Radix* (huang qi), *Pheretima* (di long) and *Carthami Flos* (hong hua).

（2）风湿痹痛，肢体麻木，半身不遂。本品能养血活血、舒筋活络。治风湿痹痛、肢体麻木，常与牛膝、杜仲等同用。治中风瘫痪，常与黄芪、地龙、红花等配伍。

Usage and dosage Apply 9～15 g in decoction.

用法用量 煎服，9～15克。

Curcumae Rhizoma (e zhu)

莪术

It is the dried product from the tuberous root of the perennial herbage *Curcuma phaeocaulis* Val., or *Curcuma kwangsiensis* S. G. Lee et C. F. Liang., or *Curcuma Wenyujin* Y. H. Chen et C. Ling., family Zingiberaceae. The medicinal herb is collected in winter, applied in crude form or vinegar-prepared form.

为姜科植物蓬莪术、广西莪术或温郁金的干燥根茎。冬季采挖。生用或醋制用。

Features Flavor: pungent and bitter. Property: warm. Meridian tropism: the Liver Meridian and the Spleen Meridian.

性味归经 辛、苦，温。归肝、脾经。

Actions Move qi, break blood, dissolve stagnation and stop pain.

功效 行气破血，消积止痛。

Application

应用

(1) Blood stasis pattern manifested by amenorrhea, abdominal masses, chest pain and cardiac

（1）瘀血经闭，癥瘕积聚，胸痹心痛。本品活血祛

pain. The medicinal herb strongly acts to activate blood, dissolve stasis, break blood and move qi. In the treatment of amenorrhea due to blood stasis, it is combined with *Chuanxiong Rhizoma* (chuan xiong) and *Carthami Flos* (hong hua). In the treatment of abdominal masses, it is combined with *Sparganii Rhizoma* (san leng) and *Trionycis Carapax* (bie jia). In the treatment of chest pain and cardiac pain, it is combined with *Salviae Miltiorrhizae Radix et Rhizoma* (dan shen) and *Cinnamomi Ramulus* (gui zhi).

瘀力强，具破血之功，且能行气。治瘀滞经闭，可与川芎、红花等同用。治癥瘕积聚，常与三棱、鳖甲等同用。治胸痹心痛，可配伍丹参、桂枝等同用。

(2) Abdominal distension and pain due to food retention. The medicinal herb acts to move qi and dissolve stagnation. In the treatment of abdominal distension and pain due to food retention, it is combined with *Aucklandiae Radix* (mu xiang) and *Aurantii Fructus Immaturus* (zhi shi).

(2) 食积胀痛。本品行气消积，常与木香、枳实等同用，治食积胀痛。

Usage and dosage Apply 6～9 g in decoction. The medicinal herb acts to break blood, move qi and dissolve stagnation in crude form, and strongly acts to stop pain in vinegar-calcined form.

用法用量 煎服，6～9克。生用破血行气、消积，醋炙后止痛力强。

Precautions for use It is prohibited to apply for pregnant women or those with heavy flow of blood in menstruation.

使用注意 孕妇及月经过多者忌用。

Sparganii Rhizoma **(san leng)**

三棱

It is the dried product from the tuber of *Sparganium stoloniferum* Buch.-Ham., family Sparganiaceae. The medicinal herb is collected in winter and next spring, applied in crude form or in vinegar-calcined form.

为黑三棱科植物黑三棱的干燥块茎。冬季至次春采挖。生用或醋炙用。

Features Flavor: pungent and bitter. Property: neutral. Meridian tropism: the Liver Meridian and the Spleen Meridian.

性味归经 辛、苦，平。归肝、脾经。

Actions Break blood, move qi, dissolve stagnation and stop pain.

Application

(1) Amenorrhea, abdominal pain, abdominal masses, chest pain and cardiac pain. The medicinal herb acts to break blood. In the treatment of amenorrhea due to blood stasis, it is combined with *Carthami Flos* (hong hua) and *Persicae Semen* (tao ren). In the treatment of abdominal masses, it is combined with *Curcumae Rhizoma* (e zhu) in mutual reinforcement. In the treatment of chest pain and cardiac pain, it is combined with *Salviae Miltiorrhizae Radix et Rhizoma* (dan shen) and *Notoginseng Radix et Rhizoma* (san qi).

(2) Abdominal pain due to food retention. The medicinal herb acts to move qi and dissolve stagnation. In the treatment of food retention manifested by indigestion, distension and fullness at epigastria and abdomen, it is combined with *Citri Reticulatae Pericarpium Viride* (qing pi) and *Hordei Fructus Germinatus* (mai ya).

Usage and dosage Apply 5～10 g in decoction. The medicinal herb acts to break blood, move qi and dissolve stagnation in crude form, and strongly acts to stop pain in vinegar-calcined form.

Precautions for use It is prohibited to apply for those with heavy flow of blood in menstruation or pregnant women.

功效 破血行气，消积止痛。

应用

（1）经闭腹痛，癥瘕积聚，胸痹心痛。本品为破血之品。治瘀滞经闭，常与红花、桃仁等同用。治癥瘕积聚，可与莪术相须为用。治胸痹心痛，可与丹参、三七等同用。

（2）食积腹痛。本品能行气消积。常与青皮、麦芽等同用，治食积不消，脘腹胀满。

用法用量 煎服，5～10克。生用破血行气、消积，醋炙后止痛力增。

使用注意 月经过多者及孕妇忌用。

Hirudo (shui zhi)

It is the dried product from the whole body of *Whitmania Pigra* Whitman, *Hirudo nipponica* Whitman, *Whitmania acranulata* Whitman, family Hirudinidae. The medicinal herb is collected and

水蛭

为水蛭科动物蚂蟥、水蛭或柳叶蚂蟥的干燥全体。夏、秋两季捕捉。生用或用滑石粉制用。

dried in summer and autumn, applied in crude form or prepared form with *Talcum* (hua shi) powder.

Features Flavor: salty and bitter. Property: neutral and slightly poisonous. Meridian tropism: the Liver Meridian.

性味归经 咸、苦，平；有小毒。归肝经。

Actions Break blood, dredge meridians, dissolve stasis and dissipate masses.

功效 破血通经，逐瘀消癥。

Application

Amenorrhea due to blood stasis, abdominal masses and traumatic injury. The medicinal herb strongly acts to break blood and dissolve stasis. In the treatment of amenorrhea due to blood stasis, it is combined with *Carthami Flos* (hong hua), *Persicae Semen* (tao ren) and *Sparganii Rhizoma* (san leng). In the treatment of abdominal masses, it is combined with *Trionycis Carapax* (bie jia) and *Curcumae Rhizoma* (e zhu). In the treatment of traumatic injury, it is combined with *Olibanum* (ru xiang) and *Myrrha* (mo yao) or combined with *Rhei Radix et Rhizoma* (da huang).

应用

血瘀经闭，癥瘕积聚及跌打损伤。本品破血逐瘀力猛。治瘀滞经闭，常与红花、桃仁、三棱同用。治癥瘕积聚，可与鳖甲、莪术等同用。治跌打损伤，常与乳香、没药或大黄等配伍。

Usage and dosage Apply 1～3 g in decoction.

用法用量 煎服，1～3克。

Precautions for use It is prohibited to apply for pregnant women.

使用注意 孕妇忌用。

Brief summary

All *Chuanxiong Rhizoma* (chuan xiong), *Corydalis Rhizoma* (yan hu suo), *Curcumae Radix* (yu jin) and *Curcumae Longae Rhizoma* (jiang huang) act to activate blood, move qi and stop pain, applied to treat blood stasis and qi stagnation pattern manifested by various pains. Chuan xiong is pungent and warm in property and acts to activate blood and

小　结

川芎、延胡索、郁金、姜黄，均能活血行气止痛，治疗血瘀气滞所致的诸痛证。其中川芎味辛性温，为活血行气要药，善调月经；且能上行头目，祛风止痛，善治头痛，又活血通脉，治风湿痹痛。

move qi, applied to regulate menstruation. It is ascending in property and moves to head and eyes, and acts to eliminate wind and stop pain, applied to treat headache. It also acts to activate blood and dredge meridians, applied to Bi (Obturation) Pattern due to wind-damp. Yan hu suo is pungent, bitter and warm in property and strongly acts to activate blood and stop pain, applied to treat blood stasis and qi stagnation pattern manifested by various pains in the upper and lower body. Yu jin is pungent, bitter and cold in property and acts to activate blood, cool blood, move qi and relieve stagnation, applied to treat blood stasis and qi stagnation pattern with heat or heat in blood manifested by hematemesis, epistaxis and retrograde menstruation. It is attributive to the Heart Meridian and acts to purify heart and open aperture, applied to treat febrile disease with loss of consciousness, and epilepsy due to phlegm blockage. It also acts to benefit gallbladder and treat jaundice, applied to treat jaundice due to damp-heat. Jiang huang is pungent and warm in property and acts to break blood, move qi, move into arms and dredge blood vessels, applied to treat pain at shoulder and arm.

延胡索味辛苦性温，活血止痛力强，凡一身上下血瘀气滞诸痛证，皆可用之。郁金味辛苦性寒，能活血凉血、行气解郁，善治血瘀气滞挟热者，以及血热吐血、衄血、倒经等证；入心经能清心开窍，治热病神昏、癫痫痰闭之证；且能利胆退黄，治湿热黄疸。姜黄味辛性温，具破血行气之功，长于行肢臂而通血脉，常用于肩臂疼痛。

Both *Olibanum* (ru xiang) and *Myrrha* (mo yao) are made of medicinal resin, fragrant, pungent and moving in property, and act to activate blood, stop pain, subside swell and engender flesh, applied to treat blood stasis and qi stagnation pattern manifested by various pains at chest and abdomen, carbuncle, furuncle and ulcer, and traumatic injury. They are applied for oral administration and external use. Ru xiang more acts to activate blood and relax tendons, while mo yao more acts to dissolve

乳香、没药，均药用树脂，气香味浊，辛散走窜，能活血止痛、消肿生肌。既治血瘀气滞心腹诸痛，又疗痈疽疮肿，跌打损伤。内服外敷并用。其中乳香长于活血伸筋，没药善于散瘀止痛。

stasis and stop pain.

All *Salviae Miltiorrhizae Radix et Rhizoma* (dan shen), *Carthami Flos* (hong hua) and *Persicae Semen* (tao ren) act to activate blood and dredge meridians, applied to treat menstrual and obstetrical diseases due to blood stasis, and blood stasis pattern manifested by chest pain, cardiac pain and traumatic injury. Dan shen is cool in property and acts to activate blood and regulate menstruation, applied to treat irregular menstruation. It acts to activate blood, dissolve stasis and stop pain, applied to treat chest pain and cardiac pain due to blood stasis. It also acts to purify heart, relieve restlessness, cool blood and dissolve carbuncle, applied to treat restlessness, insomnia, carbuncle and furuncle with swelling and pain. Hong hua is warm in property and acts to activate blood, dredge meridians, dissolve stasis and stop pain, applied to treat various pains due to blood stasis. It is also applied to treat heat accumulation and blood stasis pattern manifested by macula in purple and dark color. Tao ren is neutral and moist in property and acts to activate blood, break blood, dissolve carbuncle and drain purulence, applied to treat pulmonary abscess and acute appendicitis. It acts to moisturize intestines and promote defecation, applied to treat constipation due to dryness in intestines. It also acts to stop cough and soothe panting, applied to treat cough and panting.

丹参、红花、桃仁，均能活血通经，为瘀滞所致的经产诸证，胸痹心痛、跌打损伤等瘀血证所常用。其中丹参性凉，功善活血调经，为调经要药；且能活血化瘀止痛，善治瘀滞胸痹心痛；并能清心除烦、凉血消痈，可用于心烦不眠、疮痈肿痛。红花性温，功专活血通经、散瘀止痛，为多种瘀滞疼痛证所常用，且治热郁血滞之斑疹紫暗。桃仁性平质润，活血力强，有破血之功，兼消痈排脓，故常治肺痈、肠痈；且润肠燥而通便，治肠燥便秘；并能止咳平喘，治咳喘常用之。

Both *Leonuri Herba* (yi mu cao) and *Achyranthis Bidentatae Radix* (niu xi) act to activate blood and regulate menstruation. Yi mu cao is slightly cold in property and acts to activate blood and regulate menstruation, applied to various menstrual and

益母草、牛膝，均能活血调经。其中益母草性微寒，为活血调经要药，为治经产诸证之常用；且能利水消肿，治水瘀互结的水肿、小便不

obstetrical diseases. It acts to promote water flow and subside swell, applied to treat water retention and blood stasis pattern manifested by edema and difficult urination. It also acts to clear heat and relieve toxin, applied to treat carbuncle, furuncle and skin itch. Niu xi is neutral in property and acts to activate blood and regulate menstruation, applied to treat dysmenorrhea and amenorrhea. It is attributive to the Liver and Kidney Meridians and acts to reinforce liver and kidney and strengthen tendons and bones, applied to treat liver and kidney deficiency pattern manifested by aching and pain at low back and knees, and weakness of lower limbs. It acts to guide fire or heat to go downwards, applied to treat fire or heat in the upper or bleeding in the upper. It also acts to promote water flow and treat stranguria, applied to treat stranguria due to heat and edema.

利;还能清热解毒,治疮痈、皮肤痒疹。牛膝性平,功能活血通经,善治痛经经闭;入肝肾经,且能补肝肾、强筋骨,治肝肾不足的腰膝酸痛、下肢无力;其性下行,又能引火或引热下行,治上部火热或出血证;还能利尿通淋,治淋证、水肿。

Spatholobi Caulis (ji xue teng) is sweet, bitter and warm in property and acts to activate blood, reinforce blood, regulate menstruation and stop pain, termed as the blood-reinforcing herb among the category of blood-activating herbs, and applied to treat irregular menstruation, dysmenorrhea and amenorrhea. It also acts to nourish blood, activate blood, relax tendons and dredge collaterals, applied to treat Bi (Obturation) Pattern due to wind-damp, spasm and pain at tendons and vessels, and hemiplegia.

鸡血藤,甘苦性温,功能活血补血、调经止痛,为活血药中活血、补血两者兼能的药物,可治月经不调、痛经经闭;且能养血活血、舒筋通络,故风湿痹痛筋脉不舒,或半身不遂皆可选用。

Both *Curcumae Rhizoma* (e zhu) and *Sparganii Rhizoma* (san leng) act to break blood, move qi, dissolve stagnation and stop pain, applied together for mutual reinforcement. They are applied to treat abdominal masses, distension and pain at chest and

莪术、三棱,均破血行气、消积止痛,常相须为用。可用治癥瘕痞块,胸腹胀痛,食积不消,血滞经闭等证。其区别在于,三棱功偏破血,

abdomen, food retention due to indigestion, and amenorrhea due to blood stasis. San leng acts more to break blood, while e zhu acts more to break qi.

莪术功偏破气。

Whitmania pigra Whitman (shui zhi), an animal herb, is neutral and slightly poisonous in property, and attributive to the Liver Meridian and the Xue (Blood) Phase. It acts to break blood, dredge meridians, dissolve stasis and relieve masses, applied to treat amenorrhea due to blood stasis and abdominal masses.

水蛭，为动物药，性平有毒，专入肝经血分，善破血通经、逐瘀消癥，可治血瘀经闭、癥瘕积聚等。

Chapter 12 Phlegm-Dissolving, Cough-Stopping and Pant-Relieving Herbs

第12章 化痰止咳平喘药

The medicinal herbs acting to dissipate phlegm or acting to eliminate phlegm are called the phlegm-dissolving herbs. The medicinal acting to stop and reduce cough and pant are called the cough-stopping and pant-relieving herbs.

以消痰或祛痰为主要作用的药物，称化痰药。以制止或减轻咳嗽喘息为主要作用药物，称止咳平喘药。

The phlegm-dissolving herbs are mostly pungent, bitter or sweet in flavor, and cold or warm in property. The phlegm-dissolving herbs in warm property mostly act to desiccate damp and dissolve phlegm, to warm lung and eliminate phlegm, and to subdue qi and dissolve phlegm, applied to treat cold-phlegm pattern or damp-phlegm pattern manifested by cough with white sputum and white-sticky tongue coating, and dizziness and epilepsy due to phlegm, such as *Pinelliae Rhizoma* (ban xia), *Arisaematis Rhizoma* (tian nan xing), *Sinapis Semen Albae* (jie zi), *Inulae Flos* (xuan fu hua) and *Cynanchi Stauntonii Rhizoma et Radix* (bai qian). The phlegm-dissolving herbs in cold-cool property mostly act to clear heat and dissolve phlegm, and to moisture lung and dissolve phlegm, applied to treat heat-phlegm pattern or dryness-phlegm pattern manifested by cough with yellow sputum or with scanty sputum, and phlegm and fire accumulation pattern manifested by scrofula and goiter, such as *Peucedani Radix* (qian hu), *Trichosanthis Fructus* (gua lou), *Fritillariae Cirrhosae Bulbus*

化痰药大多味辛、苦或甘，药性寒温不一。药性偏温的化痰药大多具有燥湿化痰、温肺祛痰、降气化痰等作用，主要用于寒痰、湿痰的咳痰色白，舌苔白腻，以及因痰所致的眩晕、癫痫。如半夏、天南星、芥子、旋覆花、白前。药性偏寒凉的化痰药大多具有清化痰热、润燥化痰的作用，主要用于热痰、燥痰所致的咳嗽痰黄或少痰，以及痰火互结的瘰疬、瘿瘤。如前胡、瓜蒌、川贝母、浙贝母、竹茹等。

(chuan bei mu), *Bulbus Fritillariae Thunbergii* (zhe bei mu) and *Bambusae Caulis in Taenias* (zhu ru).

The cough-stopping and pant-relieving herbs are cold or warm in property, and act to stop cough and relieve pant, applied to treat cough and panting. Some of them act to subdue qi, disperse lung and stop cough, such as *Armeniacae Amarum Semen* (ku xing ren) and *Perillae Fructus* (zi su zi). Some of them act to moisturize lung and stop cough, such as *Stemonae Radix* (bai bu), *Aster Radix et Rhizoma* (zi wan) and *Farfarae Flos* (kuan dong hua). Some of them act to purify lung and stop cough, such as *Eriobotryae Folium* (pi pa ye). Some of them act to disperse lung and relieve panting, such as *Cortex Mori Albae Radicis* (sang bai pi) and *Descurainiae Semenlepidii Semen* (ting li zi). The medicinal herbs are applied according to the patterns and symptoms.

止咳平喘药寒温不一，以制止咳嗽、平定气喘为主要作用，用于咳嗽气喘病证。其中或功偏降气、宣肺止咳，如杏仁、紫苏子。或润肺止咳，如百部、紫菀、款冬花。或清肺止咳，如枇杷叶。或泻肺平喘，如桑白皮、葶苈子。可随证选用。

In the application of the medicinal herbs, it is important to notify that it is not advisable to apply the phlegm-dissolving herbs in bitter and warm property to treat cough with dry sputum or bloody sputum. Cough and pant vary in exterior and interior, in cold and heat and in deficiency and excess. It is necessary to choose relevant herbs and to combine proper herbs according to different types of etiology and pathogenesis.

使用本类药物时需注意，味苦性温的化痰药不宜用于燥痰或咳嗽兼有咯血者。咳喘有表里、寒热、虚实的不同，必须针对不同病因、病机，选用相应的药物，并作适当的配伍。

Section 1 Phlegm-dissolving herbs

第1节 化痰药

Pinelliae Rhizoma (ban xia)

半夏

It is the dried product from the rhizome of

为天南星科植物半夏的

Pinellia ternate (Thunb.) Breit, family Araceae. The medicinal herb is collected in summer and autumn. The products include *Pinelliae Rhizoma* Cruda (sheng ban xia), *Pinelliae Rhizoma Preparatum* (fa ban xia), *Pinelliae Rhizoma Preparata* (qing ban xia) and ginger-processed *Pinelliae Rhizoma* (jiang ban xia).

干燥块茎。夏、秋二季采挖。炮制品有生半夏、法半夏、清半夏、姜半夏。

Features Flavor: pungent. Property: warm and poisonous. Meridian tropism: the Spleen Meridian, the Stomach Meridian and the Lung Meridian.

性味归经 辛，温；有毒。归脾、胃、肺经。

Actions Desiccate damp, dissolve phlegm, subdue up-reverse flow of qi, stop vomiting, dissipate masses, relieve stagnation, subside swell and stop pain.

功效 燥湿化痰，降逆止呕，消痞散结，消肿止痛。

Application

(1) Damp-phlegm pattern or cold-phlegm pattern. The medicinal herb is warm and dry in property and acts to warm and dissolve cold phlegm and to desiccate and dissolve damp phlegm, and acts to stop cough, applied to treat cold-phlegm pattern and damp-phlegm pattern. In the treatment of damp-phlegm pattern manifested by cough with white sputum, it is combined with *Exocarpium Citri Leiocarpae* (ju pi) and *Poria* (fu ling), to form up Double Vintage Decoction (Er Chen Tang). In the treatment of cold-phlegm pattern manifested by cough with excessive, thin and clear sputum, it is combined with *Zingiberis Rhizoma* (gan jiang) and *Asari Radix et Rhizoma* (xi xin), to form up Minor Green Dragon Decoction (Xiao Qing Long Tang). In the treatment of damp-phlegm disturbing the upper manifested by headache and dizziness, it is combined with *Atractylodis Macrocephalae Rhizoma*

应用

（1）湿痰或寒痰证。本品性温燥，善温化寒痰、燥化湿痰，并有止咳作用，为治寒痰、湿痰之要药。治湿聚为痰，咳嗽气逆，痰多色白者，常配橘皮、茯苓等，如二陈汤。治寒痰咳嗽，痰多清稀者，配干姜、细辛等，如小青龙汤。治湿痰上扰，头痛眩晕者，则与白术、天麻等同用，如半夏白术天麻汤。

(bai zhu) and *Gastrodiae Rhizoma* (tian ma), to form up Pinellia, Atractylodes and Gastrodia Decoction (Ban Xia Bai Zhu Tian Ma Tang).

(2) Vomiting. The medicinal herb acts to subdue up-reverse flow of qi and harmonize stomach, applied to treat vomiting. In the treatment of vomiting due to cold in stomach, it is combined with *Zingiberis Rhizoma Recens* (sheng jiang), to form up Minor Pinellia Decoction (Xiao Ban Xia Tang). In the treatment of vomiting due to heat in stomach, it is combined with *Coptidis Rhizoma* (huang lian) and *Bambusae Caulis in Taenias* (zhu ru). In the treatment of vomiting due to stomach deficiency, it is combined with *Ginseng Radix et Raizoma* (ren shen).

（2）呕吐。本品又能降逆和胃，为止呕要药。尤宜于胃寒呕吐，常与生姜同用，即小半夏汤。治胃热呕吐，与黄连、竹茹等同用。治胃虚呕吐，可与人参等同用。

(3) Chest pain, cardiac pain, stuffy chest, globus hystericus (Plum Pit Qi), scrofula and goiter. The medicinal herb is pungent and dispersing in property and acts to dissolve masses, warm and dissolve phlegm, and dissipate phlegm accumulation. In the treatment of chest pain and cardiac pain due to phlegm-turbidity, it is combined with *Trichosanthis Fructus* (gua lou) and *Alli Macrostemi Bulbus* (xie bai), to form up Snakegourd, Longstaner Onion Bulb and Pinellia Decoction (Gua Lou Xie Bai Ban Xia Tang). In the treatment of phlegm-heat blocking chest, it is combined with gua lou and huang lian, to form up Minor Chest-Bind Decoction (Xiao Xian Xiong Tang). In the treatment of stuffy chest, it is combined with gan jiang, ren shen and huang lian, to form up Pinellia Heart-Reducing Decoction (Ban Xia Xie Xin Tang). In the treatment of globus hystericus (Plum Pit Qi), it is combined with *Magnoliae Officinalis Cortex* (hou po) and

（3）胸痹心痛，心下痞满，梅核气，瘿瘤痰核。本品有辛散消痞、温燥化痰之功，能散痰结。治痰浊胸痹心痛，可与瓜蒌、薤白同用，即瓜蒌薤白半夏汤。治痰热互结之结胸，可与瓜蒌、黄连同用，即小陷胸汤。治心下痞满，可与干姜、人参、黄连等同用，如半夏泻心汤。治痰气所致的梅核气，与厚朴、紫苏等同用。治瘿瘤痰核，与连翘、浙贝母等同用。

Perillae Folium (zi su zi). In the treatment of scrofula and goiter, it is combined with *Forsythiae Fructus* (lian qiao) and *Bulbus Fritillariae Thunbergii* (zhe bei mu).

(4) Carbuncle and furuncle due to heat-toxin. The medicinal herb acts to subside swell and stop pain for external use. In the treatment of carbuncle with unhealed ulcer, furuncle with swelling and pain, it is combined singly by grinding into powder for external use.

（4）痈疽肿毒。本品外用能消肿止痛。治痈疽发背、无名肿毒，可用生品研末调敷。

Usage and dosage Apply 3～9 g in decoction. Apply a proper amount for external use. The medicinal herb is poisonous in crude form and acts to subside swell and stop pain for external use. The prepared forms have different actions. Fa ban xia and qing ban xia act to desiccate damp and dissolve phlegm, while jiang ban xia acts to subdue up-reverse flow of qi and stop vomiting.

用法用量 煎服，3～9克。外用适量。生用有毒，消肿止痛，多作外用。炮制后作用有异，其中法半夏、清半夏功偏燥湿化痰，姜半夏功偏降逆止呕。

Precautions for use The medicinal herb is incompatible to *Aconiti Radix* (wu tou). It is cautious to apply for those with dry cough due to yin deficiency, or cough due to heat-phlegm, or cough with dryness-phlegm.

使用注意 反乌头。阴虚燥咳，热痰，燥痰应慎用。

Arisaematis Rhizoma (tian nan xing)

天南星

It is the dried product from the tuber of the perennial herbage *Arisaema erubescens* (Wall.) Schott, *Arisaema heterophyllum* Bl., or *Arisaema amurense* Maxim., family Araceae. The medicinal herb is collected in autumn and winter, applied in crude form or prepared form.

为天南星科植物天南星、异叶天南星或东北天南星的干燥块茎。秋、冬二季采挖。生用或制用。

Features Flavor: bittern and pungent. Property: warm and poisonous. Meridian tropism: the Lung Meridian, the Liver Meridian and the Spleen

性味归经 苦、辛，温；有毒。归肺、肝、脾经。

Meridian.

Actions Desiccate damp, dissolve phlegm, eliminate wind and relieve convulsion, and subside swell and stop pain for external use.

功效 燥湿化痰,祛风止痉,外用消肿止痛。

Application

(1) Cough with intractable sputum. The medicinal herb is bitter, pungent and warm in property and strongly acts to desiccate damp and dissolve phlegm. In the treatment of cough with intractable sputum, it is combined with *Pinelliae Rhizoma* (ban xia) and *Aurantii Fructus Immaturus* (zhi shi), to form up Phlegm-Abducting Decoction (Dao Tan Tang).

(2) Dizziness due to wind-phlegm, hemiplegia due to wind stroke, epilepsy and tetanus. The medicinal herb is attributive to the meridians and collaterals and acts to eliminate wind-phlegm and relieve convulsion. In the treatment of dizziness due to wind-phlegm, it is combined with ban xia and *Gastrodiae Rhizoma* (tian ma). In the treatment of wind stroke or hemiplegia due to wind-phlegm, it is combined with *Aconiti Radix* (chuan wu). In the treatment of tetanus manifested by convulsion and lockjaws, it is combined with tian ma and *Saposhnikoviae Radix* (fang feng).

(3) Carbuncle and furuncle with swelling and pain, snake-bites or insect-bites. The medicinal herb acts to subside swell and stop pain. In the treatment of carbuncle and furuncle with swelling and pain or snake-bites and insect-bites, it is applied singly by grinding into powder for external use.

应用

(1)顽痰咳嗽。本品苦温辛烈,有较强的燥湿祛痰作用。治顽痰咳喘,常与半夏、枳实等同用,如导痰汤。

(2)风痰眩晕,中风半身不遂,癫痫,破伤风。本品善走经络、祛风痰,且能止痉。治风痰眩晕,与半夏、天麻等同用。治风痰所致的中风、半身不遂,可与川乌等同用。治破伤风抽搐,牙关紧闭,可与天麻、防风等同用。

(3)痈疽肿痛,蛇虫咬伤。本品能消肿止痛。治痈疽肿痛或蛇虫咬伤,可研末调敷。

Usage and dosage Apply 3～9 g in decoction. Apply a proper amount for external use. The medicinal herb in crude form is poisonous and acts to sub-

用法用量 煎服,3～9克。外用适量。生用有毒,消肿止痛,多作外用,内服宜

side swell and stop pain for external use, so it is cautious to apply for oral administration. The medicinal herb in prepared form acts to desiccate damp, dissolve phlegm, eliminate wind and relieve spasm.

慎。制用燥湿化痰、祛风止痉。

Precautions for use It is prohibited to apply for those with yin deficiency or those with dryness-phlegm or for pregnant women.

使用注意 阴虚燥痰及孕妇忌用。

Sinapis Semen (jie zi)

芥子

It is the dried product from the seed of *Sinapis alba* L. or *Brassica juncea* (L.) Czern. et Coss., family Cruciferaceae. It is also called "*Sinapis Semen Albae* (bai jie zi)". The medicinal herb is collected in late summer and early autumn, applied in crude form or in stir-fried form.

为十字花科植物白芥或芥的干燥成熟种子。又名"白芥子"。夏末秋初时采收。生用或炒用。

Features Flavor: pungent. Property: warm. Meridian tropism: the Lung Meridian.

性味归经 辛,温。归肺经。

Actions Warm lung, dissolve phlegm, promote qi flow, dissipate stagnation, dredge collaterals and stop pain.

功效 温肺祛痰利气,散结通络止痛。

Application

(1) Cold-phlegm blocking lung, and distension and pain at chest and hypochondria. The medicinal herb is pungent and warm and acts to warm lung, dissolve phlegm, promote qi flow and dilate diaphragm. In the treatment of cold-phlegm blocking lung manifested by excessive sputum and stuffy chest, it is combined with *Perillae Folium* (zi su zi) and *Raphani Semen* (lai fu zi), to form up Three Seed Filial Devotion Decoction (San Zi Yang Qin Tang). In the treatment of phlegm-rheum retention manifested by distension and pain at chest and hypochondria, it is combined with *Kansui Radix* (gan sui) and *Euphorbiae Pekinensis Radix* (jing da ji).

应用

(1)寒痰壅肺,胸胁胀痛。本品辛温善行,能温肺祛痰、利气畅膈。治寒痰壅肺,痰多胸闷,可与紫苏子、莱菔子等同用,如三子养亲汤。治痰饮停滞,胸胁胀痛,可与甘遂、大戟等同用。

(2) Phlegm blocking meridians and collaterals manifested by numbness of joint, dorsal furuncle and deep multiple abscesses. The medicinal herb acts to dissolve phlegm in meridians and collaterals, and also acts to promote qi flow, dredge collaterals, stop pain and dissipate stagnation. In the treatment of phlegm blocking meridians and collaterals manifested by numbness or swelling and pain of joints, it is combined with *Myrrha* (mo yao) and *Cinnamomi Cortex* (rou gui). In the treatment of cold-phlegm stagnation manifested by dorsal furuncle and deep multiple abscesses, it is combined with *Colla Cornus Cervi* (lu jiao jiao), *Ephedrae Herba* (ma huang) and *Rehmanniae Radix Praeparata* (shu di huang), to form up Yang-Harmonizing Decoction (Yang He Tang).

（2）痰滞经络的关节麻木，阴疽流注。本品既善去经络之痰，又能利气通络止痛散结。治痰滞经络所致的关节麻木或肿痛，常与没药、肉桂等同用。治寒痰凝滞的阴疽流注，可与鹿角胶、麻黄、熟地黄等同用，如阳和汤。

Furthermore, the medicinal herb is combined with *Corydalis Rhizoma* (yan hu suo) and *Asari Radix et Rhizoma* (xi xin) by grinding into powder and mixed with *Zingiberis Rhizoma Recens* (sheng jiang) juice to make into paste, applied topically at Point Feishu (BL 13) in summer to treat chronic asthma.

此外，本品与延胡索、细辛等研末，生姜汁调糊，夏令时节外敷肺俞等穴，治喘哮日久不愈。

Usage and dosage Apply 3～9 g in decoction. Apply a proper amount for external use.

用法用量 煎服，3～9克。外用适量。

Precautions for use It is prohibited to apply for those chronic cough due to lung deficiency or those with yin deficiency and fire hyperactivity. It may cause gastroenteritis manifested by abdominal pain and diarrhea in large dose for oral administration, so it is prohibited to apply for those with gastrointestinal ulcer or hemorrhage. It may cause skin blisters for external use, so it is prohibited to apply for those with skin allergy.

使用注意 久咳肺虚及阴虚火旺者忌用。内服量大易致胃肠炎，产生腹痛、腹泻。消化道溃疡或出血者忌用。外用易使皮肤起泡，皮肤过敏者忌用。

Inulae Flos (xuan fu hua)

It is the dried product from the capitulum of *Inula japonica* Thunb. or *Inula britannica L.*, family Compositae. The medicinal herb is collected in summer and autumn when it is flowering, applied in crude form or honey-prepared form.

Features Flavor: bitter, pungent and salty. Property: slightly warm. Meridian tropism: the Lung Meridian, the Spleen Meridian, the Stomach Meridian and the Large Intestine Meridian.

Actions Subdue qi, dissolve phlegm, promote water flow and stop vomiting.

Application

(1) Cough and panting with excessive sputum. The medicinal herb is pungent, bitter, opening and descending in property, and acts to subdue up-reverse flow of lung qi, dissolve phlegm and rheum and dissipate masses. In the treatment of cough and panting with excessive sputum due to phlegm blockage and up-reverse flow of qi, and stuffiness at chest and diaphragm, it is combined with *Perillae Folium* (zi su zi) and *Pinelliae Rhizoma* (ban xia).

(2) Belching and vomiting. The medicinal herb acts to subdue stomach qi and stop vomiting and belching. In the treatment of phlegm and up-reverse flow of qi manifested by belching, vomiting and stuffy chest, it is combined with *Haematitum* (zhe shi), ban xia and *Zingiberis Rhizoma Recens* (sheng jiang), to form up Inula and Hermatitum Decoction (Xuan Fu Dai Zhe Tang).

Usage and dosage Apply 3～9 g in decoction by wrapping.

Precautions for use It is prohibited to apply

旋覆花

为菊科植物旋覆花或欧亚旋覆花的干燥头状花序。夏、秋二季花开时采收。生用或蜜炙用。

性味归经 苦、辛、咸，微温。归肺、脾、胃、大肠经。

功效 降气消痰行水，降逆止呕。

应用

（1）咳喘痰多。本品辛开苦降，能降上逆之肺气、消痰化饮除痞。治痰壅气逆的咳喘痰多，胸膈痞闷，常与紫苏子、半夏等同用。

（2）嗳气，呕吐。本品善降胃气、止呕逆。治痰阻气逆的嗳气、呕吐，心下痞满，常与代赭石、半夏、生姜等配伍，如旋覆代赭汤。

用法用量 煎服，3～9克。宜包煎。

使用注意 阴虚劳嗽，

for those with cough due to lung yin deficiency or dry cough due to body fluid consumption.

津伤燥咳者忌用。

Cynanchi Stauntonii Rhizoma et Radix (bai qian)

It is the dried product from the root and rhizome of *Cynanchum stauntonni* (Decne.) Schltr. ex levl. or *Cynanchum glaucescens* (Decne.) Hand-Mazz., family Asclepiadaceae. The medicinal herb is collected in autumn, applied in crude form or honey-prepared form.

Features Flavor: pungent and bitter. Property: slightly warm. Meridian tropism: the Lung Meridian.

Actions Subdue qi, dissolve phlegm and stop cough.

Application

Cough with excessive sputum, and panting due to up-reverse flow of qi. The medicinal herb is slightly warm without dryness in property, especially attributive to the Lung Meridian, and acts to subdue qi, dissolve phlegm, stop cough and relieve panting, applied to treat cough and panting of excess pattern. In the treatment of cough due to wind-cold, it is combined with *Schizonepetae Herba* (jing jie), *Platycodonis Radix* (jie geng) and *Citri Reticulatae Pericarpium* (chen pi), to form up Cough-Stopping Powder (Zhi Sou San). In the treatment of heat-phlegm in lung manifested by panting, it is combined with *Cortex Mori Albae Radicis* (sang bai pi) and *Scutellariae Radix* (huang qin). In the treatment of internal retention of phlegm-rheum manifested by cough, panting and edema, it is combined with *Euphorbiae Pekinensis Radix* (jing da ji) and *Aster Radix et Rhizoma* (zi wan), to form up

白前

为萝摩科植物柳叶白前或芫花叶白前的干燥根茎及根。秋季采挖。生用或蜜炙用。

性味归经 辛、苦，微温。归肺经。

功效 降气，消痰，止咳。

应用

咳嗽痰多，气逆喘促。本品微温不燥，专入肺经，能降气祛痰、止咳平喘，多用于咳喘实证。治风寒咳嗽，常配伍荆芥、桔梗、陈皮等同用，如止嗽散。治肺热痰喘，常与桑白皮、黄芩等同用。治痰饮内停，咳喘浮肿，可与大戟、紫菀等同用，如白前汤。

White Swallowwort Decoction (Bai Qian Tang).

Usage and dosage Apply 3～10 g in decoction. The medicinal herb acts to subdue qi and dissolve phlegm in crude form, and acts to moisturize lung and stop cough in honey-prepared form.

用法用量 煎服，3～10克。生用降气消痰，蜜炙润肺止咳。

Precautions for use It is not advisable to apply for those with dry cough due to lung deficiency.

使用注意 肺虚干咳不宜。

Platycodonis Radix (jie geng)

桔梗

It is the dried product from the root of *Platycodon grandiflorum* (Jacq.) A. DC., family Campanulaceae. The medicinal herb is collected in spring and autumn, applied in crude form.

为桔梗科植物桔梗的干燥根。春、秋二季采挖。生用。

Features Flavor: bitter and pungent. Property: neutral. Meridian tropism: the Lung Meridian.

性味归经 苦、辛，平。归肺经。

Actions Disperse lung, dissolve phlegm, drain purulence and benefit throat.

功效 宣肺，祛痰，排脓，利咽。

Application

应用

(1) Cough with excessive sputum. The medicinal herb acts to disperse lung, promote qi flow, dissolve phlegm and dilate chest. In the treatment of cough due to wind-cold, it is combined with *Perillae Folium* (zi su ye) and *Armeniacae Amarum Semen* (ku xing ren). In the treatment of cough with yellow sputum due to wind-heat, it is combined with *Mori Folium* (sang ye), *Chrysanthemi Flos* (ju hua) and ku xing ren. In the treatment of qi stagnation and phlegm blockage pattern manifested by stuffy chest, it is combined with *Aurantii Fructus* (zhi qiao) and *Trichosanthis Fructus* (gua lou).

（1）咳嗽痰多。本品能宣开肺气，祛痰宽胸。治风寒咳嗽，常与紫苏、杏仁等同用。治风热咳嗽痰黄，可与桑叶、菊花、杏仁等同用。治气滞痰阻，胸闷不舒，与枳壳、瓜蒌皮等同用。

(2) Pulmonary abscess. The medicinal herb acts to promote lung qi flow, drain purulence and dissipate carbuncle. In the treatment of pulmonary abscess with purulent sputum, it is combined with

（2）肺痈。本品善利肺气、排脓消痈。治肺痈吐脓，常与芦根、鱼腥草等同用，以清肺排脓。

Phragmitis Rhizoma (lu gen) and *Houttuyniae Herba* (yu xing cao) for the purpose to purify lung and drain purulence.

(3) Sore throat and hoarseness of voice. The medicinal herb acts to disperse lung, promote qi flow, benefit throat and ease up voice. In the treatment of sore throat and loss of voice due to wind-heat, it is combined with *Glycyrrhizae Radix et Rhizoma* (gan cao), to form up Platycodon Decoction (Jie Geng Tang). In the treatment of hoarseness of voice due to wind-cold, it is combined with *Saposhnikoviae Radix* (fang feng), *Schizonepetae Herba* (jing jie) and *Ephedrae Herba* (ma huang). In the treatment of sore throat due to heat-toxin, it is combined with *Belamecandae Rhizoma* (she gan), *Isatidis Radix* (ban lan gen).

（3）咽痛音哑。本品能宣肺气、利咽开音。治风热咽痛失声，与甘草同用，即桔梗汤。治风寒音哑，与防风、荆芥、麻黄等同用。治热毒咽痛，与射干、板蓝根等同用。

Furthermore, the medicinal herb is ascending in property and acts to guide other herbs to go upwards, as the meridian-guiding herb of the Lung Meridian.

此外，其性上行，能载药上行，为肺经之引经药。

Usage and dosage Apply 3～10 g in decoction.

用法用量 煎服，3～10克。

Precautions for use It is possible to cause nausea and vomiting in large dose.

使用注意 用量过大，易致恶心呕吐。

Peucedani Radix (qian hu)

前胡

It is the dried product from the root of *Peucedanum praeruptorum* Dunn., family Umbelliferae. The medicinal herb is collected in winter and next spring when stems and leaves are withered or before it is sprouting, applied in crude form or in honey-calcined form.

为伞形科植物白花前胡的干燥根。冬季至次春茎叶枯萎或未抽花茎时采挖。生用或蜜炙用。

Features Flavor: bitter and pungent. Property: slightly cold. Meridian tropism: the Lung Me-

性味归经 苦、辛，微寒。归肺经。

ridian.

Actions Subdue qi, dissolve phlegm and eliminate wind-heat.

Application

(1) Cough and panting due to phlegm-heat. The medicinal herb acts to purify lung, subdue qi and dissolve phlegm. In the treatment of cough and panting with thick-yellow sputum due to phlegm-heat, it is combined with *Cortex Mori Albae Radicis* (sang bai pi), *Armeniacae Amarum Semen* (ku xing ren) and *Bulbus Fritillariae Thunbergii* (zhe bei mu).

(2) Exterior wind-heat pattern. The medicinal herb acts to eliminate wind-heat, dissolve phlegm and stop cough. In the treatment of exterior wind-heat pattern manifested by aversion to cold, fever and cough with yellow sputum, it is combined with *Mori Folium* (sang ye), *Menthae Haplocalycis Herba* (bo he) and *Platycodonis Radix* (jie geng).

Usage and dosage Apply 3～10 g in decoction. The medicinal herb acts to eliminate wind-heat, subdue qi and dissolve phlegm in crude form, and acts to moisturize lung and stop cough in honey-calcined form.

功效 降气化痰，宣散风热。

应用

（1）痰热咳喘。本品具清肺降气化痰之功。治痰热咳喘，痰稠色黄，常与桑白皮、苦杏仁、浙贝母等同用。

（2）外感风热证。本品既宣散风热，又祛痰止咳。以外感风热，恶寒发热，兼见咳嗽痰黄者最宜，常与桑叶、薄荷、桔梗等同用。

用法用量 煎服，3～10克。生用宣散风热、降气化痰，蜜炙润肺止咳。

Trichosanthis Fructus (gua lou)

It is the dried product from the ripe fruit of *Trichosanthes kirilowii* Maxim. or *Trichosanthes* rosthornii Harms, family Cucurbitaceae. The medicinal herb is collected in autumn when the fruits are ripe, applied in crude form.

Features Flavor: sweet, slightly bitter. Property: cold. Meridian tropism: the Lung Meridian, the Stomach Meridian and the Large Intestine Meridian.

瓜蒌

为葫芦科植物栝楼或双边栝楼的干燥成熟果实。秋季果实成熟时采收。生用。

性味归经 甘、微苦，寒。归肺、胃、大肠经。

Actions Clear heat, dissolve phlegm, dilate chest, dissipate stagnation, moisturize intestines and promote defecation.

功效 清热化痰,宽胸散结,润肠通便。

Application

(1) Cough and panting due to phlegm-heat. The medicinal herb is sweet, cold and moist in property, and acts to purify and moisturize lung, dissolve phlegm and stop cough. In the treatment of cough with yellow-thick sputum due to phlegm-heat, it is combined with *Scutellariae Radix* (huang qin), *Arisaema cum Bile* (dan nan xing) and *Aurantii Fructus Immaturus* (zhi shi). In the treatment of dryness-heat damaging lung manifested by difficult spitting of sputum, it is combined with *Fritillariae Cirrhosae Bulbus* (chuan bei mu), *Trichosanthis Radix* (tian hua fen) and *Platycodonis Radix* (jie geng).

(2) Chest pain and phlegm-heat accumulation in chest. The medicinal herb acts to dissolve phlegm, dissipate stagnation, promote qi flow and dilate chest. In the treatment of phlegm-qi stagnation manifested by chest pain and cardiac pain, it is combined with *Alli Macrostemi Bulbus* (xie bai), to form up Snakegourd, Longstaner Onion Bulb and Liquor (Gua Lou Xie Bai Bai Jiu Tang). In the treatment of phlegm-heat accumulation in chest manifested by stuffy chest, it is combined with *Coptidis Rhizoma* (huang lian) and *Pinelliae Rhizoma* (ban xia), to form up Minor Chest-Bind Decoction (Xiao Xian Xiong Tang).

(3) Acute mastitis, pulmonary abscess and acute appendicitis. The medicinal herb acts to dissipate stagnation and dissolve abscess, applied to treat both external and internal abscesses. In the treat-

应用

(1)痰热咳喘。本品甘寒,清润相兼,功善清肺润燥,化痰止咳。治痰热咳痰黄稠,可与黄芩、胆南星、枳实等同用。治燥热伤肺,咯痰不爽,常与川贝母、天花粉、桔梗等同用。

(2)胸痹,结胸。本品既化痰散结,又利气宽胸。治痰气痹阻的胸痹心痛,常与薤白同用,如瓜蒌薤白白酒汤。治痰热互结的结胸痞满,可与黄连、半夏等药同用,如小陷胸汤。

(3)乳痈,肺痈,肠痈。本品能散结消痈,内外痈皆宜。治乳痈红肿,可与蒲公英、金银花等同用。治肺痈

ment of acute mastitis manifested by local redness and swelling, it is combined with *Taraxaci Herba* (pu gong ying) and *Lonicerae Japonicae Flos* (jin yin hua). In the treatment of pulmonary abscess manifested by cough with purulent or bloody sputum, it is combined with *Phragmitis Rhizoma* (lu gen), *Houttuyniae Herba* (yu xing cao) and *Persicae Semen* (tao ren). In the treatment of acute appendicitis manifested by abdominal pain, it is combined with *Coicis Semen* (yi yi ren), *Patriniae Herba* (bai jiang cao) and *Sargentodoxae Caulis* (hong teng).

咳吐脓血，配伍芦根、鱼腥草、桃仁等同用。治肠痈腹痛，可与薏苡仁、败酱草、红藤等同用。

(4) Constipation due to dryness in intestines. The medicinal herb acts to moisturize intestines and promote defecation. In the treatment of constipation due to dryness in intestines, it is combined with *Cannabis Fructus* (huo ma ren) and *Pruni Semen* (yu li ren).

（4）肠燥便秘。本品能润肠通便。治肠燥便秘，配伍火麻仁、郁李仁等同用。

Usage and dosage Apply 9～15 g in decoction.

用法用量 煎服，9～15克。

Precautions for use It is prohibited to apply for those with loose feces due to spleen deficiency, or those with damp-phlegm pattern or cold-phlegm pattern. The medicinal herb is incompatible to *Aconiti Radix* (wu tou).

使用注意 脾虚便溏及湿痰、寒痰者忌用。反乌头。

Remarks *Trichosanthis Fructus* (quan gua lou), *Pericarpium Trichosanthis* (gua lou pi), *Semen Trichosanthis* (gua lou ren) and *Trichosanthis Radix* (tian hua fen)

按语 全瓜蒌与瓜蒌皮、瓜蒌仁、天花粉

All the four herbs are the products from *Trichosanthes kirilowii* Maxim. or *Trichosanthes uniflora* Hao, family Cucurbitaceae. Quan gua lou is the product from the fruit and acts to purify lung, dissolve phlegm, dilate chest, dissipate stagnation,

四药均来源于栝楼。不同的是以果实入药者为全瓜蒌，具有清肺化痰、宽胸散结、润燥通便作用。以果皮入药为瓜蒌皮，功能清肺化

moisturize intestines and promote defecation. Gua lou pi is the product from the peel of fruit and acts to purify lung, dissolve phlegm, promote qi flow and dilate chest. Gua lou ren is the product from the seed and acts to moisturize lung, dissolve phlegm, moisturize intestines and promote defecation. Tian hua fen is the product from the root and acts to clear heat, reduce fire, produce body fluid, subside swell and drain purulence.

痰，利气宽胸。以种子入药为瓜蒌子，又称瓜蒌仁，功能润肺化痰，润肠通便。以根入药为天花粉，功能清热泻火、清热生津、消肿排脓。

Fritillariae Cirrhosae Bulbus (chuan bei mu)

It is the dried product from the bulb of *Fritillaria cirrhosa* D. Don, *Fritillaria unibracteata* Hsiao et K. C. Hsia and *Fritillaria Przewalskii* Maxim., *Fritillaria delavayi* Franch or *Fritillaria taipaiensis* P. Y. Li., family Liliaceae. The medicinal herb is collected in summer and autumn or in winter when the snow is melting, applied in crude form.

Features Flavor: bitter and sweet. Property: slightly cold. Meridian tropism: the Lung Meridian and the Heart Meridian.

Actions Clear heat, purify lung, dissolve phlegm, stop cough, dissipate stagnation and subside swell.

Application

(1) Dry cough with scanty sputum, and cough due to yin deficiency. The medicinal herb is cold, sweet and moist in property, and acts to eliminate and dissolve phlegm, applied to treat dry cough and chronic cough. In the treatment of cough due to dryness in lung, it is combined with *Anemarrhenae Rhizoma* (zhi mu) in mutual reinforcement, to form up Anemarrhena and Fritillary Pills (Er Mu Wan), or combined with *Ophiopogonis Radix* (mai dong)

川贝母

为百合科植物川贝母、暗紫贝母、甘肃贝母、梭砂贝母、太白贝母等的干燥鳞茎。夏、秋二季或积雪融化时采挖。生用。

性味归经 苦、甘，微寒。归肺、心经。

功效 清热润肺，化痰止咳，散结消肿。

应用

（1）燥咳少痰，阴虚咳嗽。本品性凉味甘质润，具有清润化痰之功，尤宜于燥咳、久咳。治肺燥咳嗽，可与知母相须为用，即二母丸，或与麦冬、紫菀等同用。治阴虚久咳，可与百合、麦冬、熟地黄等同用。若劳嗽痰血，可与百部、阿胶、沙参等同

and *Aster Radix et Rhizoma* (zi wan). In the treatment of chronic cough due to yin deficiency, it is combined with *Bulbus Lilii* (bai he), mai dong and *Rehmanniae Radix Praeparata* (shu di huang). In the treatment of cough with bloody sputum in pulmonary tuberculosis, it is combined with *Stemonae Radix* (bai bu), *Asini Corii Colla* (e jiao) and *Glehniae Radix* (bei sha shen).

用。

(2) Scrofula, acute mastitis and pulmonary abscess. The medicinal herb acts to clear heat, dissolve phlegm, dissipate stagnation and subside swell. In the treatment of scrofula due to phlegm-fire, it is combined with *Scrophulariae Radix* (xuan shen) and *Ostreae Concha* (mu li). In the treatment of acute mastitis and pulmonary abscess due to heat-toxin, it is combined with the heat-clearing and toxin-relieving herbs.

（2）瘰疬，乳痈，肺痈。本品能清热化痰、散结消肿。治痰火瘰疬，与玄参、牡蛎等同用。治热毒乳痈、肺痈，可与清热解毒之品同用。

Usage and dosage Apply 3～10 g in decoction. Apply 1～2 g powder.

用法用量 煎服，3～10克。研末冲服，每次1～2克。

Precautions for use It is not advisable to apply to treat cold-phlegm pattern or damp-phlegm pattern. The medicinal herb is incompatible to *Aconiti Radix* (wu tou).

使用注意 寒痰、湿痰不宜。反乌头。

Fritillariae Thunbergii Bulbus (zhe bei mu)

浙贝母

It is the dried product from the bulb of *Fritillaria thunbergii* Miq., family Liliaceae. The medicinal herb is collected in early summer when it is withered, applied in crude form.

为百合科植物浙贝母的干燥鳞茎。初夏植株枯萎时采挖。生用。

Features Flavor: bitter. Property: cold. Meridian tropism: the Lung Meridian and the Heart Meridian.

性味归经 苦，寒。归肺、心经。

Actions Clear heat, dissolve phlegm, stop

功效 清热化痰止咳，

cough, relieve toxin, dissipate stagnation and reduce carbuncle.

解毒散结消痈。

Application

(1) Cough due to wind-heat or phlegm-fire. The medicinal herb is bitter and cold and acts to purify lung, clear heat, dissolve phlegm and stop cough. In the treatment of cough due to wind-heat, it is combined with *Mori Folium* (sang ye) and *Peucedani Radix* (qian hu). In the treatment of cough with yellow-thick sputum due to phlegm-heat, it is combined with *Trichosanthis Fructus* (gua lou), *Scutellariae Radix* (huang qin) and *Anemarrhenae Rhizoma* (zhi mu).

(2) Scrofula, goiter, carbuncle and furuncle, and pulmonary abscess. The medicinal herb is bitter, cold and dispersing in property and acts to reduce fire and dissipate stagnation. In the treatment of scrofula due to phlegm-fire accumulation, it is combined with *Scrophulariae Radix* (xuan shen) and *Ostreae Concha* (mu li). In the treatment of goiter, it is combined with the accumulation-relieving and goiter-treating herbs. In the treatment of carbuncle and furuncle due to heat-toxin, it is combined with *Forsythiae Fructus* (lian qiao) and *Taraxaci Herba* (pu gong ying). In the treatment of pulmonary abscess, it is combined with *Houttuyniae Herba* (yu xing cao) and *Phragmitis Rhizoma* (lu gen).

Usage and dosage Apply 5～10 g in decoction.

Precautions for use The medicinal herb is incompatible to *Aconiti Radix* (wu tou).

应用

（1）风热、痰火咳嗽。本品苦寒，能清泄肺热、化痰止咳。治风热咳嗽，与桑叶、前胡等同用。治痰热咳嗽，咯痰黄稠，配伍瓜蒌、黄芩、知母等同用。

（2）瘰疬，瘿瘤，疮痈，肺痈等。本品苦寒开泄，清火散结力大。治痰火郁结的瘰疬结核，可与玄参、牡蛎等同用。治瘿瘤，可配伍散结消瘿药同用。治热毒疮痈，可与连翘、蒲公英等配伍。治肺痈，可与鱼腥草、芦根等同用。

用法用量 煎服，5～10克。

使用注意 反乌头。

Bambusae Caulis in Taenias (zhu ru)

It is the dried product from the culm shavings of *Bambusa tuldoides* Munro, *Sinocalamus beecheyanus* (Munro) McClure var. *pubescens* P. F. Li or *Phyilostachys nigra* (Lodd.) Munro var. *henonis* (mits.) Stapf ex Rendlle, family Gramineae. The medicinal herb is collected all over the year, by peeling the fresh culm and taking the greenish middle part, applied in crude form or in prepared form with ginger juice.

Features Flavor: sweet. Property: slightly cold. Meridian tropism: the Lung Meridian, the Stomach Meridian, the Heart Meridian and the Gallbladder Meridian.

Actions Clear heat, dissolve phlegm, relieve restlessness and stop vomiting.

Application

(1) Cough due to heat in lung. The medicinal herb is cool and moist and acts to purify lung and dissolve phlegm. In the treatment of cough with yellow-thick sputum due to heat in lung, it is combined with *Trichosanthis Fructus* (gua lou) and *Cortex Mori Albae Radicis* (sang bai pi).

(2) Phlegm-fire disturbing the internal pattern. The medicinal herb acts to reduce fire, dissolve phlegm, and relieve depression and restlessness. In the treatment of fire-phlegm in gallbladder or phlegm-fire disturbing the internal manifested by pavor, restlessness and insomnia, it is combined with *Pinelliae Rhizoma* (ban xia), *Poria* (fu ling) and *Aurantii Fructus Immaturus* (zhi shi), to form up Gallbladder-Warming Decoction (Wen Dan Tang).

竹茹

为禾本科植物青杆竹、大头典竹或淡竹的茎杆的干燥中间层。全年均可采制，取新鲜茎，除去外皮，取稍带绿色的中间层。生用或姜汁炙用。

性味归经 甘，微寒。归肺、胃、心、胆经。

功效 清热化痰，除烦，止呕。

应用

（1）肺热咳嗽。本品性凉而润，善于清肺化痰。治肺热咳嗽，痰黄稠者，配伍瓜蒌、桑白皮等同用。

（2）痰火内扰证。本品能清火化痰、开郁除烦。治胆火夹痰，痰火内扰所致的惊悸不宁、心烦不眠，常与半夏、茯苓、枳实等同用，如温胆汤。

(3) Vomiting due to heat in stomach. The medicinal herb acts to eliminate heat in stomach and stop vomiting. In the treatment of vomiting due to heat in stomach, or phlegm-heat in stomach, or failure of stomach qi in harmonizing and descending, it is combined with *Coptidis Rhizoma* (huang lian), *Citri Reticulatae Pericarpium* (chen pi) and ban xia, to form up Coptis, Bamboo Shavings, Tangerine Peel and Pinellia Decoction (Huang Lian Zhu Ru Ju Pi Ban Xia Tang). In the treatment of vomiting due to heat in stomach with deficiency, it is combined with *Ginseng Radix et Raizoma* (ren shen), chen pi and *Zingiberis Rhizoma Recens* (sheng jiang), to form up Tangerine Peel and Bamboo Shavings Decoction (Ju Pi Zhu Ru Tang).

(3) 胃热呕吐。本品能清胃热、止呕吐。治胃热或胃有痰热,胃失和降的呕吐,配伍黄连、陈皮、半夏等,如黄连竹茹橘皮半夏汤。治胃虚有热而呕者,可配伍人参、陈皮、生姜等,如橘皮竹茹汤。

Usage and dosage Apply 5～10 g in decoction. The medicinal herb acts to clear heat and dissolve phlegm in crude form, and acts to stop vomiting in prepared form with ginger juice.

用法用量 煎服,5～10克。生用清化痰热,姜汁炙止呕。

Section 2 Cough-stopping and pant-relieving herbs

第2节 止咳平喘药

Armeniacae Amarum Semen (ku xing ren)

苦杏仁

It is the dried product from the ripe seed of *Prunus armeniaca* L. var. *ansu* Maxim., or *Prunus sibirica* L. *Prunus mandshurica* (Maxim.) Koehne or *Prunus armeniaca* L., family Rosaceae. The medicinal herb is collected in summer by taking out the seed from the ripe fruit, applied in crude form or stir-fried form.

为蔷薇科植物山杏、西伯利亚杏、东北杏或杏的干燥成熟种子。夏季采收成熟果实,取出种子。生用或炒用。

Features Flavor: bitter. Property: slightly

性味归经 苦,微温;有

warm and slight poisonous. Meridian tropism: the Lung Meridian and the Large Intestine Meridian.

小毒。归肺、大肠经。

Actions Subdue qi, stop cough, soothe panting, moisturize intestine and promote defecation.

功效 降气止咳平喘，润肠通便。

Application

应用

(1) Cough and panting. The medicinal herb is bitter and reducing in property and acts to subdue qi, stop cough and soothe panting, as the major herb to treat various types of cough, panting and stuffy chest due to cold or heat, with combination of other medicinal herbs according to different patterns. In the treatment of cough and panting due to wind-cold, it is combined with *Ephedrae Herba* (ma huang) and *Glycyrrhizae Radix et Rhizoma* (gan cao), to form up Three Disobediences Decoction (San Ao Tang). In the treatment of cough due to wind-heat, it is combined with *Mori Folium* (sang ye) and *Chrysanthemi Flos* (ju hua), to form up Mulberry and Chrysanthemum Drink (Sang Ju Yin). In the treatment of cough due to dryness in lung, it is combined with sang ye, *Fritillariae Cirrhosae Bulbus* (chuan bei mu) and *Glehniae Radix* (bei sha shen), to form up Mulberry and Almond Decoction (Sang Xing Tang) or Dryness-Eliminating and Lung-Rescuing Decoction (Qing Zao Jiu Fei Tang). In the treatment of cough and panting due to heat in lung, it is combined with *Gypsum Fibrosum* (shi gao) and gan cao, to form up Ephedra, Apricot, Gypsum and Liquorice Decoction (Ma Xing Shi Gan Tang).

（1）咳嗽气喘。本品苦泄不热，功善降气止咳平喘，兼宣肺气，为肺家要药，咳嗽喘满，无论新久寒热，均可随证配伍应用。治风寒咳喘，配伍麻黄、甘草同用，即三拗汤。治风热咳嗽，配伍桑叶、菊花等，如桑菊饮。治肺燥咳嗽，与桑叶、川贝母、沙参同用，如桑杏汤、清燥救肺汤。治肺热咳喘，常与石膏、甘草同用，如麻杏石甘汤。

(2) Constipation due to dryness in intestines. The medicinal herb is moist and fatty in property and acts to subdue qi, moisturize intestines and promote defecation. In the treatment of constipation due to dryness in intestines, it is combined with

（2）肠燥便秘。本品质润多脂，能降气润肠，通利大便。治肠燥便秘，配伍柏子仁、郁李仁等同用，如五仁丸。

Platycladi Semen (bai zi ren) and *Pruni Semen* (yu li ren), to form up Five Seeds Pills (Wu Ren Wan).

Usage and dosage Apply 5～10 g in decoction, decocting later.

用法用量 煎服，5～10克。生品入煎剂宜后下。

Precautions for use The medicinal herb is slightly poisonous. It is not advisable to apply in large dose.

使用注意 有小毒，用量不宜过大。

Perillae Fructus (zi su zi)

紫苏子

It is the dried product from the ripe fruit of *Perilla frutescens* (L.) Britt. var. acuta (Thunb.) Kudo, family Labiatae, also called su zi. The medicinal herb is collected in autumn, applied in crude form or mild-fried form.

为唇形科植物紫苏的干燥成熟果实。又名苏子。秋季采收。生用或微炒。

Features Flavor: pungent. Property: warm. Meridian tropism: the Lung Meridian and the Large Intestine Meridian.

性味归经 辛，温。归肺、大肠经。

Actions Subdue qi, dissolve phlegm, stop cough, soothe panting, moisturize intestines and promote defecation.

功效 降气化痰，止咳平喘，润肠通便。

Application

(1) Cough and panting. The medicinal herb is pungent, warm, moist and descending in property, and acts to subdue qi, dissolve phlegm, stop cough and soothe panting. In the treatment of cough and panting with excessive sputum due to phlegm accumulation and up-reverse flow of qi, it is combined with *Sinapis Semen Albae* (bai jie zi) and *Raphani Semen* (lai fu zi), to form up Three Seed Filial Devotion Decoction (San Zi Yang Qin Tang). In the treatment of chronic cough and panting with sputum due to excess in the upper and deficiency in the lower, it is combined with *Cinnamomi Cortex* (rou gui), *Magnoliae Officinalis Cortex* (hou po) and

应用

（1）咳嗽气喘。本品辛温不燥，质润下降，善下气化痰、止咳定喘。善治痰壅气逆的咳喘痰多，常与白芥子、莱菔子同用，即三子养亲汤。若治上盛下虚之久咳痰喘，可配伍肉桂、厚朴、当归等同用，如苏子降气汤。

Angelicae Sinensis Radix (dang gui), to form up Perilla Fruit Qi-Downbearing Decoction (Su Zi Jiang Qi Tang).

(2) Constipation due to dryness in intestines. The medicinal herb is moist and fatty and acts to moisturize intestine and promote defecation. In the treatment of constipation due to dryness in intestines, it is combined with *Armeniacae Amarum Semen* (ku xing ren), *Cannabis Fructus* (huo ma ren) and *Trichosanthis Fructus* (gua lou).

（2）肠燥便秘。本品质润多脂，能滑肠通便，常与杏仁、火麻仁、瓜蒌仁等同用。

Usage and dosage Apply 3～10 g in decoction.

用法用量 煎服，3～10克。

Precautions for use It is cautious to apply for those with loose feces due to spleen deficiency.

使用注意 脾虚便溏者慎用。

Remarks *Perillae Folium* (zi su ye), *Perillae Caulis* (zi su geng) and *Perillae Fructus* (zi su zi)

按语 紫苏叶、紫苏梗与紫苏子

All the three medicinal herbs are the products from *Perilla frutescens* (L.) Britt. var. acuta (Thunb.) Kudo, family Labiatae, and pungent and warm in property. Zi su ye acts to make sweating, relieve exterior pattern, promote qi flow, tranquilize fetus and relieve toxin from fish and crab. Zi su geng acts to regulate qi flow, dilate middle energizer, tranquilize fetus and stop pain. Zi su zi acts to subdue qi, dissolve phlegm, stop cough, soothe panting and moisturize intestines.

三药均来源于唇形科植物紫苏，均辛温。不同的是紫苏叶药用叶，功能发汗解表、行气安胎、解鱼蟹毒。紫苏梗药用茎，功能理气宽中、安胎、止痛。紫苏子药用果实，功能降气化痰、止咳平喘，且能润肠。

Eriobotryae Folium (pi pa ye)

枇杷叶

It is the dried product from the leaf of *Eriobotrya japonica* (Thunb.) Lindl., family Rosaceae. The medicinal herb is collected all over the year, applied in crude form or honey-prepared form.

为蔷薇科植物枇杷的干燥叶。全年均可采收。生用或蜜炙用。

Features Flavor: bitter. Property: slightly

性味归经 苦，微寒。

cold. Meridian tropism: the Lung Meridian and the Stomach Meridian.

归肺、胃经。

Actions Purify lung, stop cough, subdue up-reverse flow of qi and stop vomiting.

功效 清肺止咳,降逆止呕。

Application

应用

(1) Cough due to heat in lung. The medicinal herb is descending and dispersing in property, and acts to purify lung, clear heat, dissolve phlegm and stop cough. In the treatment of heat in lung manifested by cough with yellow-thick sputum, dry throat and bitter taste in mouth, it is combined with *Cortex Mori Albae Radicis* (sang bai pi), *Peucedani Radix* (qian hu) and *Scutellariae Radix* (huang qin). In the treatment of dryness-heat damaging lung manifested by cough with scanty sputum or dry cough without sputum, it is combined with *Mori Folium* (sang ye), *Armeniacae Amarum Semen* (ku xing ren) and *Ophiopogonis Radix* (mai dong).

(1) 肺热咳嗽。本品性善降泄,能清肃肺热,化痰止咳。治肺热咳嗽,咳痰黄稠,咽干口苦,可与桑白皮、前胡、黄芩等同用。治燥热伤肺,咳嗽少痰或干咳无痰,可与桑叶、苦杏仁、麦冬等同用。

(2) Vomiting and hiccup due to heat in stomach. The medicinal herb acts to purify stomach, clear heat, subdue stomach qi and stop vomiting and hiccup. In the treatment of heat in stomach manifested by vomiting, hiccup, restlessness, feverish sensation and thirst, it is combined with *Coptidis Rhizoma* (huang lian), *Bambusae Caulis in Taenias* (zhu ru) and *Citri Reticulatae Pericarpium* (chen pi).

(2) 胃热呕逆。本品能清胃热、降胃气、止呕逆。治胃热呕吐、呃逆,烦热口渴,可与黄连、竹茹、陈皮等同用。

Usage and dosage Apply 6～10 g in decoction. The medicinal herb acts to eliminate heat in lung and stomach in crude form, and acts to stop cough in honey-calcined form.

用法用量 煎服,6～10克。生用清肺胃热,蜜炙止咳。

Stemonae Radix (bai bu)

百部

It is the dried product from the root tuber of *Stemona sessilifolia* (Miq.) Miq., *Stemona*

为百部科植物直立百部、蔓生百部或对叶百部的

japonica (Bl.) Miq., or *Stemona tuberose* Lour., family Stemonaleae. The medicinal herb is collected in spring and autumn, applied in crude form or honey-calcined form.

干燥块根。春、秋二季采挖。生用或蜜炙用。

Features Flavor: sweet and bitter. Property: slightly warm. Meridian tropism: the Lung Meridian.

性味归经　甘、苦,微温。归肺经。

Actions Moisturize lung, stop cough, and kill worms and lice.

功效　润肺止咳,杀虫灭虱。

Application

(1) Acute cough, chronic cough, paroxysmal cough, and cough due to pulmonary tuberculosis. The medicinal herb is sweet, moist, bitter and descending in property and attributive to the Lung Meridian, and acts to moisturize lung, subdue qi and stop cough, applied to treat various types of cough, as cough due to exogenous factors or due to endogenous factors, paroxysmal cough and chronic cough, as the major herb to treat chough due to pulmonary tuberculosis, chronic cough or cough due to deficiency. In the treatment of cough due to wind-cold, it is combined with *Schizonepetae Herba* (jing jie), *Platycodonis Radix* (jie geng) and *Aster Radix et Rhizoma* (zi wan). In the treatment of cough due to wind-heat, it is combined with *Puerariae Lobatae Radix* (ge gen), *Bulbus Fritillariae Thunbergii* (zhe bei mu) and *Gypsum Fibrosum* (shi gao). In the treatment of paroxysmal cough, it is combined with *Armeniacae Amarum Semen* (ku xing ren), jie geng and *Ophiopogonis Radix* (mai dong). In the treatment of cough due to pulmonary tuberculosis and cough with bloody sputum, it is combined with *Asini Corii Colla* (e jiao) and *Fritillariae Cirrhosae Bulbus* (chuan bei mu).

应用

(1)新久咳嗽,顿咳,肺痨咳嗽。本品甘润苦降,性质平和,主入肺经,善润肺下气止咳,无论外感、内伤、暴咳、久嗽,皆可用之,尤为肺痨咳嗽、久咳虚嗽的要药。治风寒咳嗽,配伍荆芥、桔梗、紫菀等同用。治风热咳嗽,配伍葛根、浙贝母、石膏等。治顿咳,配伍苦杏仁、桔梗、麦冬等。治肺痨咳嗽、痰中带血,与阿胶、川贝母等药同用。

(2) Pinworm, head louse and body louse. The medicinal herb acts to kill worms and kill lice. In the treatment of pinworm, the medicinal herb is applied singly by decocting and applying retention enema before sleep. In the treatment of head louse and body louse, it is applied singly by decocting for external use.

（2）蛲虫，头虱，体虱。本品能杀虫灭虱。治蛲虫，以本品浓煎，睡前保留灌肠。治头虱、体虱，水煎外用涂搽。

Usage and dosage Apply 3～9 g in decoction. Apply a proper amount for external use. The medicinal herb acts to stop cough and kill worms and lice in crude from, and acts to moisturize lung and stop cough in honey-calcined form.

用法用量 煎服，3～9克。外用适量。生用止咳、杀虫灭虱，蜜炙润肺止咳。

Aster Radix et Rhizoma (zi wan)

紫菀

It is the dried product from the root and rhizome of Tatarian Aster, *Aster tataricus* L. f., family Compositae. The medicinal herb is collected in spring and autumn, applied in crude form and honey-calcined form.

为菊科植物紫菀的干燥根及根茎。春、秋二季采挖。生用或蜜炙用。

Features Flavor: pungent and bitter. Property: warm. Meridian tropism: the Lung Meridian.

性味归经 辛，苦，温。归肺经。

Actions Moisturize lung, subdue qi, dissolve phlegm and stop cough.

功效 润肺下气，化痰止咳。

Application

应用

Acute and chronic cough. The medicinal herb is warm but not hot, moist but not dry, and neutral in property. It acts to moisturize lung, subdue qi, dissolve phlegm and stop cough, applied to treat acute cough and chronic cough. In the treatment of cough due to wind-cold, it is combined with *Schizonepetae Herba* (jing jie) and *Platycodonis Radix* (jie geng). In the treatment of cough with yellow-thick sputum due to heat in lung, it is combined with *Bulbus Fritillariae Thunbergii* (zhe bei mu), *Scutellariae Radix*

新久咳嗽。本品温而不热，润而不燥，性质平和，长于润肺下气、化痰止咳，且化痰力强，新久痰嗽皆宜。治风寒咳嗽，与荆芥、桔梗等同用。治肺热咳嗽，痰黄黏稠，与浙贝母、黄芩、桑白皮等同用。治阴虚劳嗽，痰中带血，与川贝母、阿胶等同用。

(huang qin) and *Cortex Mori Albae Radicis* (sang bai pi). In the treatment of cough with bloody sputum due to pulmonary tuberculosis or yin deficiency, it is combined with *Fritillariae Cirrhosae Bulbus* (chuan bei mu) and *Asini Corii Colla* (e jiao).

Usage and dosage Apply 5～10 g in decoction. The medicinal herb acts to treat acute cough due to exogenous factors in crude form, and acts to treat chronic cough due to lung deficiency in honey-calcined form.

用法用量 煎服,5～10克。生用,用于外感暴咳;蜜炙,用于肺虚久咳。

Farfarae Flos (kuan dong hua)

款冬花

It is the dried product from the flower-bud of *Tussilago farfara* L., family Compositae. The medicinal herb is collected in December when the ground is not freezing and before it is flowering, applied in crude form or honey-calcined form.

为菊科植物款冬的干燥花蕾。12月或地冻前当花尚未出土时采挖。生用或蜜炙用。

Features Flavor: pungent and slightly bitter. Property: warm. Meridian tropism: the Lung Meridian.

性味归经 辛,微苦,温。归肺经。

Actions Moisturize lung, subdue qi, stop cough and dissolve phlegm.

功效 润肺下气,止咳化痰。

Application

Acute and chronic cough. The medicinal herb acts to moisturize lung, subdue qi, stop cough and dissolve phlegm, applied to treat acute cough and chronic cough. In the treatment of cough due to wind-cold, it is combined with *Ephedrae Herba* (ma huang) and *Asari Radix et Rhizoma* (xi xin). In the treatment of unceasing cough due to cold, it is combined with *Aster Radix et Rhizoma* (zi wan) and *Fritillariae Cirrhosae Bulbus* (chuan bei mu). In the treatment of cough and panting due to heat in lung, it is combined with *Trichosanthis Fructus* (gua lou)

应用

新久咳嗽。本品功善润肺下气、止咳化痰,尤善止咳,适用于新久咳嗽。治风寒咳痰,与麻黄、细辛等同用。治寒嗽不止,可与紫菀、川贝母等同用。治肺热咳喘,配伍瓜蒌、桑白皮等同用。肺虚久咳,与人参、黄芪等同用。治阴虚燥咳,与沙参、麦冬等同用。若咳久痰中带血,常与百合同用,如百

and *Cortex Mori Albae Radicis* (sang bai pi). In the treatment of chronic cough due to lung deficiency, it is combined with *Ginseng Radix et Raizoma* (ren shen) and *Astragali Radix* (huang qi). In the treatment of dry cough due to yin deficiency, it is combined with *Glehniae Radix* (bei sha shen) and *Ophiopogonis Radix* (mai dong). In the treatment of chronic cough with bloody sputum, it is combined with *Bulbus Lilii* (bai he), to form up Lily and Coltsfoot Flower Poultice (Bai Hua Gao).

花膏。

Usage and dosage Appy 5～10 g in decoction. The medicinal herb acts to treat acute cough due to exogenous factors in crude form, and acts to treat chronic cough due to endogenous factors in honey-baked form.

用法用量 煎服，5～10克。生用，用于外感暴咳；蜜炙，用于内伤久咳。

Cortex Mori Albae Radicis (sang bai pi)

桑白皮

It is the dried product from the root bark of *Morus alba*. L., family Moraceae. The medicinal herb is collected from late autumn when the leaf falls to the next spring before it is sprouting by peeling the root, applied in crude form or honey-baked form.

为桑科植物桑的干燥根皮。秋末叶落时至次春发芽前采挖根部，刮去黄色粗皮，剥取根皮。生用或蜜炙用。

Features Flavor: sweet. Property: cold. Meridian tropism: the Lung Meridian.

性味归经 甘，寒。归肺经。

Actions Reduce lung, soothe panting, promote water flow and subside swell.

功效 泻肺平喘，利水消肿。

Application

应用

(1) Cough and panting due to heat in lung. The medicinal herb is cold in property and acts to reduce lung, clear heat, subdue qi and soothe panting. In the treatment of cough and panting due to heat in lung, it is combined with *Lycii Cortex* (di gu pi), *Glycyrrhizae Radix et Rhizoma* (gan cao) and *Semen Oryza Sativae* (jing mi), to form up White

(1) 肺热咳喘。本品性寒，善清泻肺热、降气平喘。治肺热咳喘，常与地骨皮、甘草、粳米同用，即泻白散。

Lung-Reducing Powder (Xie Bai San).

(2) Edema and scanty urine. The medicinal herb acts to subdue lung qi, dredge water passage, promote water flow and subside swell. In the treatment of lung qi failing to disperse and water failing to flow pattern manifested by general edema, puffy face and difficult urination, it is combined with *Poriae Cutis* (fu ling pi), *Arecae Pericarpium* (da fu pi) and *Zingiberis Rhizoma Recens* (sheng jiang) peel, to form up Five Cortices Drink (Wu Pi Yin).

（2）水肿尿少。本品能肃降肺气，通调水道、利水消肿。治肺气不宣，水气不行，全身水肿，面目肌肤浮肿，小便不利，配伍茯苓皮、大腹皮、生姜皮等，如五皮饮。

Usage and dosage Apply 12～15 g in decoction. The medicinal herb acts to reduce lung and promote water flow in crude form, and its cold property decreases in honey-baked form.

用法用量 煎服，12～15克。生用泻肺、利水，蜜炙寒性得减。

Precautions for use It is cautious to apply for those with edema of deficiency type.

使用注意 水肿属虚者慎用。

Remarks *Mori Folium* (sang ye) and *Cortex Mori Albae Radicis* (sang bai pi)

按语 桑叶与桑白皮

Both medicinal herbs are the products from *Morus alba*, family Moraceae, cold-cool in property, and act to clear heat in lung. Sang ye is attributive to the Lung and Liver Meridians, and acts to eliminate wind-heat, purify lung and moisturize lung, and purify liver and brighten eyes, applied to treat exterior wind-heat pattern and dry cough due to heat in lung. Sang bai pi is attributive to the Lung Meridian, and acts to reduce heat in lung and soothe panting, and also acts to promote water flow and subside swell as well.

二药均来源于桑科植物桑，性寒凉，善清肺热。不同的是桑叶药用桑的叶，入肺肝经，能发散风热，清肺润肺，清肝明目，为治风热表证、肺热燥咳多用。桑白皮药用桑的根皮，专入肺经，能泻肺热、平喘息，且能利水消肿。

Descurainiae Semenlepidii *Semen* (ting li zi)

葶苈子

It is the dried product from the ripe seed of *Descurainia sophia* (L.) Webb ex Prantl, or *Lepidum apetalum* Willd., family Cruciferae. The former is

为十字花科植物播娘蒿或独行菜的干燥成熟种子。前者习称“南葶苈子”，后者

often called "nan ting li zi", while the latter is often called "bei ting li zi". The medicinal herb is collected in summer, applied in crude form or stir-fried form.

习称"北葶苈子"。夏季采收。生用或炒用。

Features Flavor: pungent and bitter. Property: extremely cold. Meridian tropism: the Lung Meridian and the Bladder Meridian.

性味归经 辛、苦,大寒。归肺、膀胱经。

Actions Reduce lung, soothe panting, promote water flow and subside swell.

功效 泻肺平喘,利水消肿。

Application

应用

(1) Cough and panting due to excessive phlegm. The medicinal herb is pungent and dispersing, bitter and descending, and extremely cold in property, and acts to reduce lung and treat excess rheum pattern. In the treatment of excessive phlegm-rheum pattern manifested by cough with excessive sputum and severe panting with failure to lie flat, it is combined with *Fructus Ziziphi Jujubae* (da zao), to form up Pepperweed Seed and Jujube Lung-Reducing Decoction (Ting Li Da Zao Xie Fei Tang).

(1) 痰涎壅盛咳喘。本品辛散苦降,其性大寒,专泻肺之实饮。治痰涎壅盛,咳逆痰多,喘息不得卧,与大枣同用,即葶苈大枣泻肺汤。

(2) Hydrothorax and ascites of excess pattern. The medicinal herb acts to reduce lung qi, promote flow and subside swell. In the treatment of lung qi accumulation and excess pattern and water-rheum retention pattern manifested by edema, distension, fullness and difficult urination, it is applied singly or combined with *Pharbitidis Semen* (qian niu zi) and *Semen Zanthoxyli* (jiao mu).

(2) 胸腹积水实证。本品能泻肺气之闭、利水消肿。治肺气壅实、水饮停聚,水肿胀满,小便不利,可单用,或与牵牛子、椒目等同用。

Usage and dosage Apply 3～10 g in decoction by wrapping. The cold property of the medicinal herb decrease in stir-fried form.

用法用量 煎服,3～10克,宜包煎。炒后寒性得减。

Precautions for use It is prohibited to apply for those with panting due to lung deficiency or

使用注意 肺虚喘促、脾虚水肿忌服。

those with edema due to spleen deficiency.

Brief summary

1 Phlegm-dissolving herbs

Both *Pinelliae Rhizoma* (ban xia) and *Arisaematis Rhizoma* (tian nan xing) are pungent, warm and poisonous in property, and act to desiccate damp dissolve phlegm, and also act to subside swell and stop pain for external use as well. Ban xia is attributive to the Spleen and Stomach Meridians, and acts dissolve damp-phlegm or cold-phlegm in spleen and stomach. It acts to subdue up-reverse flow of qi and stop vomiting, as the major herb to treat vomiting. It also acts to dissolve masses and dissipate stagnation, applied to treat stuffiness and fullness at chest and epigastria, and globus hystericus. Tian nan xing is attributive to the Liver Meridian, warm and dry in property and good at treating intractable phlegm, and acts to be attributed to meridians and collaterals, eliminate wind-phlegm and stop convulsion, applied to treat hemiplegia due to wind stroke and tetanus with convulsion.

Sinapis Semen (jie zi), also called "*Sinapis Semen Albae* (bai jie zi)", is pungent and warm in property and attributive to the Lung Meridian, and acts to warm lung, dissolve phlegm, promote qi flow and dilate diaphragm, applied to treat cold-phlegm blocking lung pattern or phlegm-rheum retaining in chest and hypochondria pattern. It also acts to eliminate phlegm in meridians, promote qi flow, dredge collaterals and dissipate stagnation, applied to treat phlegm blocking meridians and col-

小　结

1 化痰药

半夏、天南星，均辛温有毒，均能燥湿化痰，外用消肿止痛。其中半夏主入脾胃经，善除脾胃湿痰、寒痰；还能降逆止呕，为治呕吐要药；并能消痞散结，治胸脘痞闷、梅核气等证。天南星主入肝经，温燥之性强，善治顽痰；又善走经络、祛风痰、止痉挛，常治中风半身不遂、破伤风抽搐等证。

芥子，又名“白芥子”，味辛性温，专入肺经，能温肺祛痰、利气畅膈，善治寒痰壅肺或痰饮停滞胸胁之证；又善祛经络之痰、利气通络散结，治痰阻经络的肢体麻木、阴疽流注等证。

laterals pattern manifested by numbness in body and limbs, dorsal furuncle and deep multiple abscesses.

Both *Inulae Flos* (xuan fu hua) and *Cynanchi Stauntonii Rhizoma et Radix* (bai qian) are pungent and slightly warm in property and attributive to the Lung Meridian, and act to subdue qi and dissolve phlegm, applied to treat cough and panting with excessive sputum. Xuan fu hua acts to eliminate phlegm, dissolve rheum and relieve masses. It is attributive to the Stomach Meridian, and acts to subdue stomach qi, applied to treat up-reverse flow of stomach qi manifested by belching and vomiting. Bai qian acts to subdue qi, dissolve phlegm and stop cough, applied to treat cough, panting, excessive sputum and shortness of breath.

旋覆花、白前，均味辛微温，归肺经，能降气化痰，治咳嗽气急痰多。其中旋覆花善消痰水、化饮除痞；归胃经，又能降胃气，治胃气上逆之噫气、呕吐等。白前功专降气化痰止咳，为咳喘痰多气急多用。

Both *Platycodonis Radix* (jie geng) and *Peucedani Radix* (qian hu) are attributive to the Lung Meridian, and act to dissolve phlegm. Jie geng is bitter, pungent and neutral in property, and acts to disperse lung qi, dissolve phlegm and benefit throat, applied to treat cough due to exogenous factors or cough and panting with excessive sputum, and also acts to treat sore throat, loss of voice or hoarseness of voice. It also acts to drain purulence, applied to treat pulmonary abscess manifested by cough with purulent or bloody sputum. Qian hu is bitter, pungent and slightly cold in property, and acts to subdue qi, dissolve phlegm and eliminate wind-heat, applied to treat cough due to phlegm-heat and exterior wind-heat pattern.

桔梗、前胡，均专入肺经，功能化痰。其中桔梗苦辛性平，功以宣肺为主，能开宣肺气、祛痰、利咽，既治外感咳嗽或痰多咳喘，又治咽喉肿痛，失声音哑；还能排脓，治肺痈咳吐脓血。前胡苦辛微寒，功以宣降并用，既降气化痰，又宣散风热，治痰热咳嗽、风热外感。

Both *Fritillariae Cirrhosae Bulbus* (chuan bei mu) and *Bulbus Fritillariae Thunbergii* (zhe bei mu) are cold-cool in property and acts to clear heat, dissolve phlegm, stop cough, dissipate stagnation and

川贝母、浙贝母，均药性寒凉，具清热化痰止咳、散结消肿之功，善治痰热咳嗽、瘰疬疮痈等证。其中川贝母味

subside swell, applied to treat cough due to phlegm-heat, scrofula, carbuncle and carbuncle. Chuan bei mu is sweet and moist in property and acts to moisturize lung and stop cough, applied to treat cough due to dryness in lung, chronic cough or cough in deficiency pattern. Zhe bei mu is bitter, cold and dispersing in property and acts to dissolve phlegm, clear heat and dissipate stagnation, applied to treat exterior wind-heat pattern, cough due to phlegm-heat or cough in excess pattern, and also applied to treat phlegm-fire accumulation pattern or heat-toxin accumulation pattern manifested by scrofula, carbuncle and furuncle.

甘质润，功善润肺止咳，治肺燥咳嗽及久咳虚咳多用。浙贝母苦寒清泄，苦泄化痰、清热散结力强，常用于外感风热或痰热实证咳嗽，以及痰火、热毒郁结的瘰疬疮痈。

Both *Trichosanthis Fructus* (gua lou) and *Bambusae Caulis in Taenias* (zhu ru) are cold in property and acts to clear heat and dissolve phlegm, applied to treat cough due to phlegm-heat. Gua lou is clear and moist and acts to purify lung and dissolve phlegm, and also acts to moisturize lung and eliminate dryness, applied to treat cough due to phlegm-heat or dry cough due to heat in lung. It acts to promote qi flow and dilate chest, applied to treat chest pain due to phlegm blocking chest or due to phlegm-heat accumulation. It also acts to dissipate stagnation, relieve abscess, moisturize intestines and promote defecation, applied to treat pulmonary abscess, acute appendicitis, acute mastitis and constipation due to dryness in intestines. Zhu ru acts to clear heat, dissolve phlegm, dissipate stagnation and relieve restlessness, applied to treat phlegm-fire disturbing the internal manifested by palpitation, restlessness and insomnia. It also acts to purify stomach and stop vomiting, applied to treat vomiting due to heat in stomach.

瓜蒌、竹茹，均性寒，功能清热化痰，治痰热咳嗽。其中瓜蒌清润相兼，既清肺化痰，又清润肺燥，痰热咳嗽、肺热燥咳并治；且利气宽胸，治痰气痹阻之胸痹、痰热互结之结胸；又散结消痈、润肠通便，治肺痈、肠痈、乳痈、肠燥便秘。竹茹善清痰热，且能开郁除烦，常治痰火内扰的惊悸、心烦失眠等证；又善清胃止呕，常治胃热呕吐。

2 Cough-stopping and pant-relieving herbs

Both *Armeniacae Amarum Semen* (ku xing ren) and *Perillae Fructus* (zi su zi) are warm in property and attributive to the Lung and Large Intestine Meridians, and act to stop cough, soothe panting, moisturize intestines and promote defecation, applied to treat cough and panting due to up-reverse flow of qi, and constipation due to dryness in intestines. Ku xing ren is bitter and dispersing in property and acts to subdue qi, stop cough and disperse lung, as the major herb to treat cough and panting, applied to treat various types of cough and panting by combining with other medicinal herbs. Zi su zi acts to subdue qi and dissolve phlegm, applied to treat cough and panting with excessive sputum due to up-reverse flow of qi, and chronic cough and panting with excessive sputum due to excess in the upper and deficiency in the lower.

Eriobotryae Folium (pi pa ye) is bitter and cool in property and attributive to the Lung and Stomach Meridians, and acts to reduce heat in lung, dissolve phlegm and stop cough, and also acts to purify stomach, subdue qi and stop vomiting. As the major herb to purify lung and stomach and subdue qi of lung and stomach, it is applied to treat cough due to heat in lung, and vomiting due to heat in stomach.

All *Stemonae Radix* (bai bu), *Aster Radix et Rhizoma* (zi wan) and *Farfarae Flos* (kuan dong hua) are attributive to the Lung Meridian and act to moisturize lung and stop cough, applied to treat acute or chronic cough. Bai bu is sweet, bitter, moist, descending and neutral in property, applied to treat cough due to pulmonary tuberculosis and

2 止咳平喘药

苦杏仁、紫苏子，均性温，入肺与大肠经，能止咳平喘、润肠通便，治咳喘气逆、肠燥便秘。其中苦杏仁苦泄不热，降气止咳兼能宣肺，为治咳喘要药，经配伍可治各种咳喘。紫苏子功善降气消痰，既治咳喘痰多气逆，又治上盛下虚之久咳痰喘。

枇杷叶，味苦性凉，入肺胃二经，性善降泄，既清泄肺热、化痰止咳，又清胃降气、以止呕逆，故枇杷叶为清肺胃、降肺胃逆气之品，治肺热咳嗽、胃热呕逆。

百部、紫菀、款冬花，均归肺经，功能润肺止咳，无论新久咳嗽皆可应用。其中百部甘润苦降，药性平和，善治肺痨咳嗽及百日咳；又能杀虫灭虱，治蛲虫、头虱等。紫菀温而不热，润而不燥，功善

whooping cough, it also acts to kill worms and kill lice, applied to treat pinworm, body louse and head louse. Zi wan is warm but not hot, moist but not dry, and acts to dissolve phlegm, applied to treat cough with excessive sputum. Kuan dong hua acts to moisturize lung, subdue qi and stop cough, applied to treat cough with excessive sputum. It is often combined with zi wan in mutual reinforcement.

于化痰,凡咳嗽痰多者多用。款冬花功善润肺下气,长于止咳,治咳嗽痰多,常与紫菀相须为用。

Both *Cortex Mori Albae Radicis* (sang bai pi) and *Descurainiae Semenlepidii Semen* (ting li zi) are cold in property and act to reduce lung, soothe panting, promote water flow and subside swell, applied to treat cough and panting due to phlegm-rheum blocking lung, edema and difficult urination in excess pattern. Sang bai pi is sweet and cold in property and acts to reduce heat in lung, subdue qi and soothe panting, applied to treat cough and panting due to heat in lung. Ting li zi is bitter and cold in property and acts to reduce rheum of excess type in lung, applied to treat phlegm-rheum blocking lung manifested by cough with excessive sputum and panting with failure to lie flat.

桑白皮、葶苈子,均性寒,功能泻肺平喘,利水消肿,治痰涎壅肺的咳嗽喘满,以及水肿、小便不利属实证者。其中桑白皮味甘性寒,善泻肺热、降气平喘,常用于肺热喘咳之证。葶苈子味苦性寒,专泻肺之实饮,善治痰涎壅盛、咳逆痰多、喘息不得平卧等。

Chapter 13 Mind-Tranquilizing Herbs

第13章 安神药

The medicinal herbs acting to quiet spirit and calm mind are called the mind-tranquilizing herbs.

以安定神志为主要作用的药物,称为安神药。

The medicinal herbs are attributive to the Heart and Liver Meridians, and acting to treat restlessness, fearful throbbing, palpitation, insomnia, poor memory, dream-disturbed sleep, convulsion, epilepsy and mental disorders. The medicinal herbs of minerals and shells in heavy quality act to calm mind, applied to treat restlessness of excess type due to heart fire flaming and hyperactivity or pathogenic heat disturbing the internal. The medicinal herbs of plant seeds are moist in property and acts to nourish heart and calm mind, applied to treat restlessness of deficiency type due to heart and liver blood deficiency or heart and liver yin deficiency.

本类药入心、肝二经,主要用于心神不宁,惊悸、失眠、健忘、多梦及惊风、癫痫、癫狂等神志异常的病证。其中,质重的矿石、贝壳类药物功能重镇安神,适用于心火炽盛或邪热内扰所致的心神不宁之实证。植物种子类药物质润滋养,功能养心安神,适用于心肝血虚或心肝阴虚所致的心神不宁之虚证。

In the application of the medicinal herbs, it is necessary to notice that the medicinal herbs of minerals may damage spleen and stomach, so it is not advisable to apply them for long time. In the decoction, it is necessary to smash them and decoct them first for long time. Some of the medicinal herbs are poisonous, so it is not advisable to apply them in overdose, so as to prevent poisoning.

使用本类药需注意,矿石类安神药易伤脾胃,不宜长期服用;入煎剂时,应打碎先煎、久煎。部分有毒性的药物,不宜过量,以防中毒。

Cinnabaris (zhu sha)

朱砂

It is the product from the cinnabar of sulfide

为硫化物类矿物辰砂族

type, mainly containing mercuric sulfide (HgS). After mining, the mineral is smashed and refined. Then the magnet is applied to absorb the iron particles, and the water is applied to wash away the miscellaneous stones, mud and sand. In the end, the medicinal herb is refined into powder with water.

辰砂，主要成分为硫化汞。采挖后，选取纯净者，用磁铁吸净含铁的杂质，再用水淘去杂石和泥沙，研细水飞。

Features Flavor: sweet. Property: slightly cold and poisonous. Meridian tropism: the Heart Meridian.

性味归经 甘，微寒；有毒。归心经。

Actions Tranquilize heart, calm mind, reduce heat and relieve toxin.

功效 镇惊安神，清热解毒。

Application

应用

(1) Heart fire flaming and hyperactivity manifested by restlessness and insomnia. The medicinal herb is sweet, cold and heavy in property and attributive to the Heart Meridian, and acts to reduce heart fire and calm mind. In the treatment of heart fire flaming and hyperactivity manifested by restlessness and insomnia, it is combined with *Coptidis Rhizoma* (huang lian) and *Glycyrrhizae Radix et Rhizoma* (gan cao). In the treatment of the above condition complicated by heart blood deficiency, it is combined with *Angelicae Sinensis Radix* (dang gui) and *Rehmanniae Radix Praeparata* (shu di huang), to form up Cinnabar and Spirit-Calming Pills (Zhu Sha An Shen Wan). In the treatment of yin blood insufficiency manifested by palpitation, insomnia and dream-disturbed sleep, it is combined with *Ziziphi Spinosae Semen* (suan zao ren), *Platycladi Semen* (bai zi ren) and dang gui.

（1）心火亢盛，烦躁失眠。本品甘寒质重，专入心经。能清心火、镇惊安神，最宜于心火亢盛之心神不宁、烦躁不眠，常与黄连、甘草等同用。若兼心血虚者，可与当归、熟地黄等同用，如朱砂安神丸。阴血不足所致的心悸、失眠多梦，常与酸枣仁、柏子仁、当归等配伍。

(2) Convulsion and epilepsy. The medicinal herb acts to tranquilize heart and calm mind. In the treatment of infantile acute convulsion, it is combined with *Bovis Calculus* (niu huang), *Scorpio*

（2）惊风，癫痫。本品能重镇安神。治小儿急惊风，多与牛黄、全蝎、钩藤等配伍。治癫痫，常与磁石、神曲

(quan xie) and *Uncariae Ramulus cum Uncis* (gou teng). In the treatment of epilepsy, it is combined with *Magnetitum* (ci shi) and *Massa Medicata Fermentata* (shen qu).

同用。

(3) Carbuncle and furuncle, sore throat, mouth ulcer and ulcer on tongue. The medicinal herb is cold in property and acts to clear heat and relieve toxin for both oral administration and external use. In the treatment of carbuncle and furuncle, it is combined with the heat-clearing and toxin-relieving herbs. In the treatment of sore throat, mouth ulcer and ulcer on tongue, it is combined with *Borneolum Syntheticum* (bing pian) and *Borax* (peng sha), to form up Borneol and *Borax* Powder (Bing Peng San).

（3）疮疡肿毒，咽喉肿痛，口舌生疮。本品性寒，内服外用均有较强的清热解毒作用。治疮疡肿毒，多与清热解毒之品同用。治咽喉肿痛、口舌生疮，多与冰片、硼砂等配伍，如冰硼散。

Usage and dosage Apply 0.1～0.5 g in pills or powder, it is not applied in decoction. Apply a proper amount for external use.

用法用量 0.1～0.5克，多入丸散服，不入煎剂。外用适量。

Precautions for use The medicinal herb is poisonous, so it is not advisable to apply in overdose or for long time. It is prohibited to apply for those for pregnant women or those with hepatic and renal dysfunction.

使用注意 本品有毒，不宜多服久服。孕妇及肝肾功能不全者忌用。

Magnetitum (ci shi)

磁石

It is the product from the magnetic iron ore magnetite, mainly containing ferriferous oxide (Fe_3O_4). After mining, remove the impurities, applied in crude form or calcined form.

为氧化物类矿物尖晶石族磁铁矿，主要成分为四氧化三铁。采挖后，除去杂质。生用或煅用。

Features Flavor: salty. Property: cold. Meridian tropism: the Liver Meridian, the Heart Meridian and the Kidney Meridian.

性味归经 咸，寒。归肝、心、肾经。

Actions Tranquilize heart, calm mind, soothe liver, subdue yang, improve hearing, brighten

功效 镇惊安神，平肝潜阳，聪耳明目，纳气定喘。

eyes, accept qi and relieve panting.

Application

(1) Palpitation and insomnia. The medicinal herb is salty, cold, descending and heavy in property, and attributive to the Heart and Kidney Meridians, and acts to tranquilize heart, calm mind, benefit kidney and subdue yang. In the treatment of restlessness, palpitation and insomnia caused by kidney deficiency and liver hyperactivity to disturb heart mind, or by fear and fright causing qi disturbance to lead to derangement, it is combined with *Cinnabaris* (zhu sha), to form up Magnetite and Cinnabar Pill (Ci Zhu Wan).

(2) Dizziness and blurring of vision. The medicinal herb is attributive to the Liver and Kidney Meridians, and acts to benefit kidney, soothe liver and subdue yang. In the treatment of liver yang hyperactivity manifested by dizziness, blurring of vision, irritability and anger, it is combined with *Ostreae Concha* (mu li), *Haliotidis Concha* (shi jue ming) and *Paeoniae Radix Alba* (bai shao).

(3) Blurring of vision and deafness. The medicinal herb acts to benefit kidney, improve hearing and brighten eyes. In the treatment of tinnitus and deafness due to kidney deficiency, it is combined with *Rehmanniae Radix Praeparata* (shu di huang), *Corni Fructus* (shan zhu yu) and *Schisandrae Chinensis Fructus* (wu wei zi). In the treatment of blurring of vision due to liver and kidney insufficiency, it is combined with *Lycii Fructus* (gou qi zi), *Whellote Chrysanthemum* (bai ju hua) and *Ligustri Lucidi Fructus* (nü zhen zi).

(4) Panting due to kidney deficiency. The medicinal herb acts to benefit kidney, accept qi and

应用

（1）惊悸失眠。本品咸寒，质重沉降，入心肾经，能镇心安神、益肾镇潜，可用于肾虚肝旺，扰动心神或惊恐气乱，神不守舍所致的心神不宁、惊悸、失眠，常与朱砂等同用，如磁朱丸。

（2）头晕目眩。本品入肝肾经，具益肾、平肝潜阳之功。治肝阳上亢的头晕目眩、急躁易怒，常与牡蛎、石决明、白芍等同用。

（3）目暗耳聋。本品能益肾聪耳明目。治肾虚耳鸣、耳聋，多配伍熟地黄、山茱萸、五味子等同用。治肝肾不足，目暗不明，可与枸杞子、白菊花、女贞子等同用。

（4）肾虚喘促。本品能益肾纳气而平喘。治肾虚摄

soothe pant. In the treatment of panting of deficiency type due to deficiency of kidney which fails to accept qi, it is combined with the lung-reinforcing and kidney-benefiting herbs.

纳无权的虚喘，常与补肺益肾之品同用。

Usage and dosage Apply 15～30 g in decoction. Decoct it first in crude form. The medicinal herb acts to tranquilize heart, calm mind, soothe liver and subdue yang in crude form, and acts to improve hearing, brighten eyes, accept qi and relieve panting in calcined form.

用法用量 煎服，15～30克。生用宜先煎。生用镇惊安神、平肝潜阳，煅用聪耳明目、纳气平喘。

Os Draconis (long gu)

龙骨

It is the product from the fossil of the skeleton of ancient large mammals, such as Hipparion Christol, Rhinocerotidae, Cervidae, Bovine, Elephantoidea, etc. The medicinal herb is collected all over the year, applied in crude form or calcined form.

为古代哺乳动物如三趾马、犀类、鹿类、牛类、象类等的骨骼化石或象类门齿的化石。全年均可采挖。生用或煅用。

Features Flavor: sweet and astringent. Property: neutral. Meridian tropism: the Heart Meridian, the Liver Meridian and the Kidney Meridian.

性味归经 甘、涩，平。归心、肝、肾经。

Actions Tranquilize heart, calm mind, soothe liver and subdue yang by astringing and consolidating.

功效 镇惊安神，平肝潜阳，收敛固涩。

Application

应用

(1) Palpitation, insomnia, convulsion, epilepsy and mental disorder. The medicinal herb is heavy in property and acts to tranquilize heart and calm mind. In the treatment of restlessness, palpitation, insomnia, poor memory and dream-disturbed sleep, it is combined with *Cinnabaris* (zhu sha), *Ziziphi Spinosae Semen* (suan zao ren) and *Platycladi Semen* (bai zi ren). In the treatment of convulsion, spasm due to epilepsy and attack of mental disorder, it is combined with other mind-tranquilizing herbs.

（1）心悸失眠，惊痫癫狂。本品质重镇惊，为重镇安神之要药。治心神不宁、心悸失眠、健忘多梦等症，常与朱砂、酸枣仁、柏子仁等同用。治疗惊痫抽搐、癫狂发作，可与镇惊息风药配伍同用。

(2) Dizziness and blurring of vision. The medicinal herb is heavy in property and acts to soothe liver and subdue yang. In the treatment of liver yang hyperactivity manifested by dizziness, blurring of vision, irritability and anger, it is combined with *Haematitum* (zhe shi), *Ostreae Concha* (mu li) and *Achyranthis Bidentatae Radix* (niu xi).

(2) 头晕目眩。本品质重镇潜，能平肝潜阳。治肝阳上亢所致的头晕目眩、烦躁易怒，常与赭石、牡蛎、牛膝等配伍。

(3) Leakage and prolapse patterns. The medicinal herb acts to astringe in calcined form and consolidate the liquid substances, applied to treat various leakage and prolapse pattern. In the treatment of seminal emission and nocturnal emission due to kidney deficiency, it is combined with mu li, *Astragali Complanati Semen* (sha yuan zi) and *Euryales Semen* (qian shi). In the treatment of frequency of urination due to heart and kidney deficiency, it is combined with *Mantidis OÖTheca* (sang piao xiao), *Testudinis Carapax et Plastrum* (gui jia) and *Poria cum Radix pini* (fu shen). In the treatment of metrorrhagia, metrostaxis and morbid leucorrhea due to qi failing to check liquid substances or Thoroughfare and Conception Vessels failing to hold liquid substances, it is combined with *Astragali Radix* (huang qi), *Schisandrae Chinensis Fructus* (wu wei zi) and *Halloysitum Rubrum* (chi shi zhi). In the treatment of spontaneous sweating due to qi deficiency or nocturnal sweat due to yin deficiency, it is combined with *Astragali Radix* (huang qi), *Fructus Tritici Levis* (fu xiao mai) and *Schisandrae Chinensis Fructus* (wu wei zi).

(3) 滑脱诸证。本品煅用性涩，具收敛固涩之功，治滑脱诸证。治肾虚遗精、滑精，常与牡蛎、沙苑子、芡实等配伍。治心肾两虚，小便频数者，常与桑螵蛸、龟甲、茯神等配伍。治气虚不摄，冲任不固之崩漏、带下，可与黄芪、五味子、赤石脂等同用。治表虚自汗或阴虚盗汗，可与黄芪或浮小麦、五味子等同用。

(4) Eczema, impetigo and unhealed ulcer. The medicinal herb in calcined form acts to absorb damp, heal ulcer and engender flesh for external use. It is combined with dried *Alumen* (bai fan) in

(4) 湿疹湿疮，疮疡久溃不敛。煅龙骨外用，有吸湿敛疮，生肌之效。可与枯矾等份，共为细末，掺敷患处。

equal proportions by grinding into fine powder and topically applying.

Usage and dosage Apply 15～30 g in decoction, by decocting first in crude form. Apply a proper amount for external use. The medicinal herb acts to astringe and consolidate in calcined form, and acts to treat other disease in crude form.

用法用量 煎服，15～30 克；生用宜先煎；外用适量。煅用收敛固涩，余皆生用。

Succinum (hu po)

琥珀

It is the product from the resin of ancient pines buried in the earth for a long period of time. The medicinal herb is collected all over the year, applied in powdered form.

古代松科松属植物的树脂，埋藏地下经年久转化而成。全年均可采收。研末用。

Features Flavor: sweet. Property: neutral. Meridian tropism: the Heart Meridian, the Liver Meridian and the Bladder Meridian.

性味归经 甘，平。归心、肝、膀胱经。

Actions Tranquilize heart, calm mind, activate blood, dissolve stasis, promote urination and treat stranguria.

功效 镇惊安神，活血散瘀，利尿通淋。

Application

(1) Palpitation, insomnia, convulsion and epilepsy. The medicinal herb is heavy in property and acts to tranquilize heart and calm mind. In the treatment of restlessness, palpitation, insomnia, poor memory and dream-disturbed sleep, it is combined with *Ziziphi Spinosae Semen* (suan zao ren) and *Polygalae Radix* (yuan zhi). In the treatment of infantile convulsion, high fever, spasm or epilepsy seizure, it is combined with *Arisaematis Rhizoma* (tian nan xing), *Cinnabaris* (zhu sha) and *Concretio Siliceae Bambusae* (tian zhu huang).

应用

（1）心悸失眠，惊风癫痫。本品质重，能镇心定惊、安神。治心神不宁、惊悸失眠、健忘多梦，常与酸枣仁、远志等配伍。治小儿惊风，高热抽搐或癫痫发作，可与天南星、朱砂、天竺黄等同用。

(2) Blood stasis blockage pattern. The medicinal herb is attributive to the Heart and Liver Meridian and the Xue (Blood) Phase, and acts to activate

（2）瘀血阻滞证。本品入心、肝血分，能活血通经、散瘀消癥。治瘀滞经闭、痛

blood, dredge meridians, dissolve stasis and relieve masses. In the treatment of amenorrhea and dysmenorrhea due to blood stasis, it is combined with *Angelicae Sinensis Radix* (dang gui), *Curcumae Rhizoma* (e zhu) and *Linderae Radix* (wu yao). In the treatment of stuffy chest and cardiac pain, it is combined with *Notoginseng Radix et Rhizoma* (san qi) by grinding into fine powder for oral administration. In the treatment of abdominal masses, it is combined with *Sparganii Rhizoma* (san leng), *Trionycis Carapax* (bie jia) and *Rhei Radix et Rhizoma* (da huang).

经，可与当归、莪术、乌药等同用。治胸痹心痛，可与三七共研末服。治癥瘕痞块，与三棱、鳖甲、大黄等同用。

(3) Stranguria. The medicinal herb acts to promote urination and treat stranguria and also to dissolve stasis and stanch blood as well. In the treatment of stranguria, such as stranguria with bleeding, stranguria with stones and stranguria with burning sensation, it is applied singly by grinding into fire powder for oral administration with *Medulla Junci* (deng xin cao) decoction, or combined with other medicinal herbs.

(3) 淋证。本品既利尿通淋、又散瘀止血。治淋证，尤宜于血淋，亦治石淋、热淋，可单用本品为散，灯心汤送服。或与其他药物配伍同用。

Usage and dosage Apply 1.5～3 g in powdered form. It is prohibited to decoct it.

用法用量 研末冲服，每次 1.5～3 克。不入煎剂。

Ziziphi Spinosae Semen (suan zao ren)

酸枣仁

It is the dried product from the ripe seed of *Ziziphus jujuba* Mill. var. *spinosa* (Bunge) Hu ex H. F. Chow, family Rhamnaceae. The medicinal herb is collected in late autumn and early winter when the fruit is ripe, applied in crude form or stir-fried form.

为鼠李科植物酸枣的干燥成熟种子。秋末冬初果实成熟时采收。生用或炒用。

Features Flavor: sweet and sour. Property: neutral. Meridian tropism: the Liver Meridian, the Gallbladder Meridian and the Heart Meridian.

性味归经 甘、酸，平。归肝、胆、心经。

Actions Nourish heart, benefit liver, tranquilize heart, calm mind, astringe sweat and produce fluid.

Application

(1) Palpitation and insomnia. The medicinal herb is sweet and neutral in property and attributive to the Heart and Liver Meridians, and acts to nourish blood in heart and liver, nourish heart and calm mind. In the treatment of palpitation and insomnia due to heart and spleen deficiency, it is combined with *Angelicae Sinensis Radix* (dang gui), *Astragali Radix* (huang qi) and *Codonopsis Radix* (dang shen). In the treatment of restlessness and poor sleep due to false heat in liver, it is combined with *Anemarrhenae Rhizoma* (zhi mu), *Poria* (fu ling) and *Glycyrrhizae Radix et Rhizoma* (gan cao), to form up Wild Jujube Seed Decoction (Suan Zao Ren Tang).

(2) Profuse sweating due to weak body. The medicinal herb is sour and astringent in property. In the treatment of spontaneous sweating and nocturnal sweat due to weak body, it is combined with huang qi, *Schisandrae Chinensis Fructus* (wu wei zi) and *Corni Fructus* (shan zhu yu).

(3) Thirst due to consumption of body fluid. The medicinal herb is sour in flavor and acts to produce fluid. In the treatment of thirst due to consumption of body fluid, it is combined with *Dendrobii Herba* (shi hu) and *Trichosanthis Radix* (tian hua fen).

Usage and dosage Apply 10～15 g in decoction. The medicinal herb in crude form is neutral and cool in property, applied to treat insomnia due to yin deficiency. The medicinal herb in stir-fried form is warm in property, applied to treat palpitation and in-

功效 养心益肝，宁心安神，敛汗，生津。

应用

（1）心悸失眠。本品味甘性平，入心、肝经，能养心肝之血而安神，为养心安神之要药。治心脾两虚的心悸失眠，常与当归、黄芪、党参等同用。治肝虚有热之虚烦不眠，常与知母、茯苓、甘草等配伍，如酸枣仁汤。

（2）体虚多汗。本品味酸收敛。治体虚自汗、盗汗，常与黄芪、五味子、山茱萸等同用。

（3）津伤口渴。本品味酸生津。治津伤口渴，可与石斛、天花粉等同用。

用法用量 煎服，10～15克。生用性平而偏凉，宜用于阴虚失眠；炒用性偏温，宜用于心脾两虚的心悸失眠。

somnia due to heart and spleen deficiency.

Platycladi Semen (bai zi ren)

It is the dried product from the ripe seed of *Platycladus orientalis* (L.) Franco, family Cupressaceae. The medicinal herb is collected in autumn and winter by peeling the fruit and taking out the seed, applied in crude form or frost-prepared form.

Features Flavor: sweet. Property: neutral. Meridian tropism: the Heart Meridian, the Kidney Meridian and the Large Intestine Meridian.

Actions Nourish heart, calm mind, moisturize intestines and promote defecation.

Application

(1) Palpitation and insomnia. The medicinal herb is sweet, moist and neutral in property, and acts to nourish heart and calm mind. In the treatment of palpitation, fearful throbbing, restlessness and insomnia due to yin-blood insufficiency or loss of nourishment of heart spirit, it is combined with *Schisandrae Chinensis Fructus* (wu wei zi), *Poria* (fu ling) and *Ziziphi Spinosae Semen* (suan zao ren).

(2) Constipation due to dryness in intestines. The medicinal herb is sweet, moist and fatty in property and acts to moisturize intestines and promote defecation. In the treatment of constipation due to dryness in intestines in those with old age or weak body, it is combined with *Cannabis Fructus* (huo ma ren) and *Pruni Semen* (yu li ren), to form up Five Seeds Pills (Wu Ren Wan).

Usage and dosage Apply 3～10 g in decoction, in crude form. The medicinal herb in frost-prepared form is applied for those with loose feces.

Precautions for use It is cautious to apply for

柏子仁

为柏科植物侧柏的干燥成熟种仁。秋、冬二季采收成熟种子，去除种皮，收集种仁。生用或制霜用。

性味归经 甘，平。归心、肾、大肠经。

功效 养心安神，润肠通便。

应用

（1）心悸失眠。本品甘润性平，能养心安神，多用治阴血不足，心神失养的心悸怔忡、虚烦不眠，常与五味子、茯苓、酸枣仁等同用。

（2）肠燥便秘。本品甘润多脂，能润肠通便。治年老体弱的肠燥便秘，常与火麻仁、郁李仁等同用，如五仁丸。

用法用量 煎服，3～10克。一般生用，制霜后宜于大便溏薄者。

使用注意 便溏及多痰

those with loose feces or profuse phlegm.

者慎用。

Polygalae Radix (yuan zhi)

远志

It is the dried product from the root of the perennial herbage *Polygala tenuifolia* Wild., or *Polygala sibirica* L., family Polygalaceae. The medicinal herb is collected in spring and autumn, applied in crude form or in stir-baked form.

为远志科植物远志或卵叶远志的干燥根。春、秋二季采挖。生用或炙用。

Features Flavor: bitter and pungent. Property: warm. Meridian tropism: the Heart Meridian, the Kidney Meridian and the Lung Meridian.

性味归经 苦、辛，温。归心、肾、肺经。

Actions Calm mind, improve intelligence, harmonize heart and kidney, dissolve phlegm and eliminate carbuncle.

功效 安神增智，交通心肾，祛痰，消散痈肿。

Application

应用

(1) Fearful throbbing, poor memory, insomnia, dream-disturbed sleep. The medicinal herb is attributive to the Heart and Kidney Meridians and acts to harmonize heart and kidney, tranquilize heart and calm mind. In the treatment of disharmony between heart and kidney manifested by restlessness, fearful throbbing, insomnia and poor memory, it is combined with *Ginseng Radix et Raizoma* (ren shen), *Os Draconis* (long gu) and *Poria cum Radix pini* (fu shen), to form up Spirit-Calming and Mind-Quieting Pills (An Shen Ding Zhi Wan).

(1) 惊悸健忘，失眠多梦。本品主入心肾，能交通心肾，安定神志。治心肾不交的心神不宁，惊悸不安，失眠健忘，常与人参、龙骨、茯神等同用，如安神定志丸。

(2) Vagrancy. The medicinal herb is pungent in property and acts to eliminate phlegm and open heart aperture. In the treatment of phlegm blocking heart aperture manifested by vagrancy, epilepsy and mania, it is combined with *Acori Tatarinowii Rhizoma* (shi chang pu) and *Curcumae Radix* (yu jin).

(2) 神志恍惚。本品味辛通利，既祛痰，又利心窍，治痰阻心窍的神志恍惚、癫痫发狂，可与石菖蒲、郁金等同用。

(3) Cough with profuse sputum. The medicinal herb acts to eliminate phlegm and stop cough. In

(3) 咳嗽痰多。本品能祛痰、止咳。治痰多黏稠、咳

the treatment of cough with excessive and sticky sputum, it is combined with *Fritillariae Cirrhosae Bulbus* (chuan bei mu), *Armeniacae Amarum Semen* (ku xing ren) and *Platycodonis Radix* (jie geng).

吐不爽者,可与川贝母、苦杏仁、桔梗等同用。

(4) Carbuncle and furuncle, swelling and pain at breasts. The medicinal herb is bitter, warm and dredging, and acts to dissolve qi and blood stagnation and relieve carbuncle and swelling. In the treatment of carbuncle, furuncle and acute mastitis, it is applied singly by grinding into powder and taken with millet wine for oral administration or external use.

(4) 痈疽疮毒,乳房肿痛。本品苦泄温通,善疏通气血壅滞,能消痈散肿。治疮痈、乳痈,可单味研末,黄酒送服或外用调敷。

Usage and dosage Apply 3～10 g in decoction. Apply a proper amount for external use. The medicinal herb acts to dissolve phlegm and relieve carbuncle in crude form, and acts to calm mind and improve intelligence in prepared form.

用法用量 煎服,3～10克。外用适量。生用祛痰、消痈,制用安神增智。

Precautions for use It is cautious to apply for those with gastritis or gastric ulcer.

使用注意 有胃炎及胃溃疡者慎用。

Albiziae Cortex (he huan pi)

合欢皮

It is the dried product from the bark of *Albizzia julibrissin* Durazz, family Legminosae. The medicinal herb is collected by peeling in spring and autumn, applied in crude form.

为豆科植物合欢的干燥树皮。夏、秋二季剥取。生用。

Features Flavor: sweet. Property: neutral. Meridian tropism: the Heart Meridian, the Liver Meridian and the Lung Meridian.

性味归经 甘,平。归心、肝、肺经。

Actions Calm mind, relieve melancholy, activate blood and desiccate swell.

功效 安神解郁,活血消肿。

Application

应用

(1) Melancholy and insomnia. The medicinal herb acts to soothe liver, relieve melancholy, nourish heart and calm mind. In the treatment of restlessness, insomnia and dream-disturbed sleep due to

(1) 忧郁失眠。本品能疏解肝郁、悦心安神,尤宜于情志不遂、忿怒忧郁而致的烦躁不宁、失眠多梦,可单用

emotional depression or anger, it is combined with *Platycladi Semen* (bai zi ren), *Polygoni Multiflori Caulis* (ye jiao teng) and *Curcumae Radix* (yu jin).

或与柏子仁、夜交藤、郁金等同用。

(2) Traumatic injury, pulmonary abscess, carbuncle and furuncle. The medicinal herb acts to activate blood, dissolve stasis, desiccate swell and relieve pain. In the treatment of traumatic injury and fracture with swelling and pain, it is combined with *Carthami Flos* (hong hua), *Persicae Semen* (tao ren) and *Angelicae Sinensis Radix* (dang gui). In the treatment of pulmonary abscess, it is combined with *Phragmitis Rhizoma* (lu gen) and *Houttuyniae Herba* (yu xing cao). In the treatment of carbuncle and furuncle, it is combined with *Taraxaci Herba* (pu gong ying) and *Violae Herba* (zi hua di ding).

（2）跌打伤痛，肺痈，疮痈。本品能活血祛瘀，消肿止痛。治跌打损伤、骨折肿痛，常与红花、桃仁、当归等配伍。治肺痈，与芦根、鱼腥草等同用。治疮痈肿痛，与蒲公英、紫花地丁等同用。

Usage and dosage Apply 6～12 g in decoction.

用法用量 煎服，6～12克。

Precautions for use It is cautious to apply for pregnant women.

使用注意 孕妇慎用。

Brief summary

Both *Cinnabaris* (zhu sha) and *Succinum* (hu po) are heavy in quality and act to tranquilize heart and calm mind, applied to treat restlessness. Zhu sha is cold-cool in property and attributive to the Heart Meridian, and acts to tranquilize heart and calm mind, and also to reduce heart fire, applied to treat palpitation and insomnia due to heart fire flaming and hyperactivity. It also acts to clear heat and relieve toxin, applied to treat heat-toxin pattern. Hu po is neutral and heavy in property and attributive to the Heart and Liver Meridians and Xue (Blood) Phase, and acts to activate blood and dis-

小　结

朱砂、琥珀，均质重，功能镇惊安神，治心神不安之证。其中朱砂药性寒凉，专入心经，既重镇安神，又善清心火，最宜心火亢盛之心悸失眠；又清热解毒，治多种热毒之证。琥珀药性平和，质重镇惊，又入心肝血分，能活血化瘀，治瘀滞诸证；且能利尿通淋、散瘀止血，尤适用于血淋等证。

solve stasis, applied to treat stagnation and stasis patterns. It also acts to promote urination, treat stranguria, dissolve stasis and stanch blood, applied to treat stranguria with bleeding.

Both *Os Draconis* (long gu) and *Magnetitum* (ci shi) are attributive to the Heart and Liver Meridians and act to tranquilize heart, calm mind, soothe liver and subdue yang, applied to treat irritable spirit in heart manifested by fearful throbbing and mental disorder, and also to treat dizziness and blurring of vision due to liver yang hyperactivity. Long gu is sweet, neutral and heavy in property, and acts to relieve irritability and calm mind. Furthermore, the medicinal herb in calcined form is astringent in property and acts to absorb damp, astringe carbuncle and engender flesh, applied to treat leakage and prolapse patterns, and also to treat eczema, impetigo and unhealed ulcer as well. Ci shi is salty and heavy in property, and acts to benefit kidney yin, subdue floating yang and calm heart mind, applied to treat fearful throbbing and insomnia due to kidney deficiency and liver hyperactivity, or due to heart spirit disturbance. It also acts to benefit kidney, improve hearing, brighten eyes, accept qi and soothe panting, applied to treat blurring of vision and hearing decrease due to liver and kidney deficiency, and panting due to kidney deficiency.

龙骨、磁石，均入心、肝经，能镇惊安神、平肝潜阳，可用治心神不宁的惊悸、癫狂，以及肝阳眩晕。其中龙骨甘平质重，镇惊安神效佳，为镇惊安神之要药。煅用性涩，善收敛固涩、收湿敛疮生肌，治滑脱诸证，以及湿疮痒疹、疮疡不溃不愈等证。磁石咸寒质重，善益肾阴、镇浮阳而安心神，尤宜于肾虚肝旺，扰动心神的惊悸失眠；又善益肾聪耳明目、纳气平喘，治肝肾亏虚之目暗耳聋、肾虚喘促等证。

Both *Ziziphi Spinosae Semen* (suan zao ren) and *Platycladi Semen* (bai zi ren) are sweet and neutral in property, and act to nourish heart and calm mind, applied in mutual reinforcement to treat palpitation and insomnia due to yin-blood insufficiency or loss of nourishment of heart spirit. Suan zao ren is also attributive to the Liver Meridian and

酸枣仁、柏子仁，均味甘性平，有养心安神之效，常相须为用，治阴血不足，心神失养之心悸、失眠。其中酸枣仁兼入肝经，具养心益肝之功，多用于心肝血虚之心神不宁；又酸收敛汗，治疗自

acts to nourish heart and benefit liver, applied to treat restlessness due to heart and liver blood deficiency. It is sour in flavor and acts to astringe sweating, applied to treat spontaneous sweating and nocturnal sweat. It is also sour in flavor and acts to produce fluid, applied to treat thirst due to consumption of body fluid. Bai zi ren is fatty in property and acts to moisturize intestines and promote defecation, applied to treat constipation due to dryness in intestines.

汗、盗汗;味酸生津,治津伤口渴。柏子仁富含油脂,能润肠通便,治疗肠燥便秘。

Polygalae Radix (yuan zhi) is pungent, bitter and warm in property and attributive to the Heart and Kidney Meridians, and acts to promote heart qi flow and kidney qi flow, and to harmonize heart and kidney, applied to treat disharmony between heart and kidney manifested by fearful throbbing, poor memory, insomnia and dream-disturbed sleep. It acts to dissolve phlegm and open heart aperture, applied to treat cough with excessive sputum, and vagrancy and epilepsy due to phlegm blocking heart aperture. It also acts to desiccate swell and stop pain, applied to treat carbuncle, furuncle, and swelling and pain in breasts.

远志,味辛苦性温,入心肾经,能开心气、通肾气,具交通心肾之长,善治心肾不交之惊悸健忘、失眠多梦;兼祛痰、开心窍之功,可治咳嗽痰多,痰阻心窍的神志恍惚、癫痫等证;又消散痈肿,治疮痈、乳房肿痛。

Albiziae Cortex (he huan pi) is sweet and neutral in property, and acts to soothe liver, relieve melancholy, nourish heart and calm mind, applied to treat emotional depression, anger and restlessness. It also acts to activate blood and dissolve stasis, applied to treat traumatic injury, fracture, carbuncle and furuncle.

合欢皮,味甘性平,能疏肝解郁、悦心安神,善治情志不遂、忿怒忧郁之烦躁不宁;又活血散瘀,治疗跌打骨折、痈肿疮毒。

Chapter 14 Liver-Soothing and Wind-Eliminating Herbs

第 14 章 平肝息风药

The medicinal herbs acting to soothe liver yang and eliminate liver wind are called the liver-soothing and wind-eliminating herbs.

The medicinal herbs are mostly attributive to the Liver Meridian. The medicinal herbs of minerals and shells are heavy in quality and act to soothe liver and subdue yang or to inhibit liver yang, and act to reduce liver heat and calm heart mind, applied to treat liver yang hyperactivity manifested by dizziness and blurring of vision, and to treat liver fire manifested by redness of eyes, headache, dizziness, irritability and anger. The medicinal herbs of insects act to eliminate liver wind and relieve spasm, applied to treat internal movement of liver wind manifested by blurring of vision, dizziness, giddiness, spasm and convulsion, or applied to treat phlegm-heat pattern manifested by epilepsy, convulsion and spasm, or applied to treat tetanus and opisthotonus.

It is necessary to notice in the application of the medicinal herbs that the medicinal herbs are cold or warm in property and should be applied distinctively. It is not advisable to apply the medicinal herbs of insects or minerals for long time for those with spleen deficiency, chronic convulsion, yin deficiency or blood insufficiency, so as to avoid damage of

以平肝阳、息肝风为主要作用的药物,称平肝息风药。

本类药物大多入肝经。其中,以质重的贝壳矿石类为主的药物,具有平肝潜阳或平抑肝阳的功效,兼能清肝热、安心神,主要用治肝阳上亢之头晕目眩,或肝火目赤、头痛头昏、烦躁易怒等证。以虫类药为主的药物,具有息肝风、止痉挛的作用,主要用于肝风内动的眩晕欲仆、痉挛抽搐等证。或用治痰热癫痫、惊风抽搐,以及破伤风角弓反张等证。

使用本类药需注意,本类药物寒温不一,应区别使用。脾虚慢惊以及阴虚血亏者,不宜长期使用虫类或矿石类药物,以便影响脾胃、损伤正气。

spleen and stomach and injury of Zheng (Anti-Pathogenic) Qi.

Haliotidis Concha (shi jue ming)

石决明

It is the dried product from the shell of *Haliotis diversicolor* Reeve, *Haliotis discus hannai* Ino, *Haliotis ovina* Gmelin, *Haliotis ruber* (Leach), *Haliotis asimins* Linnacus or *Haliotis laevigata* (Donovan), family Haliotidae. The medicinal herb is collected in summer and autumn, applied in crude form and calcined form.

为鲍科动物杂色鲍、皱纹盘鲍、羊鲍、澳洲鲍、耳鲍或白鲍的贝壳。夏、秋二季捕捞。生用或煅用。

Features Flavor: salty. Property: cold. Meridian tropism: the Liver Meridian.

性味归经 咸,寒。归肝经。

Actions Soothe liver, subdue yang, purify liver and brighten eyes.

功效 平肝潜阳,清肝明目。

Application

应用

(1) Dizziness and blurring of vision. The medicinal herb is attributive to the Liver Meridian and cold and heavy in property, and acts to reduce heat and subdue yang, as the major herb to sedate liver and cool liver. In the treatment of dizziness and blurring of vision due to liver and kidney yin deficiency or liver yang hyperactivity, it is combined with *Rehmanniae Radix* (sheng di huang), *Paeoniae Radix Alba* (bai shao) and *Ostreae Concha* (mu li). In the treatment of liver yang hyperactivity with liver fire, it is combined with *Saigae Tataricae Cornu* (ling yang jiao), *Prunellae Spica* (xia ku cao) and *Uncariae Ramulus cum Uncis* (gou teng).

(1) 头晕目眩。本品专入肝经,性寒清热,质重潜阳,为镇肝、凉肝之要药。治肝肾阴虚,阳亢眩晕,常与生地黄、白芍、牡蛎等同用。若肝阳上亢兼肝火者,可与羚羊角、夏枯草、钩藤等同用。

(2) Redness of eyes, cataract and blurring of vision. The medicinal herb acts to purify liver, brighten eyes and treat cataract, as the major herb to treat eye diseases. In the treatment of redness, swelling and pain of eyes due to liver fire flaming

(2) 目赤翳障,视物昏花。本品能清肝明目退翳,为目疾常用药。治肝火上炎的目赤肿痛,可与夏枯草、决明子、菊花等配伍。治风热

upwards, it is combined with xia ku cao, *Cassiae Semen* (jue ming zi) and *Chrysanthemi Flos* (ju hua). In the treatment of cataract due to wind-heat, it is combined with the wind-eliminating and heat-clearing herbs. In the treatment of blurring of vision due to liver blood deficiency, it is combined with *Rehmanniae Radix Praeparata* (shu di huang), *Lycii Fructus* (gou qi zi) and *Cuscutae Semen* (tu si zi).

翳障,可与疏风清热药配伍。治肝虚血少,目暗不明,可与熟地黄、枸杞子、菟丝子等同用。

Usage and dosage Apply 15～30 g in decoction and decoct first. The medicinal herb acts to soothe liver and purify liver in crude form, and acts as eye drop in calcined form after water-refining.

用法用量 煎服,15～30 克。生用宜先煎。生用平肝、清肝,煅后水飞外用点眼。

Ostreae Concha (mu li)

牡蛎

It is the dried product from the shell of *Ostrea gigas* Thunberg, *Ostrea talienwhanensis* Crosse or *Ostrea rivularis* Gould, family Ostreidae. The medicinal herb is collected all over the year, applied in crude form or calcined form.

为牡蛎科动物长牡蛎、大连湾牡蛎或近江牡蛎的贝壳。全年均可捕捞。生用或煅用。

Features Flavor: salty. Property: slightly cold. Meridian tropism: the Liver Meridian, the Gallbladder Meridian and the Kidney Meridian.

性味归经 咸,微寒。归肝、胆、肾经。

Actions Tranquilize, calm mind, nourish yin, subdue yang, soften the hard and dissolve stasis. It acts to astringe and hold the liquid in calcined form, and also acts to relieve acid and stop pain as well.

功效 重镇安神,益阴潜阳,软坚散结,煅用收敛固涩,制酸止痛。

Application

(1) Fearful throbbing, insomnia, dizziness and blurring of vision. The medicinal herb is heavy in quality and acts to tranquilize, calm mind, nourish yin and subdue yang. In the treatment of restlessness, fearful throbbing and insomnia, it is combined with *Os Draconis* (long gu) and *Succinum* (hu po). In the treatment of yin deficiency and yang hyper-

应用

(1) 惊悸失眠,头晕目眩。本品质重,既镇惊安神,又益阴潜阳。治心神不宁、惊悸失眠,常与龙骨、琥珀等同用。治阴虚阳亢,眩晕耳鸣,常与龟甲、龙骨等同用。

activity, it is combined with *Testudinis Carapax et Plastrum* (gui jia) and *Os Draconis* (long gu).

(2) Globus hystericus, scrofula and abdominal masses. The medicinal herb is salty in flavor and acts to soften the hard. In the treatment of globus hystericus and scrofula due to phlegm-fire, it is combined with *Bulbus Fritillariae Thunbergii* (zhe bei mu) and *Scrophulariae Radix* (xuan shen). In the treatment of abdominal masses, it is combined with *Trionycis Carapax* (bie jia), *Salviae Miltiorrhizae Radix et Rhizoma* (dan shen) and *Curcumae Rhizoma* (e zhu).

（2）痰核瘰疬，癥瘕积聚。本品味咸软坚。治痰火所致的痰核瘰疬，常与浙贝母、玄参等配伍。治癥瘕痞块，多与鳖甲、丹参、莪术等配伍。

(3) Leakage and prolapse patterns. The medicinal herb in calcined form is astringent in property and acts to astringe and hold liquids. In the treatment of leakage and prolapse patterns, it is combined with other astringing herbs according to pattern identification.

（3）滑脱诸证。本品煅后性涩，具收敛固涩之功。治体虚滑脱诸证，可与其他收敛药随证配伍应用。

(4) Gastric pain and acid regurgitation. The medicinal herb in calcined form acts to relieve acid and stop pain. In the treatment of gastric pain and acid regurgitation, it is combined with *Bulbus Fritillariae Thunbergii* (zhe bei mu) by grinding into fine powder for oral administration.

（4）胃痛泛酸。本品煅用制酸止痛。治胃痛泛酸，常与浙贝母等共为细末服用。

Usage and dosage Apply 10～30 g in decoction and decoct first in crude form. The medicinal herb acts to astringe and hold liquids, relieve acid and stop pain in calcined form, and acts to treat other diseases in crude form.

用法用量 煎服，10～30克。生用宜先煎。煅用收敛固涩、制酸止痛，余皆生用。

***Haematitum* (zhe shi)**

赭石

It is the dried product from the red iron of trigonal system, containing ferric oxide (Fe_2O_3), also called dai zhe shi. After mining and removing mis-

为氧化物类矿物刚玉族赤铁矿，主含三氧化二铁。又名代赭石。采挖后，除去

cellaneous stones, the mineral is smashed and refined. The medicinal herb is applied in crude form and calcined form.

杂石,打碎。生用或煅用。

Features Flavor: bitter. Property: cold. Meridian tropism: the Liver Meridian, the Heart Meridian, the Lung Meridian and the Stomach Meridian.

性味归经 苦,寒。归肝、心、肺、胃经。

Actions Soothe liver, subdue yang, tranquilize liver, subdue up-reverse flow of qi, cool blood and stanch blood.

功效 平肝潜阳,重镇降逆,凉血止血。

Application

应用

(1) Dizziness and blurring of vision. The medicinal herb is heavy, sinking and descending in property and acts to tranquilize liver and subdue yang. It is bitter and cold in property and acts to reduce liver fire. In the treatment of liver yang hyperactivity or liver fire flaming and excess manifested by dizziness, blurring of vision, irritability and anger, it is combined with *Haliotidis Concha* (shi jue ming), *Prunellae Spica* (xia ku cao) and *Achyranthis Bidentatae Radix* (niu xi). In the treatment of liver and kidney yin deficiency or liver yang hyperactivity, it is combined with *Testudinis Carapax et Plastrum* (gui jia), *Paeoniae Radix Alba* (bai shao) and *Ostreae Concha* (mu li).

(1) 头晕目眩。本品质重沉降,长于镇肝潜阳;味苦性寒,又清肝火。治肝阳上亢、肝火炽盛的头晕目眩、烦躁易怒,常与石决明、夏枯草、牛膝等同用。治肝肾阴虚,肝阳上亢者,常与龟甲、白芍、牡蛎等同用。

(2) Vomiting, hiccup and belching. The medicinal herb is heavy in quality and acts to subdue up-reverse flow of qi, applied to treat up-reverse flow of stomach qi. In the treatment of vomiting, hiccup and belching due to up-reverse flow of stomach qi, it is combined with *Inulae Flos* (xuan fu hua), *Pinelliae Rhizoma* (ban xia) and *Zingiberis Rhizoma Recens* (sheng jiang), to form up Inula and Hermatitum Decoction (Xuan Fu Dai Zhe Tang).

(2) 呕吐,呃逆,噫气。本品重镇降逆,善降上逆之胃气。治胃气上逆之呕吐、呃逆、噫气等,常与旋覆花、半夏、生姜等同用,如旋覆代赭汤。

(3) Panting. The medicinal herb acts to subdue

(3) 喘息。本品亦能降

up-reverse flow of lung qi and soothe panting, applied singly by grinding into fine powder for oral administration with vinegar. In the treatment of panting due to lung and kidney insufficiency, it is combined with *Codonopsis Radix* (dang shen), *Corni Fructus* (shan zhu yu) ,etc.

肺气、平喘息。可单用本品研末,米醋调服。若治肺肾不足之虚喘,常与党参、山茱萸等同用。

(4) Hemoptysis, epistaxis, metrorrhagia and metrostaxis due to heat in blood. The medicinal herb is bitter and cold and attributive to the Xue (Blood) Phase, and acts to cool blood and stanch blood. In the treatment of hemoptysis and epistaxis due to heat in blood, it is combined with *Imperatae Rhizoma* (bai mao gen) and *Cirsii Herba* (xiao ji). In the treatment of metrorrhagia and metrostaxis, it is combined with *Rubiae Radix Et Rhizoma* (qian cao) and *Typhae Pollen* (pu huang).

(4) 血热吐衄,崩漏。本品苦寒,且入血分,能凉血止血。治血热所致的吐血、衄血,可与白茅根、小蓟等同用。治崩漏下血,可与茜草、蒲黄等同用。

Usage and dosage Apply 9～30 g in decoction and decoct first after smashing. The medicinal herb acts to subdue up-reverse flow of qi and soothe liver in crude form, and acts to stanch blood in calcined form.

用法用量 煎服,9～30克。生用宜打碎先煎。生用降逆、平肝,煅用止血。

Precautions for use It is cautious to apply for pregnant women.

使用注意 孕妇慎用。

Tribuli Fructus (ji li)

蒺藜

It is the dried product from the ripe fruit of *Tribulus terrestris* L., family Zygophylaceae, also called "bai ji li" and "ci ji li". The medicinal herb is collected in autumn when the fruit is ripe, applied in stir-fried form.

为蒺藜科植物蒺藜的干燥成熟果实。又名"白蒺藜""刺蒺藜"。秋季果实成熟时采收。炒黄用。

Features Flavor: pungent and bitter. Property: slightly warm and slightly poisonous. Meridian tropism: the Liver Meridian.

性味归经 辛、苦,微温;有小毒。归肝经。

Actions Soothe liver, tranquilize liver, elimi-

功效 平肝疏肝,祛风

nate wind, brighten eyes and stop itching.

Application

(1) Dizziness and blurring of vision. The medicinal herb is bitter and descending in property and attributive to the Liver Meridian, and acts to soothe liver and subdue yang. In the treatment of dizziness and blurring of vision due to liver yang hyperactivity, it is combined with *Uncariae Ramulus cum Uncis* (gou teng) and *Chrysanthemi Flos* (ju hua).

(2) Distension and pain at chest and hypochondria, lactation deficiency, and distension and pain at breasts. The medicinal herb is pungent and dispersing in property and acts to relieve liver qi stagnation. In the treatment of liver qi stagnation, distension and pain at chest and hypochondria, it is combined with *Bupleuri Radix* (chai hu), *Cyperi Rhizoma* (xiang fu) and *Citri Reticulatae Pericarpium Viride* (qing pi). In the treatment of lactation deficiency and distension and pain at breasts due to liver qi stagnation after delivery, it is applied singly by grinding into fine powder for oral administration, or combined with *Akebiae Caulis* (mu tong).

(3) Redness of eyes and cataract. The medicinal herb acts to eliminate wind-heat, brighten eyes and treat cataract. In the treatment of redness, swelling and pain of eyes due to wind-heat, or cataract, it is combined with ju hua and *Cassiae Semen* (jue ming zi).

(4) Urticaria due to wind and skin itch. The medicinal herb acts to eliminate wind and relieve itching. In the treatment of urticaria and skin itch, it is combined with *Saposhnikoviae Radix* (fang feng), *Schizonepetae Herba* (jing jie) and *Menthae Haplocalycis Herba* (bo he).

明目,止痒。

应用

(1) 头晕目眩。本品苦降入肝,能平抑肝阳。治肝阳上亢的头晕目眩,常与钩藤、菊花等同用。

(2) 胸胁胀痛,乳闭胀痛。本品辛散,有疏肝解郁之效。治肝郁气滞,胸胁胀痛,可与柴胡、香附、青皮等配伍。治产后肝郁乳闭、乳房胀痛,常单用本品研末服,或与木通等药同用。

(3) 目赤翳障。本品能祛散风热、明目退翳。治风热目赤肿痛,或翳膜遮睛,多与菊花、决明子等同用。

(4) 风疹瘙痒。本品能祛风止痒。治风疹瘙痒,常与防风、荆芥、薄荷等同用。

Usage and dosage Apply 6～10 g in decoction.

用法用量 煎服，6～10克。

Saigae Tataricae Cornu (ling yang jiao)

羚羊角

It is the product from the horn of *Saiga tatarica* Linnaeus, family Bovidae. The medicinal herb is collected by cutting the horn and drying in sun, and cut into slices or ground into fine powder.

为牛科动物赛加羚羊的角。猎捕后锯取其角，晒干。镑片或研细粉。

Features Flavor: salty. Property: cold. Meridian tropism: the Liver Meridian and the Heart Meridian.

性味归经 咸，寒。归肝、心经。

Actions Soothe liver, eliminate wind, purify liver, brighten eyes, reduce heat and relieve toxin.

功效 平肝息风，清肝明目，清热解毒。

Application

应用

(1) Convulsion and spasm. The medicinal herb is cold in property and attributive to the Liver Meridian, and acts to reduce liver heat and eliminate liver wind, as the major herb to treat convulsion and spasm due to internal movement of liver wind. In the treatment of convulsion and spasm in high fever due to extreme heat producing wind, it is combined with *Uncariae Ramulus cum Uncis* (gou teng), *Chrysanthemi Flos* (ju hua) and *Rehmanniae Radix* (sheng di huang), to form up Antelope's Horn and Cat's Claw Decoction (Ling Jiao Gou Teng Tang).

(1) 惊痫抽搐。本品性寒入肝，功善清肝热、息肝风，为治肝风内动、惊痫抽搐之要药，治高热不退的热极生风，惊厥抽搐，常与钩藤、菊花、鲜地黄等同用，如羚角钩藤汤。

(2) Dizziness and blurring of vision. The medicinal herb acts to soothe liver and subdue yang. In the treatment of dizziness and blurring of vision due to liver yang hyperactivity, it is combined with *Haliotidis Concha* (shi jue ming), *Ostreae Concha* (mu li) and *Gastrodiae Rhizoma* (tian ma).

(2) 头晕目眩。本品能平肝阳。常与石决明、牡蛎、天麻等同用，治肝阳上亢的头晕目眩。

(3) Redness of eyes and cataract. The medicinal herb acts to reduce liver fire. In the treatment of headache, redness of eyes and cataract due to liv-

(3) 目赤翳障。本品善清肝火。治肝火上炎之头痛、目赤或翳障等，常与龙胆

er fire flaming upward, it is combined with *Gentianae Radix et Rhizoma* (long dan), *Cassiae Semen* (jue ming zi) and *Scutellariae Radix* (huang qin).

草、决明子、黄芩等同用。

(4) Macula due to heat-toxin. The medicinal herb acts to clear heat and relieve toxin. In the treatment of macula due to heat-toxin, it is combined with *Rehmanniae Radix* (sheng di huang) and *Paeoniae Radix Rubra* (chi shao).

（4）热毒发斑。本品能清热解毒。治热毒发斑，常与生地黄、赤芍等同用。

Usage and dosage Apply 1～3 g in decoction and decoct separate for over 2 hours. Milled into liquid or grind into fine powder and apply 0.3～0.6 g each time.

用法用量 煎服，1～3克。另煎2小时以上。磨汁或研粉服，每次0.3～0.6克。

Bovis Calculus (niu huang)

牛黄

It is the dried product from the stone in the gallbladder and biliary duct of *Bos taurus domesticus* Gmelin, family Bovidae. In slaughtering domestic cattle, if the medicinal herb is found, it is taken out, cleaned and dried in the shade.

为牛科动物牛干燥的胆结石。宰牛时，如发现有牛黄，应立即滤去胆汁，将牛黄取出，除去外部薄膜，阴干。

Features Flavor: sweet. Property: cool. Meridian tropism: the Liver Meridian and the Heart Meridian.

性味归经 甘，凉。归肝、心经。

Actions Purify heart, cool liver, eliminate wind, relieve spasm, dissolve phlegm, open aperture, clear heat and relieve toxin.

功效 清心凉肝，息风止痉，化痰开窍，清热解毒。

Application

应用

(1) Febrile disease manifested by loss of consciousness, convulsion and spasm. The medicinal herb acts to purify heart, cool liver, eliminate wind and relieve spasm. In the treatment of febrile disease manifested by loss of consciousness, convulsion and spasm, it is combined with *Cinnabaris* (zhu sha), *Scorpio* (quan xie) and *Uncariae Ramulus cum Uncis* (gou teng).

（1）热病神昏，惊痫抽搐。本品能清心凉肝、息风止痉。治热病神昏或惊痫抽搐，常与朱砂、全蝎、钩藤等同用。

(2) Wind stroke, epilepsy and mania due to phlegm. The medicinal herb acts to purify heart, dissolve phlegm, open aperture and wake up mind. In the treatment of wind stroke due to phlegm or epilepsy and mania due to phlegm-heat, it is applied singly by grinding into fine powder and taken with *Succus Bambosae* (zhu li), or combined with the aperture-opening and mind-waking herbs.

（2）中风痰迷，癫痫发狂。本品能清心豁痰、开窍醒神。治中风痰迷或痰热癫狂，可单用本品为末，淡竹沥化服即效，或与开窍醒神药同用。

(3) Sore throat, mouth ulcer, carbuncle and furuncle. The medicinal herb acts to reduce heat and relieve toxin. In the treatment of sore throat and mouth ulcer, it is combined with *Scutellariae Radix* (huang qin) and *Rhei Radix et Rhizoma* (da huang). In the treatment of carbuncle and furuncle, it is combined with the blood-activating and heat-clearing herbs or the swell-subsiding and pain-stopping herbs.

（3）咽痛口疮，疮痈肿痛。本品功善清热解毒。治咽痛口疮，常与黄芩、大黄等同用。用治疮痈疔毒，可与活血清热、消肿止痛之品同用。

Usage and dosage Apply 0.15～0.35 g in pills or powder. Apply a proper amount for external use.

用法用量 入丸散，0.15～0.35克。外用适量。

Precautions for use It is cautious to apply for pregnant women.

使用注意 孕妇慎用。

Uncariae Ramulus cum Uncis (gou teng)

钩藤

It is the dried product from the hooked vine of *Uncaria rhynchophylla* (Miq.) Jacks., or *Uncaria* macrophylla Wall., or *Uncaria hirsuta* Havil., or *Uncaria sinensis* (Oliv.) Havil., or *Uncaria sessiilifructus* Roxb., family Rubiaceae. The medicinal herb is collected in autumn and winter, applied in crude form.

为茜草科植物钩藤、大叶钩藤、毛钩藤、华钩藤或无柄果钩藤的干燥带钩茎枝。秋、冬二季采收。生用。

Features Flavor: sweet. Property: cool. Meridian tropism: the Liver Meridian and the Pericardium Meridian.

性味归经 甘，凉。归肝、心包经。

Actions Eliminate wind, relieve spasm, clear

功效 息风止痉，清热

heat and soothe liver.

平肝。

Application

应用

(1) Convulsion, epilepsy and spasm. The medicinal herb is sweet and cool in property and attributive to the Liver Meridian, and acts to eliminate wind, relieve spasm and purify liver. In the treatment of convulsion due to liver wind or high fever, it is combined with *Gastrodiae Rhizoma* (tian ma) and *Scorpio* (quan xie).

(1) 惊痫抽搐。本品甘凉入肝,具息风止痉之功,兼能清肝。治肝风或高热所致的抽搐,常与天麻、全蝎等同用。

(2) Headache and dizziness. The medicinal herb acts to purify liver and soothe liver. In the treatment of headache due to liver fire, it is combined with *Prunellae Spica* (xia ku cao), *Gardeniae Fructus* (zhi zi) and *Scutellariae Radix* (huang qin). In the treatment of dizziness due to liver yang hyperactivity, it is combined with tian ma, *Haliotidis Concha* (shi jue ming) and *Chrysanthemi Flos* (ju hua).

(2) 头痛眩晕。本品能清肝平肝。治肝火头痛,常与夏枯草、栀子、黄芩等同用。治阳亢眩晕,常与天麻、石决明、菊花等同用。

Furthermore, it acts to cool liver and relieve convulsion. In the treatment of morbid night cry of baby, it is combined with *Menthae Haplocalycis Herba* (bo he).

此外,本品与薄荷等同用,有凉肝止惊之效,可治小儿夜啼。

Usage and dosage Apply 3～12 g in decoction and decoct later.

用法用量 煎服,3～12克。宜后下。

Gastrodiae Rhizoma (tian ma)

天麻

It is the dried product from the tuber of *Gastrodia elata* BI., family Orchidaceae. The medicinal herb is collected from the Beginning of Winter (19th solar term) to the Pure Brightness (5th solar term) of next year, applied in crude form.

为兰科植物天麻的干燥块茎。立冬后至次年清明前采挖。生用。

Features Flavor: sweet. Property: neutral. Meridian tropism: the Liver Meridian.

性味归经 甘,平。归肝经。

Actions Eliminate wind, relieve spasm,

功效 息风止痉,平抑

soothe liver, subdue yang, eliminate wind and dredge meridians.

肝阳，祛风通络。

Application

应用

(1) Convulsion, epilepsy and spasm. The medicinal herb is sweet, moist and neutral in property and attributive to the Liver Meridian, and acts to eliminate wind and relieve spasm, applied to treat convulsion, epilepsy and spasm due to internal movement of liver wind, no matter of cold or hot type, by combining other medicinal herbs according to the patterns. In the treatment of infantile acute convulsion, it is combined with *Saigae Tataricae Cornu* (ling yang jiao), *Uncariae Ramulus cum Uncis* (gou teng) and *Scorpio* (quan xie). In the treatment of infantile chronic convulsion due to spleen deficiency, it is combined with *Ginseng Radix et Raizoma* (ren shen), *Atractylodis Macrocephalae Rhizoma* (bai zhu) and *Bombyx Batryticatus* (bai jiang can). In the treatment of convulsion and spasm due to tetanus, it is combined with *Arisaematis Rhizoma* (tian nan xing) and *Saposhnikoviae Radix* (fang feng), to form up Jade Genius Powder (Yu Zhen San).

（1）惊痫抽搐。本品甘润性平，入肝经，能息风止痉，治肝风内动，惊痫抽搐，不论寒热，皆可随证配伍应用。治小儿急惊风，常与羚羊角、钩藤、全蝎等同用。治小儿脾虚慢惊，则与人参、白术、白僵蚕等配伍。治破伤风的痉挛抽搐，常与天南星、防风等配伍，如玉真散。

(2) Headache and dizziness. The medicinal herb acts to soothe liver and subdue yang, as the major herb to relieve dizziness. In the treatment of dizziness and headache due to liver yang hyperactivity, it is combined with gou teng, *Taxilli Herba* (sang ji sheng) and *Haliotidis Concha* (shi jue ming), to form up Gastrodia and Cat's Claw Drink (Tian Ma Gou Teng Yin). In the treatment of dizziness and headache due to wind-phlegm, it is combined with *Pinelliae Rhizoma* (ban xia), bai zhu and *Poria* (fu ling), to form up Pinellia, Atrac-

（2）头痛眩晕。本品能平抑肝阳，为止眩晕之良药。治肝阳上亢之眩晕、头痛，常与钩藤、桑寄生、石决明等同用，如天麻钩藤饮。治风痰眩晕头痛，常与半夏、白术、茯苓等同用，如半夏白术天麻汤。

tylodes and Gastrodia Decoction (Ban Xia Bai Zhu Tian Ma Tang).

(3) Numbness of body and limbs, and Bi (Obturation) Pattern due to wind-damp. The medicinal herb acts to eliminate exogenous wind and dredge meridians. In the treatment of paralysis of hand and foot, numbness of body and limbs, or Bi (Obturation) Pattern, it is combined with *Gentianae Macrophyllae Radix* (qin jiao), *Notopterygii Rhizoma et Radix* (qiang huo).

（3）肢体麻木，风湿痹痛。本品能祛外风、通经络。治手足不遂、肢体麻木，或风湿痹痛，常与秦艽、羌活等同用。

Usage and dosage Apply 3～10 g in decoction.

用法用量 煎服，3～10克。

Scorpio (quan xie)

全蝎

It is the dried product from the whole body of *Buthus martensii* Karsch, family Buthidae. The medicinal herb is collected from late spring to early autumn, applied in crude form.

为钳蝎科动物东亚钳蝎的干燥体。春末至秋初捕捉。生用。

Features Flavor: pungent. Property: neutral and poisonous. Meridian tropism: the Liver Meridian.

性味归经 辛，平；有毒。归肝经。

Actions Eliminate wind, relieve spasm, attack toxin, desiccate stasis, dredge meridians and stop pain.

功效 息风止痉，攻毒散结，通络止痛。

Application

应用

(1) Spasm and convulsion. The medicinal herb is attributive to the Liver Meridian and neutral in property, and acts to soothe liver, eliminate wind and relieve spasm. In the treatment of spasm and convulsion due to various causes, it is combined with *Scolopendra* (wu gong) by grinding into fine powder, to form up Spasm-Stopping Powder (Zhi Jing San). It is applied to treat acute or chronic convulsion of baby, spasm in epilepsy due to phlegm, opis-

（1）痉挛抽搐。本品专入肝性平，具平息肝风，制止痉挛之功，善治各种原因之痉挛抽搐，常与蜈蚣同用，研细末服，如止痉散。随证配伍亦治小儿急慢惊风，以及痰迷癫痫的抽搐，破伤风的角弓反张，风中经络的口眼㖞斜等。

thotonus in tetanus, and deviation of mouth due to wind stroke of meridian attack, by combining with other herbs according to the patterns.

(2) Carbuncle, furuncle and scrofula. The medicinal herb acts to desiccate stasis and attack toxin, applied to treat carbuncle, furuncle and scrofula for oral administration or external use. In external use, the medicinal herb is baked to yellow and ground to fine powder to make ointment. In oral administration, the medicinal herb is baked to yellow and ground to fine powder, and then taken with millet wine.

（2）疮痈、瘰疬。本品有散结、攻毒之功。内服或外用，可治疮痈、瘰疬。外用多焙黄研末制膏外敷，内服可焙黄研末，黄酒送服。

(3) Stubborn Bi (Obturation) Pattern due to wind-damp, migraine and headache. The medicinal herb acts to eliminate pathogenic wind in meridians, dredge meridians and stop pain. In the treatment of unhealed Bi (Obturation) Pattern, it is combined with *Aconiti Radix* (chuan wu), *Agkistrodon* (qi she) and *Myrrha* (mo yao). In the treatment of stubborn migraine and headache, it is applied singly by grinding into fine powder or combined with *Bombyx Batryticatus* (bai jiang can) and *Chuanxiong Rhizoma* (chuan xiong).

（3）风湿顽痹，偏正头痛。本品善于搜剔经络风邪、通利经络，且止痛力强。治风湿痹痛、日久不愈，可与川乌、蕲蛇、没药等同用。治顽固性偏正头痛，可单味研末，或与白僵蚕、川芎等药同用。

Usage and dosage Apply 3～6 g in decoction. Apply a proper amount for external use.

用法用量 煎服，3～6克。外用适量。

Precautions for use It is prohibited to apply for pregnant women.

使用注意 孕妇禁用。

Scolopendra (wu gong)

蜈蚣

It is the dried product from the whole body of *Scolopendra subspinipes mutilans* L., Koch., family *Scolopendrae*. The medicinal herb is collected in spring and summer, applied in crude form.

为蜈蚣科动物少棘巨蜈蚣的干燥体。春、夏季捕捉。生用。

Features Flavor: pungent. Property: warm and

性味归经 辛，温。有

poisonous. Meridian tropism: the Liver Meridian.

Actions　Eliminate wind, relieve spasm, attack toxin, desiccate stasis, dredge meridians and stop pain.

Application

(1) Convulsion and spasm. The medicinal herb is pungent and warm and acts to connect the internal and surface, eliminate wind and relieve spasm. In the treatment of spasm and convulsion due to various causes, it is combined with *Scorpio* (quan xie) in mutual reinforcement. By proper combinations, the medicinal herb is applied to treat acute or chronic convulsion, tetanus and deviation of mouth due to wind stroke of meridian attack.

(2) Carbuncle, furuncle and scrofula. The medicinal herb acts to attack toxin with its poisonous property, desiccate stasis and subside swell. In the treatment of carbuncle, furuncle and scrofula, it is applied singly and backed to yellow by grinding into fine powder for external use. It is combined with other medicinal herbs for oral administration.

(3) Stubborn Bi (Obturation) Pattern due to wind-damp and headache. The medicinal herb acts to eliminate wind, dredge meridians and stop pain. In the treatment of stubborn Bi (Obturation) Pattern due to wind-damp, it is combined with *Saposhnikoviae Radix* (fang feng), *Angelicae Pubescentis Radix* (du huo) and *Clematidis Radix et Rhizoma* (wei ling xian). In the treatment of stubborn headache or migraine, it is combined with *Gastrodiae Rhizoma* (tian ma) and *Chuanxiong Rhizoma* (chuan xiong).

Usage and dosage　Apply 3～5 g in decoction. Apply a proper amount for external use.

毒。归肝经。

功效　息风止痉，攻毒散结，通络止痛。

应用

(1) 痉挛抽搐。本品辛温，性善走窜，通达内外，息风搜风止痉力强，治多种原因引起的痉挛抽搐，常与全蝎相须为用。经适当配伍，亦用于急慢惊风、破伤风、风中经络的口眼㖞斜等证。

(2) 疮痈、瘰疬。本品能以毒攻毒，散结消肿。治疮痈、瘰疬，内服外用均可，可单味焙黄研末外用，内服可与其他药物配伍同用。

(3) 风湿顽痹，头痛。本品能搜风通络且止痛，治风湿顽痹，可与防风、独活、威灵仙等同用。治顽固性头痛或偏正头痛，可与天麻、川芎等同用。

用法用量　煎服，3～5克。外用适量。

Precautions for use It is prohibited to apply for pregnant women.

使用注意 孕妇忌服。

Pheretima (di long)

地龙

It is the dried product from the body of *Pheretima asperygillum* (E. Perrier), or the body of *Pheretima vulgaris* Chen, or of *Pheretima guillemi* (Michaelsen), or of *Pheretima Pectinifera* Michaelsen, family Magscolecidae. The former one is commonly called "guang di long" and collected from spring to autumn. The three latter ones are commonly called "hu di long" and collected in summer. The medicinal herb is applied in crude form.

为钜蚓科动物参环毛蚓、通俗环毛蚓、威廉环毛蚓或栉盲环毛蚓的干燥体。前一种习称"广地龙",春季至秋季捕捉。后三种习称"沪地龙",夏季捕捉。生用。

Features Flavor: salty. Property: cold. Meridian tropism: the Liver Meridian, the Spleen Meridian and the Bladder Meridian.

性味归经 咸,寒。归肝、脾、膀胱经。

Actions Clear heat, eliminate wind, dredge meridians, relieve panting and promote urination.

功效 清热息风,通络,平喘,利尿。

Application

应用

(1) High fever, convulsion and epilepsy. The medicinal herb acts to clear heat, eliminate wind and relieve convulsion. In the treatment of extreme heat producing wind pattern manifested by loss of consciousness, delirium, spasm and convulsion, it is applied singly or combined with *Uncariae Ramulus cum Uncis* (gou teng), *Bovis Calculus* (niu huang) and *Bombyx Batryticatus* (bai jiang can).

(1) 高热惊痫。本品具清热、息风、定惊之功。治热极生风的神昏谵语、痉挛抽搐,可单味煎服,或与钩藤、牛黄、白僵蚕等同用。

(2) Hemiplegia. The medicinal herb acts to dredge meridians. In the treatment of qi deficiency and blood stasis pattern after wind stroke manifested by hemiplegia and deviation of mouth, it is combined with *Astragali Radix* (huang qi), *Angelicae Sinensis Radix* (dang gui) and *Chuanxiong Rhizoma* (chuan xiong), to form up Yang-Invigorating and

(2) 半身不遂。本品长于通利经络。治中风后气虚血滞的半身不遂、口眼㖞斜,常与黄芪、当归、川芎等同用,如补阳还五汤。

Recuperating Decoction (Bu Yang Huan Wu Tang).

(3) Bi (Obturation) Pattern due to wind-damp. The medicinal herb is cold in property and acts to clear heat and dredge meridians. In the treatment of heat-type Bi (Obturation) Pattern manifested by redness, swelling, pain and motor impairment of joints, it is combined with *Stephaniae Tetrandrae Radix* (fang ji), *Gentianae Macrophyllae Radix* (qin jiao) and *Lonicerae Japonicae Caulis* (ren dong teng).

（3）风湿痹痛。本品性寒清热，且能通络，善治热痹的关节红肿疼痛、屈伸不利，常与防己、秦艽、忍冬藤等同用。

(4) Panting and wheezing due to heat in lung. The medicinal herb acts to reduce heat from lung and soothe panting. In the treatment of panting due to heat in lung, it is applied singly by grinding into powder or combined with *Ephedrae Herba* (ma huang), *Gypsum Fibrosum* (shi gao) and *Armeniacae Amarum Semen* (ku xing ren).

（4）肺热哮喘。本品清肺热、平喘息。治肺热喘息，可单用研末内服，或与麻黄、石膏、苦杏仁等同用。

(5) Difficulty urination. The medicinal herb acts to clear heat and promote urination. In the treatment of difficulty urination or scanty urine due to heat accumulation in bladder, it is combined with *Plantaginis Semen* (che qian zi), *Akebiae Caulis* (mu tong) and *Alismatis Rhizoma* (ze xie).

（5）小便不利。本品能清热利水。治热蕴膀胱的小便不利，或尿少，可与车前子、木通、泽泻等同用。

Usage and dosage Apply 5～10 g in decoction.

用法用量 煎服，5～10克。

Bombyx Batryticatus (jiang can)

僵蚕

It is the dried product from the body of the larva of *Bombyx mori* Linnaeus before its spinning of silk infected (or artificially inoculated) by *Beauveria* bassiana (Bals.) Vuillent. The medicinal herb is also called "bai jiang can", collected in spring and autumn. It is applied in crude form or stir-fried form.

为蚕蛾科昆虫家蚕4～5龄的幼虫感染（或人工接种）白僵菌而致死的干燥体。又名"白僵蚕"。多于春、秋生产，将感染的白僵蚕病死的蚕干燥。生用或炒用。

Features Flavor: salty and pungent. Property: neutral. Meridian tropism: the Liver Meridian, the Lung Meridian and the Stomach Meridian.

Actions Eliminate wind, relieve spasm, remove wind, stop pain, dissolve phlegm and desiccate stasis.

Application

(1) Convulsion, epilepsy and spasm. The medicinal herb acts to eliminate liver wind, relieve spasm and dissolve phlegm. In the treatment of convulsion, epilepsy and spasm due to internal movement of liver wind or phlegm-heat accumulation, it is combined with *Scorpio* (quan xie) and *Gastrodiae Rhizoma* (tian ma). In the treatment of infantile acute or chronic convulsion, it is combined with *Codonopsis Radix* (dang shen), *Atractylodis Macrocephalae Rhizoma* (bai zhu) and *Gastrodiae Rhizoma* (tian ma). In the treatment of wind stroke of meridian attack manifested by deviation of mouth, it is combined with quan xie etc., to form up Anti-Contracture Powder (Qian Zheng San).

(2) Headache, redness of eyes, sore throat, urticaria and skin itch. The medicinal herb is pungent and dispersing in property and acts to eliminate exogenous wind, remove wind-heat and stop pain and itch. In the treatment of headache and redness of eyes due to wind-heat attacking upwards, it is combined with *Mori Folium* (sang ye), *Chrysanthemi Flos* (ju hua) and *Schizonepetae Herba* (jing jie). In the treatment of sore throat and hoarseness of voice due to wind-heat, it is combined with *Platycodonis Radix* (jie geng), *Peucedani Radix* (qian hu) and *Arctii Fructus* (niu bang zi). In the treatment of urticaria and skin itch, it is applied singly by grinding

性味归经 咸、辛，平。归肝、肺、胃经。

功效 息风止痉，祛风止痛，化痰散结。

应用

（1）惊痫抽搐。本品能息肝风、止痉挛，兼化痰，尤宜于肝风内动或痰热壅盛所致的惊痫抽搐，可与全蝎、天麻等同用。若治小儿脾虚慢惊，可与党参、白术、天麻等同用。治风中经络的口眼喎斜，常与全蝎等同用，如牵正散。

（2）头痛目赤，咽喉肿痛，风疹瘙痒。本品辛散，具祛外风、散风热、止痛止痒之功。治风热上攻的头痛、目赤，常与桑叶、菊花、荆芥等同用。治风热咽痛音哑，可与桔梗、前胡、牛蒡子等同用。治风疹瘙痒，可单用研末服，或与荆芥、薄荷等同用。

into fine powder for oral administration, or combined with jing jie and *Menthae Haplocalycis Herba* (bo he).

(3) Scrofula and goiter due to phlegm. The medicinal herb is salty in flavor and acts to soften the hard, desiccate stasis and dissolve phlegm. In the treatment of scrofula and goiter due to phlegm accumulation of phlegm-fire accumulation, it is combined with *Bulbus Fritillariae Thunbergii* (zhe bei mu), *Prunellae Spica* (xia ku cao) and *Forsythiae Fructus* (lian qiao).

Usage and dosage Apply 5～10 g in decoction. The medicinal herb acts to eliminate wind-heat in crude form, and acts to treat other diseases in stir-fried form.

(3) 瘰疬痰核。本品味咸而软坚散结，兼能化痰。治痰结或痰火互结的痰核、瘰疬等证，常与浙贝母、夏枯草、连翘等同用。

用法用量 煎服，5～10克。生用散风热，余多制用。

Brief summary

All *Haliotidis Concha* (shi jue ming), *Ostreae Concha* (mu li) and *Haematitum* (zhe shi) are heavy, sinking and descending in property and act to soothe liver and subdue yang, applied to treat liver yang hyperactivity manifested by dizziness and blurring of vision. Shi jue ming is attributive to the Liver Meridian and cold in property, and acts to purify liver and brighten eyes, applied to treat eye diseases. Mu li is cool and heavy in property and acts to tranquilize heart and calm mind, applied to treat fearful throbbing and insomnia. It also acts to soften the hard and desiccate stasis, applied to treat scrofula and goiter due to phlegm. The medicinal herb in prepared form is astringent in property and acts to astringe liquids, stop acid and relieve pain, applied to treat all types of leakage and prolapse

小　结

石决明、牡蛎、赭石，均为质重沉降之品，功能平潜肝阳，治肝阳上亢，头晕目眩。其中石决明，专入肝经，性寒清肝，且能明目，为治目疾要药。牡蛎，性凉质重，又镇惊安神，为惊悸失眠所常用；味咸软坚散结，治瘰疬、瘿瘤；制用性涩，收敛固涩、制酸止痛，治体虚滑脱诸证，以及胃痛泛酸。赭石，又名“代赭石”，味苦性寒，质重潜阳、性寒清肝，善治阳亢火旺之头痛目眩、烦躁易怒；且重镇降逆，既降肺气治喘息，又降胃气治呕逆；入血分凉血

patterns, gastric pain and acid regurgitation. Zhe shi, also called "dai zhe shi", is bitter, cold and heavy in property and acts to subdue yang and purify liver, applied to treat liver yang hyperactivity or liver fire flaming upwards manifested by headache, blurring of vision, irritability and anger. It is heavy in property and acts to subdue up-reverse flow of qi, applied to treat panting due to up-reverse flow of lung qi and vomiting and hiccup due to up-reverse flow of stomach qi. It is attributive to the Xue (Blood) Phase and acts to cool blood, reduce heat and stanch blood, applied to treat hemoptysis, epistaxis, metrorrhagia and metrostaxis.

热而止血，治血热吐衄、崩漏。

Tribuli Fructus (ji li), also called "bai ji li" and "ci ji li", is pungent, bitter and slightly warm in property and acts to soothe liver and subdue yang, applied to treat dizziness due to liver yang hyperactivity and hypochondriac pain due to liver qi stagnation. It also acts to eliminate wind, brighten eyes and stop itching, applied to treat redness of eyes, cataract, urticaria and skin itch.

蒺藜，又名"白蒺藜""刺蒺藜"，味辛苦性微温，具平肝疏肝之功，善治阳亢眩晕，肝郁胁痛；且能祛风明目、止痒，既治目赤翳障，又疗风疹瘙痒。

Both *Saigae Tataricae Cornu* (ling yang jiao) and *Bovis Calculus* (niu huang), animal durgs, are cold-cool in property and act to eliminate wind and relieve spasm, applied to treat convulsion, epilepsy and spasm due to internal movement of liver wind. Ling yang jiao is stronger in acting to clear heat, eliminate wind and relieve spasm, as the major herb to treat convulsion due to extreme heat producing wind. It acts to soothe liver and subdue yang, applied to treat dizziness and blurring of vision. It acts to purify liver and brighten eyes, applied to treat redness of eyes and cataract. It is attributive to the Heart Meridian and acts to clear heat and relieve

羚羊角、牛黄，均来源于动物，药性寒凉，均能息风止痉，治肝风内动之惊痫抽搐。其中羚羊角清热息风止痉力强，为治热极生风抽搐之要药；且能平肝阳、止眩晕；又清肝明目，治目赤翳障；入心经，清热解毒，治热毒发斑。牛黄既息肝风，又清心凉肝，常治热病神昏或抽搐；且能化痰开窍、清热解毒，治中风痰迷、癫痫发狂，以及咽痛口疮。

toxin, applied to treat macula due to heat-toxin. Niu huang acts to eliminate liver wind, purify heart and cool liver, applied to treat febrile disease manifested by loss of consciousness or convulsion. It also acts to dissolve phlegm, open aperture, clear heat and relieve toxin, applied to treat wind stroke due to phlegm misting heart, epilepsy, mania, sore throat and mouth ulcer.

Both *Uncariae Ramulus cum Uncis* (gou teng) and *Gastrodiae Rhizoma* (tian ma) act to eliminate wind, relieve spasm, soothe liver and subdue yang, applied to treat spasm due to internal movement of liver wind. Gou teng is cool in property and acts to purify liver, applied to treat headache due to liver fire. It also acts to cool liver and relieve convulsion, applied to treat morbid night cry of baby. Tian ma is sweet, moist and moderate in property, applied to treat convulsion due to internal movement of liver wind, no matter of cold or heat, or of deficiency or excess. It acts to soothe liver, as the major herb to treat dizziness due to liver yang hyperactivity. It also acts to eliminate exogenous wind and dredge meridians, applied to treat numbness of body and limbs and Bi (Obturation) Pattern of wind-damp.

钩藤、天麻，均能息风止痉、平抑肝阳，善治肝风内动之抽搐。其中钩藤性凉，兼能清肝，亦治肝火头痛，并能凉肝止惊，治小儿夜啼。天麻甘润不烈，作用平和，治肝风内动之抽搐，无论寒热虚实，皆可用之；且善平肝，又为治阳亢眩晕之要药；还能祛外风、通经络，常治肢体麻木、风湿痹痛等。

Both *Scorpio* (quan xie) and *Scolopendra* (wu gong), insect herbs, are poisonous in property and acts to eliminate wind, relieve spasm, dredge meridians, stop pain, attack toxin and desiccate stasis, applied to treat spasm and convulsion due to internal movement of liver wind, deviation of mouth due to wind stroke of meridian attack, Bi (Obturation) Pattern due to wind-damp, headache, migraine, carbuncle, furuncle and scrofula. Wu gong is warm and more poisonous in property with stronger ac-

全蝎、蜈蚣，均为虫类药，且有毒。均能息风止痉、通络止痛、攻毒散结。均治肝风内动的痉挛抽搐，风中经络的口眼㖞斜，以及风湿顽痹，偏正头痛，疮痈、瘰疬。其中蜈蚣性温，毒大而力强；全蝎性平，毒性及药力均稍缓。

tion, while quan xie is neutral and less poisonous in property with lighter action.

Both *Pheretima* (di long) and *Bombyx Batryticatus* (jiang can) are insect herbs and act to eliminate wind and relieve spasm, applied to treat convulsion, epilepsy and spasm. Di long is cold in property, applied to treat convulsion, epilepsy and spasm due to heat in liver. It also acts to clear heat, dredge meridians, soothe panting and promote urination, applied to treat Bi (Obturation) Pattern due to heat, asthma due to heat in lung, and difficulty urination. Jiang can is neutral in property and acts to dissolve phlegm, applied to treat convulsion, epilepsy and spasm due to liver wind or phlegm-heat. It acts to remove wind-heat, stop pain and relieve itching, applied to treat headache due to wind-heat, redness of eyes, urticaria and skin itch. It is salty in flavor and acts to soften the hard and desiccate stasis, applied to treat scrofula and goiter due to phlegm.

地龙、僵蚕，均为虫类药，均能息风止痉，治惊痫抽搐。其中地龙性寒，以惊痫抽搐属肝热者为宜；且能清热通络、平喘、利尿，治热痹、肺热哮喘、小便不利等。僵蚕性平，兼能化痰，多用于惊痫抽搐属肝风或痰热者；且能散风热、止痛止痒，治风热头痛目赤、风疹瘙痒；且味咸软坚散结，治瘰疬痰核。

Chapter 15 Aperture-Opening Herbs

第 15 章 开窍药

The medicinal herbs, pungent and fragrant in flavor and moving and wandering in property, acting to open aperture and wake up mind are called aperture-opening herbs.

具辛香走窜之性，以开窍醒神为主要作用的药物，称开窍药。

The medicinal herbs are pungent and fragrant in flavor, moving and wandering in property, and attributive to the Heart Meridian, and act to dredge pass, open aperture, bring back consciousness and wake up mind, applied to treat wind stroke of closure type. Wind stroke of closure type is divided into cold-closure type and heat-closure type. Wind stroke of cold-closure type, manifested by loss of consciousness, blue complexion, coolness in body, white tongue coating and slow pulse, can be treated with the medicinal herbs which are warm and opening in property, such as *Moschus* (she xiang), *Bufonis Venenum* (chan su) and *Acori Tatarinowii Rhizoma* (shi chang pu). Wind stroke of heat-closure type, manifested by loss of consciousness, red complexion, feverishness in body, yellow tongue coating and rapid pulse, can be treated with the medicinal herbs which are cool and opening in property, such as *Borneolum Syntheticum* (bing pian).

本类药物味辛、芳香，善于行窜，皆入心经，有通关开窍、回苏醒神的作用，主要用于闭证神昏。闭证有寒闭、热闭之分。寒闭者，症见神昏面青，身凉、苔白、脉迟，可选用性温的温开之品，如麝香、蟾酥、石菖蒲；热闭者，症见神昏面赤、身热、苔黄、脉数，可选用性寒的凉开之品，如冰片。

It is necessary to notice in the application of this type of herbs that the medicinal herbs are applied to treat the branch of the disease. They are

使用时需注意的是本类药为治标之品，且辛香走窜，易耗气伤正，只可暂服，不可

pungent and fragrant in flavor and moving and wandering in property, so they are easy to consume the Zheng (Anti-Pathogenic) Qi, and can only be applied temporarily and cannot be applied for long time. The medicinal herbs are mostly fragrant, so they are not applied in decoction, but only in pills and powder.

久用。本类药大多气香，一般不入煎剂，多入丸剂、散剂服用。

Moschus (she xiang)

麝香

It is the dried product from the substance secreted by a gland in the subumbilical sac of the *Moschus berezovskii* Flerov, *Moschus sifanicus* Przewalski, and *Moschus moschiferus* Linnaeus. For the wild, it is collected from winter to next spring by cutting off the musk gland to get the musk. For the homebred, it is collected by cutting off the musk gland to get the musk. The medicinal herb is dried in shade.

为鹿科动物林麝、马麝或原麝成熟雄体香囊中的干燥分泌物。野麝多在冬季至次春猎取，捕获后割取香囊。家麝直接从香囊中取出麝香仁。干燥后用。

Features Flavor: pungent. Property: warm. Meridian tropism: the Heart Meridian and the Spleen Meridian.

性味归经 辛，温。归心、脾经。

Actions Open aperture, wake up mind, activate blood, dredge meridians, subside swell and stop pain.

功效 开窍醒神，活血通经，消肿止痛。

Application

(1) Wind stroke of closure type manifested by loss of consciousness. The medicinal herb is pungent and extremely fragrant in flavor and moving and wandering in property, and acts to open aperture, dredge pass, wake up mind and bring back consciousness, as the major herb to treat wind stroke of closure type. It is warm in property, applied to treat wind stroke of cold-closure type manifested by loss of consciousness, with combination of the war-

应用

(1) 闭证神昏。本品味辛，气极香，善走窜，开窍通闭、醒神回苏之效甚佳，为治闭证要药。其性偏温，善治寒闭神昏，常与温开药同用。亦治热陷心包、痰热蒙蔽心窍等热闭神昏，可与牛黄、冰片、朱砂等同用，如安宫牛黄丸等。

ming and opening herbs. In the treatment of loss of consciousness due to heat blocking pericardium or phlegm-heat misting heart aperture, it is combined with *Bovis Calculus* (niu huang), *Borneolum Syntheticum* (bing pian) and *Cinnabaris* (zhu sha), to form up Peaceful Palace Bovine Bezoar Pills (An Gong Niu Huang Wan).

(2) Various types of blood stasis pattern. The medicinal herb acts to activate blood, dissolve stasis and dredge meridians. In the treatment of amenorrhea and abdominal masses due to blood stasis, it is combined with *Carthami Flos* (hong hua), *Persicae Semen* (tao ren) and *Chuanxiong Rhizoma* (chuan xiong). In the treatment of chest pain and cardiac pain, it is combined with *Salviae Miltiorrhizae Radix et Rhizoma* (dan shen) and *Borneolum Syntheticum* (bing pian). In the treatment of acute cardiac pain or acute abdominal pain, it is combined with *Aucklandiae Radix* (mu xiang) and tao ren. In the treatment of traumatic injury, swelling and pain due to fracture, it is combined with *Olibanum* (ru xiang), *Myrrha* (mo yao) and *Carthami Flos* (hong hua). In the treatment of stubborn and unhealed Bi (Obturation) Pattern with pain, it is combined with *Angelicae Pubescentis Radix* (du huo), *Clematidis Radix et Rhizoma* (wei ling xian) and *Taxilli Herba* (sang ji sheng).

（2）血瘀诸证。本品善行血中瘀滞，通利经脉。治瘀滞经闭、癥瘕，常与红花、桃仁、川芎等同用。治胸痹心痛，可与丹参、冰片等同用。治心腹暴痛，可与木香、桃仁等配伍。治跌打损伤、骨折肿痛，可与乳香、没药、红花等同用。治痹证疼痛，顽固不愈，可与独活、威灵仙、桑寄生等配伍。

(3) Carbuncle and furuncle due to heat-toxin, and sore throat. The medicinal herb acts to activate blood, desiccate stasis, subside swell and stop pain. In the treatment of carbuncle and furuncle due to heat-toxin, it is combined with niu huang, ru xiang and mo yao. In the treatment of sore throat, it is combined with niu huang and *Bufonis Venenum*

（3）疮疡肿毒，咽喉肿痛。本品能活血散结、消肿止痛。治疮疡肿毒，常与牛黄、乳香、没药同用。治咽喉肿痛，可与牛黄、蟾酥等配伍。

(chan su).

Usage and dosage Apply 0.03～0.1 g in pills or powder. Apply a proper amount for external use.

Precautions for use It is prohibited to apply for pregnant women.

用法用量 入丸散，0.03～0.1克。外用适量。

使用注意 孕妇忌用。

Borneolum Syntheticum **(bing pian)**

It is the dried product from *Cinnamomum camphora* (L.) Presl, family Dipterocarpceae, or crystals of evaporated trunk, called natural borneol (R-borneol). It is the dried product from crystals of leaves of *Blumea balsamifera* (L.) DC., family Compositae, called Borneolum Luodian (L-borneol). It is the product from crystals of Campher and turpentine oil by chemical synthesis, called synthetic borneol.

Features Flavor: pungent and bitter. Property: cool. Meridian tropism: the Heart Meridian, the Spleen Meridian and the Lung Meridian.

Actions Open aperture, wake up mind, clear heat and stop pain.

Application

(1) Wind stroke of closure type manifested by loss of consciousness. The medicinal herb is cold-cool in property and acts to open aperture and wake up mind, as the cool-opening herb. In the treatment of wind stroke of heat-closure type manifested by loss of consciousness, it is combined with *Bovis Calculus* (niu huang), *Moschus* (she xiang) and *Coptidis Rhizoma* (huang lian), to form up Peaceful Palace Bovine Bezoar Pills (An Gong Niu Huang Wan).

(2) Chest pain and cardiac pain. The medicinal herb acts to open heart aperture. In the treatment

冰片

冰片的来源包括樟科植物樟的新鲜枝、叶经加工提取的结晶，称天然冰片（右旋龙脑）。菊科植物艾纳香的新鲜叶经加工提取的结晶，称艾片（左旋龙脑）。用樟脑等化学合成的结晶称冰片（合成龙脑）。

性味归经 辛、苦，凉。归心、脾、肺经。

功效 开窍醒神，清热止痛。

应用

（1）闭证神昏。本品有开窍醒神之功效，性偏寒凉，为凉开之品，宜用治热闭神昏，常与牛黄、麝香、黄连等配伍，如安宫牛黄丸。

（2）胸痹心痛。本品能开心窍之闭，与丹参、红花等

of chest pain and cardiac pain, it is combined with the blood-activating herbs, such as *Salviae Miltiorrhizae Radix et Rhizoma* (dan shen), *Carthami Flos* (hong hua), etc.

活血药同用,治胸痹心痛。

(3) Redness of eyes, sore throat, mouth ulcer and purulent discharge in ear. The medicinal herb acts to clear heat, stop pain and subside swell. In the treatment of redness, swelling and pain of eyes, it is applied singly as eye droppings, or combined with other medicinal herbs to make into eye droppings. In the treatment of sore throat and mouth ulcer, it is combined with *Borax* (peng sha), *Cinnabaris* (zhu sha) and *Natrii Sulfas* Exsiccatus (xuan ming fen) by grinding into fine powder to spray at diseased area, to form up Borneol and Borax Powder (Bing Peng San). In the treatment of purulent discharge in ear, it is melted in walnut oil to drop in ear.

(3) 目赤肿痛、咽痛口疮,耳道流脓。本品有清热止痛、消肿之功。治目赤肿痛,单用点眼即效,或与其他药物配伍制成点眼药水用。治咽喉肿痛、口舌生疮,常与硼砂、朱砂、玄明粉共研细末,吹敷患处,如冰硼散。治耳道流脓,可将本品搅溶于核桃油中滴耳。

Usage and dosage Apply 0.15～0.3 g in pills or powder. Apply a proper amount for external use.

用法用量 入丸散,0.15～0.3 克。外用适量。

Precautions for use It is cautious to apply for pregnant women.

使用注意 孕妇慎用。

Acori Tatarinowii Rhizoma (shi chang pu)

石菖蒲

It is the dried product from the Rhizoma of *Acorus trtarinowii* Schott, family Araceae. The medicinal herb is collected in autumn and winter, applied in crude form.

为天南星科植物石菖蒲的干燥根茎。秋、冬二季采挖。生用。

Features Flavor: pungent and bitter. Property: warm. Meridian tropism: the Heart Meridian and the Stomach Meridian.

性味归经 辛、苦,温。归心、胃经。

Actions Open aperture, wake up mind, dissolve damp and harmonize stomach.

功效 开窍醒神,化湿和胃。

Application

(1) Loss of consciousness, epilepsy, dizziness and tinnitus. The medicinal herb is pungent, bitter and fragrant in flavor and warming and dredging in property, and acts to open aperture, dissolve damp and wake up mind. In the treatment of loss of consciousness due to phlegm-damp, it is combined with *Curcumae Radix* (yu jin) and *Pinelliae Rhizoma* (ban xia). In the treatment of epilepsy due to phlegm-heat, it is combined with *Aurantii Fructus Immaturus* (zhi shi), *Bambusae Caulis in Taenias* (zhu ru) and *Coptidis Rhizoma* (huang lian). In the treatment of dizziness, poor memory, tinnitus and deafness due to damp-turbidity blocking clear aperture, it is combined with *Poria* (fu ling), *Polygalae Radix* (yuan zhi) and *Os Draconis* (long gu).

(2) Distension and stuffiness at epigastria and abdomen, abdominal masses and pain. The medicinal herb is fragrant and acts to dissolve damp, wake up spleen and harmonize stomach. In the treatment of distension and stuffiness at epigastria and abdomen due to damp-turbidity block middle energizer, it is combined with *Amomi Fructus* (sha ren), *Atractylodis Rhizoma* (cang zhu) and *Magnoliae Officinalis Cortex* (hou po).

Usage and dosage Apply 3～10 g in decoction.

应用

（1）神昏癫痫，头晕耳鸣。本品辛香温通，苦燥除湿，开心窍、去湿浊、醒神志为其擅长，尤宜治痰湿神昏之证，常与郁金、半夏等同用。治痰热癫痫，可与枳实、竹茹、黄连等同用。治湿浊蒙蔽清窍所致的头晕健忘、耳鸣耳聋等，常与茯苓、远志、龙骨等同用。

（2）脘腹胀闷，痞塞疼痛。本品芳香化湿，醒脾开胃。治湿浊中阻，脘闷腹胀，常与砂仁、苍术、厚朴等同用。

用法用量 煎服，3～10克。

Bufonis Venenum (chan su)

It is the dried product from the secretion of *Bufo bufo gargarizans* Cantor or *Bufo melanostictus* Schneider, family Bufonidae. It is prepared by grinding into fine powder.

Features Flavor: pungent. Property: warm

蟾酥

为蟾蜍科动物中华大蟾蜍或黑眶蟾蜍的干燥分泌物。研细用。

性味归经 辛，温；有

and poisonous. Meridian tropism: the Heart Meridian.

毒。归心经。

Actions Open aperture, wake up mind, stop pain and relieve toxin.

功效 开窍醒神，止痛，解毒。

Application

应用

(1) Cholera with abdominal pain, vomiting, diarrhea, heat stroke and loss of consciousness. The medicinal herb is pungent and warm in property and acts to open aperture, wake up mind and remove turbidity. In the treatment of cholera with abdominal pain, vomiting, diarrhea and loss of consciousness due to turbid damp-heat in summer attacking body or due to unclean food, it is combined with *Moschus* (she xiang), *Caryophylli Flos* (ding xiang) and *Atractylodis Rhizoma* (cang zhu).

（1）痧胀腹痛，吐泻，中暑神昏。本品辛温走窜，有开窍醒神、辟秽之功。治夏伤暑湿秽浊之气或饮食不洁所致的痧胀腹痛、吐泻不止，甚则昏厥之证，常与麝香、丁香、苍术等同用。

(2) Stubborn ulcer, scrofula and sore throat. The medicinal herb acts to relieve toxin, subside swell and stop pain. In the treatment of stubborn ulcer and scrofula, it is applied singly for external use, or combined with dried *Alumen* (bai fan) and *Cinnabaris* (zhu sha) for oral administration. In the treatment of sore throat, it is combined with *Bovis Calculus* (niu huang), *Realgar* (xiong huang) and *Borneolum Syntheticum* (bing pian).

（2）恶疮瘰疬，咽喉肿痛。本品能解毒消肿止痛。治恶疮瘰疬，可单味外敷，或与枯矾、朱砂等配伍内服。治咽喉肿痛，常与牛黄、雄黄、冰片等同用。

Usage and dosage Apply 0.015～0.03 g in pills or powder. Apply a proper amount for external use.

用法用量 入丸散，0.015～0.03克。外用适量。

Precautions for use It is not advisable to apply in overdose. It is not allowed to contact with eyes in external use. It is prohibited to apply for pregnant women.

使用注意 不可过量。外用不可入目。孕妇忌用。

Brief summary

Both *Moschus* (she xiang) and *Borneolum Syntheticum* (bing pian) are pungent and fragrant in flavor and moving and wandering in property, attributive to the Heart and Spleen Meridians, and act to open aperture and wake up mind, applied for mutual reinforcement to treat wind stroke of closure type manifested by loss of consciousness. She xiang is warm and extremely fragrant in property and strongly acts to open aperture and wake up mind, as the major herb to treat wind stroke of closure type, no matter of cold or of heat. It is attributive to the Xue (Blood) Phase and acts to activate blood and dredge meridians, applied to treat amenorrhea due to blood stasis, chest pain, cardiac pain, abdominal masses and traumatic injury. It also acts to subside swell and stop pain, applied to treat carbuncle, furuncle and sore throat. Bing pian is cool in property, as the cool-opening herb. It is weaker than *Moschus* (she xiang) in opening aperture and waking up mind, but it is more suitable to treat wind stroke of heat-closure type, and also to treat cold-closure type as well. It also acts to clear heat and subside swell, applied to treat redness of eyes and sore throat.

Acori Tatarinowii Rhizoma (shi chang pu) is pungent, bitter and warm in property and acts to open heart aperture, dissolve damp-turbidity and wake up mind, applied to treat loss of consciousness due to phlegm blocking aperture. It also acts to dissolve damp and harmonize stomach, applied to treat distension and stuffiness at epigastria and abdomen due to damp-turbidity blocking middle energizer.

Bufonis Venenum (chan su) is pungent, warm

小　结

麝香、冰片，均辛香走窜，均入心脾经，均能开窍醒神，常相须为用，治闭证神昏。其中麝香性温，气极香，开窍醒神力强，为治闭证要药，无论寒闭、热闭皆宜；且入血分，能活血通经，治瘀滞经闭、胸痹心痛、癥瘕积聚、跌打伤痛；又消肿止痛，治疮痈咽痛。冰片性凉，为凉开之品，开窍醒神之力逊于麝香，更宜治热闭，兼治寒闭；且能清热消肿，治目赤咽痛。

石菖蒲，辛苦性温，能开心窍、去湿浊、醒神志，治痰阻窍闭之神昏；且具化湿和胃之功，亦治湿浊中阻所致的脘腹胀闷。

蟾酥，辛温有毒，能开窍

and poisonous in property and acts to open aperture, wake up mind and remove turbidity, applied to treat cholera with abdominal pain, vomiting, diarrhea and loss of consciousness due to turbid damp-heat in summer attacking body or due to unclean food. It also acts to relieve toxin, subside swell and stop pain, applied to treat stubborn ulcer, scrofula and sore throat.

醒神、辟秽，多用治夏伤暑湿秽浊不正之气或饮食不洁所致的痧胀腹痛、吐泻，甚则神昏；且能解毒消肿止痛，常用治恶疮、瘰疬、咽喉肿痛等。

Chapter 16 Reinforcing Herbs

第16章 补虚药

The medicinal herbs acting to reinforcing qi, blood, yin or yang of human body, to improve functions of zang-fu organs and to increase resistance to diseases are called the reinforcing herbs.

以补充人体气血阴阳之不足，改善脏腑功能，提高抗病能力为主要作用的药物，称为补虚药，亦称补养药或补益药。

The medicinal herbs are applied to treat deficiency pattern. The deficiency pattern is divided into qi deficiency pattern, yang deficiency pattern, blood deficiency pattern and yin deficiency pattern. The medicinal herbs, according to their actions and major indications, are divided into the qi-reinforcing herbs, the yang-reinforcing herbs, the blood-reinforcing herbs and the yin-reinforcing herbs.

本类药主要用于虚证。虚证有气虚、阳虚、血虚、阴虚之不同。本类药物根据其功效和主要适应证的不同，可分为补气药、补阳药、补血药、补阴药四类。

The qi-reinforcing herbs are mostly sweet and warm in property or sweet and neutral in property, and act to reinforce qi of zang-fu organs, especially to reinforce qi of spleen and lung, applied to treat spleen qi deficiency pattern manifested by poor appetite, distension and fullness at epigastria and abdomen, loose feces, edema, scanty urine, prolapse of internal organs, etc., and to treat lung qi deficiency pattern manifested by lack of energy, dislike of speaking, light voice, panting, shortness of breath, sweating, etc.

补气药性味大多甘温或甘平，能补益脏腑之气，尤善补脾、肺之气，主要用于脾气虚的食欲不振、脘腹胀满、大便溏薄，或水肿少尿、脏器下垂等证，以及肺气虚的少气懒言、语音低微，甚或喘促、易出虚汗等。

The yang-reinforcing herbs are mostly sweet and warm in property or pungent and hot in property, and act to warm and reinforce yang qi of human

补阳药性味大多甘温、或辛热，能温补人体之阳气，以补肾阳为主，主要用于肾

body, especially to reinforce kidney yang, applied to treat kidney yang insufficiency pattern manifested by fear of cold, chills in limbs, aching and weakness at low back and knees, impotence, seminal emission, infertility due to cold in uterus, frequency of urination, enuresis, etc., to treat panting due to kidney deficiency, applied to treat diarrhea due to spleen and kidney yang deficiency, and applied to treat kidney deficiency and essence depletion pattern manifested by early grey hair, metrorrhagia, metrostaxis and morbid leucorrhea due to cold of deficiency type in lower energizer.

阳不足的畏寒肢冷、腰膝酸软、阳痿遗精、宫冷不孕、尿频遗尿，或肾虚喘促，或脾肾阳虚的泄泻等证。还可用于肾虚精亏的须发早白、下元虚冷的崩漏带下。

The blood-reinforcing herbs are mostly sweet and warm in property or sweet and neutral in property, and moist in texture, and act to reinforce liver and nourish heart, or to benefit spleen and reinforce blood, applied to treat liver and heart blood deficiency pattern manifested by sallow-yellow complexion, pale lips and nails, dizziness, blurring of vision, tinnitus, palpitation, fearful throbbing, insomnia, poor memory, irregular menstruation with scanty volume and light color of blood, etc. They also act to moisturize and nourish liver and kidney, applied to treat liver blood and kidney essence deficiency pattern manifested by dizziness, blurring of vision, tinnitus, aching and weakness at low back and knees, early grey hair, etc.

补血药性味大多甘温或甘平，质地滋润，能补肝养心或益脾补血。主要用于心肝血虚的面色萎黄，唇爪苍白，眩晕耳鸣，心悸怔忡，失眠健忘，或月经不调，量少色淡等证。还能滋养肝肾，可用于肝肾精血亏虚所致的眩晕耳鸣、腰膝酸软、须发早白等证。

The yin-reinforcing herbs are mostly sweet and cold or cool in property, and moist in texture, and act to reinforce yin, nourish fluid and moisturize organs, applied to treat yin deficiency pattern. They are applied to treat lung yin deficiency pattern manifested by dry cough with scanty sputum or with blood sputum, to treat stomach yin deficiency pat-

补阴药性味大多甘寒或凉，且质润，能补阴滋液润燥，主要用于阴虚证。如肺阴虚的干咳少痰、痰中带血；胃阴虚的咽干口渴或嘈杂不饥、呕哕，或大便秘结；肝阴虚的两目干涩昏花、头晕目

tern manifested by dry throat, thirst, satiety with no desire for eating food, vomiting, constipation, etc., to treat liver yin deficiency manifested by dryness of eyes, dazzling, dizziness, blurring of vision, etc., and to treat kidney yin deficiency pattern manifested by aching and pain at low back and knees, feverish sensation in five centers, tidal fever, nocturnal sweats, seminal emission, etc.

眩；肾阴虚的腰膝酸痛、五心烦热、潮热盗汗，或遗精等症。

In the application of this type of medicinal herbs, it is necessary to protect the spleen and stomach, by combining with the spleen-strengthening and food-digesting herbs, so as to promote transportation and transformation and to play a better role of the reinforcing herbs. It is not advisable to apply the reinforcing herbs for those with exterior pattern due to exogenous factors, for the purpose to avoid "retention of pathogens inside". It is cautious to apply the reinforcing herbs for those with strong body constitution without deficiency. It is cautious to apply the yang-reinforcing herbs, which are warm and dry in property and may assist fire and consume yin, for those with yin deficiency and fire hyperactivity. The blood-reinforcing herbs and yin-reinforcing herbs are mostly thick and sticky, so it is cautious to apply the herbs for those with damp retention in spleen and stomach manifested by distension and fullness at epigastria and abdomen.

使用本类药需注意顾护脾胃，适当配伍健脾消食药，以促进运化，更好地发挥补虚药作用。外感表证及实邪炽盛者不宜应用，以免"闭门留寇"。体健无虚者慎用。性多温燥的补阳药，易助火伤阴，阴虚火旺者慎用。补血、滋阴药多滋腻黏滞，湿滞脾胃、脘腹胀满者亦应慎用。

Section 1 Qi-reinforcing herbs

第1节 补气药

Ginseng Radix et Raizoma (ren shen)

人参

It is the dried product from the root and rhizo-

为五加科植物人参的干

me of *Panax ginseng* C. A. Mey., family araliceae. The cultured ginseng is commonly called "garden ginseng", while the ginseng growing naturally in the mountain is commonly called "forest and mountain ginseng". The medicinal herb is collected in autumn, applied in crude form or prepared form.

燥根和根茎。栽培者俗称"园参",播种在山林野生状态下自然生长的称"林下山参"。多于秋季采挖。生用或制用。

Features Flavor: sweet and slightly bitter. Property: slightly warm. Meridian tropism: the Spleen Meridian, the Lung Meridian, the Heart Meridian and the Kidney Meridian.

性味归经 甘、微苦,微温。归脾、肺、心、肾经。

Actions Reinforce Yuan (Primary) Qi, reinforce spleen, benefit lung, produce fluid, relieve thirst, calm mind and improve intelligence.

功效 大补元气,补脾益肺,生津止渴,安神益智。

Application

(1) Qi deficiency and qi collapse. The medicinal herb is sweet and warm and acts to reinforce Yuan (Primary) Qi and rescue life from collapse. In the treatment of qi collapse pattern due to various causes, it is applied singly, to form up Ginseng Solo Decoction (Du Shen Tang), or combined with other medicinal herbs according to causes.

(2) Lung qi deficiency and spleen qi deficiency. The medicinal herb is attributive to the Lung and Spleen Meridians and acts to benefit lung qi and reinforce spleen qi. In the treatment of lung qi deficiency pattern manifested by shortness of breath and sweating on exertion, it is combined with *Astragali Radix* (huang qi) and qi-benefiting and lung-tonifying herbs. In the treatment of spleen deficiency pattern manifested by lassitude, loose feces and poor appetite, it is combined with *Atractylodis Rhizoma Macrocephalae* (bai zhu) and *Poria* (fu ling), to form up Four Nobles Decoction (Si Jun Zi Tang).

应用

(1) 气虚欲脱。本品甘温,善大补元气,有救脱扶危之良效。治各种原因所致的气脱危证,可单用本品大量浓煎服,即独参汤。或根据病因配伍其他药物同用。

(2) 肺气虚,脾气虚。本品入肺、脾经,能益肺气,补脾气。治肺虚气短,动则汗出,可与黄芪等益气补肺药同用。治脾虚乏力,便溏食少,可与白术、茯苓等同用,如四君子汤。

(3) Thirst due to fluid consumption and diabetes. The medicinal herb is sweet and warm but not dry in property, and acts to benefit qi, produce fluid and relieve thirst. In the treatment of febrile disease consuming fluid manifested by thirst, it is combined with *Gypsum Fibrosum* (shi gao) and *Anemarrhenae Rhizoma* (zhi mu), to form up White Tiger and Ginseng Decoction (Bai Hu Jia Ren Shen Tang). In the treatment of febrile disease consuming qi and yin manifested by thirst, profuse sweating, weak breath and weak pulse, it is combined with *Ophiopogonis Radix* (mai dong) and *Schisandrae Chinensis Fructus* (wu wei zi), to form up Pulse-Engendering Powder (Sheng Mai San). In the treatment of diabetes, it is combined with *Trichosanthis Radix* (tian hua fen), *Rehmanniae Radix* (sheng di huang) and *Astragali Radix* (huang qi).

(3) 津伤口渴，消渴证。本品甘温不燥，能益气生津止渴。治热病伤津口渴，常配伍石膏、知母等同用，如白虎加人参汤。治热伤气阴，口渴多汗、气虚脉弱者，可与麦冬、五味子同用，即生脉散。治消渴证，可与天花粉、生地黄、黄芪等同用。

(4) Palpitation, insomnia, dream-disturbed sleep and poor memory. The medicinal herb acts to reinforce Yuan (Primary) Qi, calm mind and improve intelligence. It is applied singly or combined with *Angelicae Sinensis Radix* (dang gui), and *Ziziphi Spinosae Semen* (suan zao ren), to form up Angelica Splenic Pills (Gui Pi Wan).

(4) 心悸失眠，多梦健忘。本品能大补元气，安神益智。可单用，亦可配伍当归、酸枣仁等同用，如归脾丸。

Usage and dosage Apply 3～9 g in decoction. Apply 15～30 g for acute and severe disease. It is advisable to decoct separately in slow fire. Apply 1.5～2 g powder.

用法用量 煎服，3～9克；用于急重证，用量可增为15～30 克。宜文火另煎兑服。研末吞服，每次 1.5～2克。

Precautions for use The medicinal herb is incompatible with *Radix et Rhizoma Veratri Nigri* (li lu). It is not advisable to apply it together with *Faeces Trogopterorum* (wu ling zhi). It is not advisable to take *Raphani Semen* (lai fu zi).

使用注意 反藜芦。不宜与五灵脂同用，不宜与莱菔子同用。

Remarks

According to the different processing methods, *Ginseng Radix et Raizoma* (ren shen) is divided into sun-dried ginseng, red ginseng and white ginseng. Sun-dried ginseng is neutral in property and acts to reinforce qi, applied to treat qi and yin insufficiency pattern. White ginseng, similar to sun-dried ginseng, is weaker in action, applied to treat mild condition of qi and yin insufficiency pattern. Red ginseng is warm in property, applied to treat qi deficiency pattern with yang deficiency.

按语

人参根据加工方法不同有生晒参、红参、白参的区分。生晒参补气作用较好，且药性平和，适用于气阴不足证。白参功似生晒参而力弱，用于气阴两虚轻证。红参性偏温，适用于气虚兼阳虚者。

Codonopsis Radix (dang shen)

党参

It is the dried product from the root of *Codonopsis pilosula* (Franch.) Nannf., *Codonopsis pilosula Nannf. var. modesta* (Nannf.) or *Codonopsis tangshen* Oliv., family Campanulaceae. The medicinal herb is collected in autumn, applied in crude form or stir-fried form.

为桔梗科植物党参、素花党参或川党参的干燥根。秋季采挖。生用或炒用。

Features Flavor: sweet. Property: neutral. Meridian tropism: the Spleen Meridian and the Lung Meridian.

性味归经 甘，平。归脾、肺经。

Actions Strengthen spleen, benefit lung, nourish blood and produce fluid.

功效 健脾益肺，养血生津。

Application

(1) Spleen deficiency pattern. The medicinal herb is sweet and neutral in property, neither dry nor sticky, and acts to reinforce middle energizer and benefit qi. In the treatment of spleen deficiency pattern manifested by fatigue, poor appetite and loose feces, it is combined with *Atractylodis Macrocephalae Rhizoma* (bai zhu), *Poria* (fu ling) and *Glycyrrhizae Radix et Rhizoma* (gan cao).

应用

（1）脾虚证。本品味甘性平，不燥不腻，善补中益气。治脾虚倦怠、食少便溏，多与白术、茯苓、甘草等同用。

(2) Lung deficiency pattern. The medicinal

（2）肺虚证。本品能益

herb acts to benefit lung qi. In the treatment of lung qi deficiency manifested by shortness of breath, cough, panting, dislike of speaking and light voice, it is combined with *Astragali Radix* (huang qi) and *Schisandrae Chinensis Fructus* (wu wei zi).

肺气。治肺气虚气短咳喘、言少声低，常与黄芪、五味子等药同用。

(3) Blood deficiency pattern. The medicinal herb acts to benefit qi and nourish blood. In the treatment of blood deficiency pattern manifested by sallow and yellow complexion, dizziness and palpitation, it is combined with *Rehmanniae Radix Praeparata* (shu di huang) and *Angelicae Sinensis Radix* (dang gui).

（3）血虚证。本品益气养血，治血虚萎黄，头晕心悸，常与熟地黄、当归等同用。

(4) Thirst due to consumption of fluid. The medicinal herb acts to benefit qi and produce fluid. In the treatment of thirst due to consumption of fluid, it is combined with *Ophiopogonis Radix* (mai dong) and *Schisandrae Chinensis Fructus* (wu wei zi).

（4）津伤口渴。本品能益气生津，治津伤口渴，常与麦冬、五味子同用。

Usage and dosage Apply 9～30 g in decoction. The medicinal herb acts to benefit lung, nourish blood and produce fluid in crude form, and acts to strengthen spleen and stop diarrhea in stir-fried form.

用法用量 煎服，9～30克。生用益肺、养血、生津，炒用健脾止泻。

Precautions for use The medicinal herb is incompatible with *Radix et Rhizoma Veratri Nigri* (li lu). It is cautious to apply for those with heat pattern of excess.

使用注意 反藜芦。实热证慎用。

Panacis Quinquefolii Radix (xi yang shen)

西洋参

It is the dried product from the root of *Panax quinquefolium*, L., family Campanulaceae. The medicinal herb is collected in autumn, applied in crude form.

为五加科植物西洋参的干燥根。秋季采挖。生用。

Features Flavor: sweet and slightly bitter. Property: cool. Meridian tropism: the Heart Meridian, the Lung Meridian and the Kidney Meridian.

性味归经 甘、微苦，凉。归心、肺、肾经。

Actions Reinforce qi, nourish yin, reduce heat and produce fluid.

Application

(1) Cough, panting and bloody sputum. The medicinal herb is sweet, moist and cool in property, and acts to benefit lung qi, nourish lung yin and reduce lung fire. In the treatment of yin deficiency and fire hyperactivity pattern manifested by cough, panting and bloody sputum, it is applied singly by grinding into fine powder for oral administration, or combined with *Anemarrhenae Rhizoma* (zhi mu), *Fritillariae Cirrhosae Bulbus* (chuan bei mu) and *Asini Corii Colla* (e jiao).

(2) Febrile disease manifested by restlessness, fatigue and thirst, and diabetes. The medicinal herb acts to reinforce qi, nourish yin, reduce fire and produce fluid. In the treatment of thirst due to febrile disease or qi and yin deficiency, it is combined with *Rehmanniae Radix* (sheng di huang), *Dendrobii Herba* (shi hu) and *Ophiopogonis Radix* (mai dong). In the treatment of diabetes due to yin deficiency, it is combined with *Astragali Radix* (huang qi), *Trichosanthis Radix* (tian hua fen) and *Schisandrae Chinensis Fructus* (wu wei zi).

Usage and dosage Apply 3～6 g in decoction. Decoct it separately.

Precautions for use It is prohibited to apply for those with yang collapse of middle energizer or cold-damp in stomach. The medicinal herb is incompatible with *Radix et Rhizoma Veratri Nigri* (li lu).

功效 补气养阴，清热生津。

应用

（1）喘咳痰血。本品甘润性凉，善益肺气，养肺阴，清肺火。治阴虚火旺的咳喘痰血，可研末单用，或与知母、川贝母、阿胶等药同用。

（2）热病烦倦口渴，消渴证。本品功善补气养阴、清火生津。治热病气阴两伤的口渴，可与生地黄、石斛、麦冬等同用。治阴虚消渴，可与黄芪、天花粉、五味子等同用。

用法用量 煎服，3～6克。另煎兑服。

使用注意 中阳衰微，胃有寒湿者忌服。反藜芦。

Pseudostellariae Radix (tai zi shen)

It is the dried product from the tuberous root of

太子参

为石竹科植物孩儿参的

Pseudostellaria heterophylla (Miq.) Pax ex Pax et Hoffm., family Caryophyllaceae. The medicinal herb is collected in summer when most of the leaves are withered, applied in crude form.

干燥块根。夏季茎叶大部分枯萎时采挖。生用。

Features Flavor: sweet, slightly bitter. Property: neutral. Meridian tropism: the Spleen Meridian and the Lung Meridian.

性味归经 甘、微苦,平。归脾、肺经。

Actions Benefit qi, strengthen spleen, produce fluid and moisturize lung.

功效 益气健脾,生津润肺。

Application

应用

(1) Spleen deficiency pattern. The medicinal herb is sweet, neutral and moderate in property and attributive to the Spleen Meridian, and acts to benefit spleen qi and nourish stomach yin, as a clearing-reinforcing herb. In the treatment of spleen qi and stomach yin deficiency pattern, it is combined with *Dioscoreae Rhizoma* (shan yao) and *Dendrobii Herba* (shi hu).

(1) 脾虚证。本品甘平入脾,有益脾气,养胃阴之功,药力较缓,为清补之品。常用治脾虚胃阴不足的病证,可与山药、石斛等药同用。

(2) Lung deficiency pattern manifested by dry cough, thirst due to consumption of fluid, palpitation and profuse sweating. The medicinal herb acts benefit qi, moisturize lung, produce fluid and stop thirst. In the treatment of lung deficiency pattern manifested by dry cough, it is combined with *Glehniae Radix* (bei sha shen), *Ophiopogonis Radix* (mai dong) and *Fritillariae Cirrhosae Bulbus* (chuan bei mu). In the treatment of yin deficiency manifested by thirst, it is combined with shi hu and *Schisandrae Chinensis Fructus* (wu wei zi). In the treatment of profuse sweating, palpitation and insomnia, it is combined with *Ziziphi Spinosae Semen* (suan zao ren) and wu wei zi.

(2) 肺虚燥咳,津伤口渴,心悸多汗。本品能益气润燥、生津止渴。治肺虚燥咳,常与北沙参、麦冬、川贝母等同用。治阴虚口渴,可与石斛、五味子等同用。若治多汗心悸不眠,可与酸枣仁、五味子等同用。

Usage and dosage Apply 9～30 g in decoction.

用法用量 煎服,9～30克。

Precautions for use　It is cautious to apply for those with excess of Xie (Pathogenic) Qi without deficiency of Zheng (Anti-Pathogenic) Qi.

使用注意　邪实正不虚者慎用。

Astragali Radix (huang qi)

黄芪

It is the dried product from the root of *Astragalus membranaceus* (Fisch.) Bunge var. *mongholicus* (Bunge) Hsiao, or *Astragalus membranaceus* (Fisch.) Bunge, family Leguminosae. The medicinal herb is collected in spring and autumn, applied in crude form or honey-baked form.

为豆科植物蒙古黄芪或膜荚黄芪的干燥根。春、秋二季采挖。生用或蜜炙用。

Features　Flavor: sweet. Property: slightly warm. Meridian tropism: the Spleen Meridian and the Lung Meridian.

性味归经　甘，微温。归脾、肺经。

Actions　Reinforce qi, uplift yang, benefit Wei (Defensive) Qi, protect body surface, promote water flow, subside swell, drain pus and engender muscle.

功效　补气升阳，益卫固表，利水消肿，托疮生肌。

Application

(1) Spleen and stomach qi deficiency and sinking of Zhong (Middle Energizer) Qi. The medicinal herb is sweet and warm in property and attributive to the Spleen Meridian, and acts to reinforce middle energizer, benefit qi, uplift yang and treat sinking, as the major herb to reinforce qi and uplift yang. In the treatment of spleen deficiency pattern manifested by poor appetite and loose feces, it is combined with *Atractylodis Macrocephalae Rhizoma* (bai zhu), to form up Astragalus and Atractylodes Ointment (Qi Zhu Gao). In the treatment of sinking of spleen yang or sinking of Zhong (Middle Energizer) Qi manifested by chronic diarrhea, prolapse of rectum or prolapse of internal organs, it is combined with *Ginseng Radix et Raizoma* (ren shen),

应用

（1）脾胃气虚，中气下陷。本品甘温入脾，功擅补中益气、升阳举陷，为补气升阳之要药。治脾虚食少便溏，常与白术同用，即芪术膏。治脾阳不升、中气下陷，症见久泻脱肛、内脏下垂，常与人参、升麻、柴胡等同用，如补中益气汤。

Cimicifugae Rhizoma (sheng ma) and *Bupleuri Radix* (chai hu), to form up Center-Supplementing Qi-Boosting Decoction (Bu Zhong Yi Qi Tang).

(2) Lung qi deficiency pattern or exterior deficiency pattern manifested by spontaneous sweating. The medicinal herb acts to reinforce lung qi, benefit Wei (Defensive) Qi, strengthen body surface and stop sweating. In the treatment of lung deficiency pattern manifested by cough, panting and shortness of breath, it is combined with *Aster Radix et Rhizoma* (zi wan) and *Schisandrae Chinensis Fructus* (wu wei zi). In the treatment of exterior deficiency pattern manifested by spontaneous sweating and being liable to catching cold, it is combined with bai zhu and *Saposhnikoviae Radix* (fang feng), to form up Jade Screen Powder (Yu Ping Feng San).

（2）肺气虚，表虚自汗。本品能补肺气、益卫气、固表止汗。治肺虚咳喘气短，常与紫菀、五味子等同用。治表虚自汗，且易外感者，常配伍白术、防风同用，即玉屏风散。

(3) Edema and difficult urination. The medicinal herb acts to reinforce qi, promote urination and subside swell. In the treatment of edema and difficult urination due to qi deficiency, it is combined with *Stephaniae Tetrandrae Radix* (fang ji) and bai zhu, to form up Tetrandrae and Astragalus Decoction (Fang Ji Huang Qi Tang).

（3）浮肿，小便不利。本品有补气利尿消肿之功，常与防己、白术等同用，治气虚浮肿、小便不利，如防己黄芪汤。

(4) Deep pitting of carbuncle and furuncle. The medicinal herb acts to reinforce qi, nourish blood, drain pus and engender muscle. In the treatment of deep pitting of carbuncle and furuncle due to qi and blood deficiency, it is combined with *Angelicae Sinensis Radix* (dang gui), etc. In the treatment of unhealed ulcer of carbuncle and furuncle, it is combined with ren shen and *Cinnamomi Cortex* (rou gui).

（4）疮疡内陷证。本品能补气养血、托毒生肌。治气血亏虚的疮疡内陷，脓成不溃，常配伍当归等同用。治疮疡久溃不敛，可与人参、肉桂等同用。

Furthermore, the medicinal herb acts to benefit qi and nourish blood, applied to treat sallow-yellow

此外，本品能益气养血，治血虚萎黄。且能行滞通

complexion due to blood deficiency. It acts to dissolve stasis and relieve blockage, applied to treat hemiplegia.

痹,治半身不遂。

Usage and dosage Apply 9～30 g in decoction. The medicinal herb acts to benefit qi and reinforce middle energizer in honey-baked form, and acts to treat other diseases in crude form.

用法用量 煎服,9～30克。蜜炙用益气补中,余皆生用。

Precautions for use It is cautious to apply for those with excess pattern.

使用注意 实证慎用。

Atractylodis Macrocephalae Rhizoma (bai zhu)

白术

It is the dried product from the rhizome of *Atractylodes macrocephala* Koidz., family Compositae. The medicinal herb is collected in winter when leaves in the lower are withered and leaves in the upper are crisped, applied in crude form or stir-fried form.

为菊科植物白术的干燥根茎。冬季下部叶枯黄、上部叶变脆时采挖。生用或炒用。

Features Flavor: bitter and sweet. Property: warm. Meridian tropism: the Spleen Meridian and the Stomach Meridian.

性味归经 苦、甘,温。归脾、胃经。

Actions Strengthen spleen, benefit qi, desiccate damp, promote water flow, stop sweating and quiet fetus.

功效 健脾益气,燥湿利水,止汗,安胎。

Application

应用

(1) Spleen deficiency pattern. The medicinal herb is sweet and warm, and bitter and dry in property, and attributive to the Spleen Meridian, and acts to strengthen spleen in transporting and benefit spleen qi. In the treatment of spleen deficiency pattern manifested by poor appetite and loose feces, it is combined with *Ginseng Radix Et Raizoma* (ren shen), *Poria* (fu ling) and *Glycyrrhizae Radix Et Rhizoma Preparata* (zhi gan cao), to form up Four Nobles Decoction (Si Jun Zi Tang). In the treatment of diarrhea due to deficiency and cold of

(1) 脾虚证。本品甘温苦燥,主入脾经,善健脾运、益脾气。治脾虚食少便溏,常配伍人参、茯苓、炙甘草等同用,即四君子汤。治脾胃虚寒的腹泻,常配伍人参、干姜、炙甘草等同用,即理中汤。治脾虚的脘腹痞满,常配伍枳实同用,即枳术丸。

spleen and stomach, it is combined with ren shen, *Zingiberis Rhizoma* (gan jiang) and zhi gan cao, to form up Center-Rectifying Decoction (Li Zhong Tang). In the treatment of epigastric and abdominal masses and distension due to spleen deficiency, it is combined with *Aurantii Fructus Immaturus* (zhi shi), to form up Immature Orange and Atractylodes Pills (Zhi Zhu Wan).

(2) Phlegm-rheum and edema. The medicinal herb acts to reinforce qi and strengthen spleen, and also desiccate damp and promote water flow as well. In the treatment of phlegm-rheum, it is combined with *Cinnamomi Ramulus* (gui zhi), fu ling and zhi gan cao, to form up Poria, Cinnamon, Atractylodes and Liquorice Decoction (Ling Gui Zhu Gan Tang). In the treatment of edema due to spleen deficiency, it is combined with *Poriae Cutis* (fu ling pi), *Arecae Pericarpium* (da fu pi) and *Alismatis Rhizoma* (ze xie).

(2) 痰饮,水肿。本品既补气健脾,又燥湿利水。治痰饮,常与桂枝、茯苓、炙甘草同用,即苓桂术甘汤。治脾虚水肿,常与茯苓皮、大腹皮、泽泻等同用。

(3) Spontaneous sweating due to qi deficiency. The medicinal herb acts to strengthen body surface and stop sweating. In the treatment of spontaneous sweating due to exterior Wei (Defensive) Qi deficiency, it is combined with *Astragali Radix* (huang qi) and *Saposhnikoviae Radix* (fang feng).

(3) 气虚自汗。本品能固表止汗。常配伍黄芪、防风等同用,治卫表不固的自汗。

(4) Irritable fetus. The medicinal herb acts to strengthen spleen and quiet fetus. In the treatment of irritable fetus due to spleen deficiency, it is combined with *Scutellariae Radix* (huang qin) if internal heat presents, or combined with *Perillae Caulis* (zi su geng), *Amomi Fructus* (sha ren) and *Citri Reticulatae Pericarpium* (chen pi) if abdominal distension due to qi stagnation presents.

(4) 胎动不安。本品有补气健脾而安胎之功。常用治脾虚胎动不安。亦可根据兼证与其他药配伍同用。兼内热者,配伍黄芩。兼气滞腹胀者,配伍紫苏梗、砂仁、陈皮等。

Usage and dosage Apply 6～15 g in decoc-

用法用量 煎服,6～15

tion. The medicinal herb acts to desiccate damp and promote water flow in crude form, and acts to strengthen spleen, reinforce qi and stop diarrhea in stir-fried form.

克。生用燥湿利水，炒用健脾补气止泻。

Precautions for use It is cautious to apply for those with yin deficiency or body fluid deficiency.

使用注意 阴虚或津亏者慎用。

Remarks *Atractylodis Rhizoma* (cang zhu) and *Atractylodis Macrocephalae Rhizoma* (bai zhu)

按语 苍术与白术

Both herbs acts to desiccate damp and strengthen spleen. Cang zhu is pungent, bitter and warm in property, and more acts to desiccate damp and strengthen spleen, and also acts to eliminate wind, dissolve damp and brighten eyes as well. Bai zhu is sweet, bitter and warm in property and more acts to reinforce spleen and desiccate damp, and also acts to promote water flow and quiet fetus as well.

二药均能燥湿、健脾。不同的是苍术辛苦性温，功偏燥湿健脾，还能辛散祛风除湿、明目。白术甘苦性温，功偏补脾燥湿，还能利水、安胎。

Dioscoreae Rhizoma (shan yao)

山药

It is the dried product from the rhizome of *Dioscorea opposite* Thunb., family Dioscoreaceae. The medicinal herb is mainly produced in Henan Province, called huai shan yao. It is collected in winter when stem leaves are withered, applied in crude form or stir-fried form.

为薯蓣科植物薯蓣的干燥根茎。主产于河南者，称怀山药。冬季茎叶枯萎后采挖。生用或炒用。

Features Flavor: sweet. Property: neutral. Meridian tropism: the Spleen Meridian, the Lung Meridian and the Kidney Meridian.

性味归经 甘，平。归脾、肺、肾经。

Actions Reinforce spleen, nourish stomach, produce fluid, benefit lung, reinforce kidney and hold essence.

功效 补脾养胃，生津益肺，补肾涩精。

Application

应用

(1) Spleen and stomach deficiency pattern. The medicinal herb is sweet, moist and neutral in property, and acts to reinforce spleen qi and benefit

(1) 脾胃虚弱证。本品甘润性平，能补脾气、益脾阴。治脾虚胃弱，食少便溏，

spleen yin. In the treatment of spleen and stomach deficiency pattern manifested by poor appetite and loose feces, it is combined with *Codonopsis Radix* (dang shen), *Atractylodis Macrocephalae Rhizoma* (bai zhu) and *Poria* (fu ling).

常与党参、白术、茯苓等同用。

(2) Lung and kidney deficiency pattern. The medicinal herb acts to reinforce qi of spleen and lung, and also acts to reinforce yin of lung and kidney as well. It also acts to reinforce kidney and hold essence. In the treatment of cough and panting due to lung deficiency, or chronic cough and chronic panting due to lung and kidney deficiency, it is combined with *Ginseng Radix et Raizoma* (ren shen), *Ophiopogonis Radix* (mai dong) and *Schisandrae Chinensis Fructus* (wu wei zi). In the treatment of kidney deficiency with failure of checking manifested by seminal emission and frequency of urination, it is combined with *Rehmanniae Radix Praeparata* (shu di huang), *Corni Fructus* (shan zhu yu) and *Cuscutae Semen* (tu si zi). In the treatment of thin-clear and unceasing leucorrhea due to kidney deficiency or damp of spleen, it is combined with the kidney-benefiting herbs or with the spleen-strengthening herbs.

（2）肺肾虚弱证。本品既补脾肺之气，又益肺肾之阴，且能固涩肾精。治肺虚咳喘，或肺肾两虚久咳久喘，常配人参、麦冬、五味子等同用。治肾虚不固的遗精、尿频等，常配熟地黄、山茱萸、菟丝子等同用。治肾虚或脾湿的带下清稀，绵绵不止，可配益肾或健脾药同用。

(3) Diabetes. The medicinal herb acts to benefit qi, nourish yin, produce fluid and stop thirst. In the treatment of diabetes due to yin deficiency, it is combined with *Astragali Radix* (huang qi), *Anemarrhenae Rhizoma* (zhi mu) and wu wei zi.

（3）消渴证。本品具益气养阴、生津止渴之功。治阴虚消渴，常与黄芪、知母、五味子等同用。

Usage and dosage Apply 15～30 g in decoction. The medicinal herb acts to reinforce yin, produce fluid, reinforce kidney and hold essence in crude form, and acts to reinforce spleen and strengthen stomach in stir-fried form.

用法用量 煎服，15～30克。生用补阴生津、补肾涩精，炒用补脾健胃。

Precautions for use It is prohibited to apply for those with excessive damp and stasis in middle energizer.

使用注意 湿盛中满而有积滞者忌服。

Glycyrrhizae Radix et Rhizoma (gan cao)

甘草

It is the dried product from the root and rhizome of *Glycyrrhiza uraleusis* Fisch., or *Glycyrrhiza inflate* Batalin, or *Glycyrrhiza grabra* L., family Leguminosae. The medicinal herb is collected in spring and autumn, applied in crude form or honey-baked form.

为豆科植物甘草、胀果甘草或光果甘草的干燥根及根茎。春、秋季采挖。生用或蜜炙用。

Features Flavor: sweet. Property: neutral. Meridian tropism: the Heart Meridian, the Lung Meridian, the Spleen Meridian and the Stomach Meridian.

性味归经 甘,平。归心、肺、脾、胃经。

Actions Reinforce spleen, benefit qi, dissolve phlegm, stop cough, relieve spasm, stop pain, clear heat, relieve toxin and harmonize other herbs.

功效 补脾益气,祛痰止咳,缓急止痛,清热解毒,调和诸药。

Application

应用

(1) Spleen qi deficiency pattern or heart qi deficiency pattern. The medicinal herb is sweet and neutral in property and attributive to the Heart and Spleen Meridians, and acts to reinforce spleen qi and benefit heart qi. In the treatment of spleen deficiency pattern manifested by fatigue, poor appetite and loose feces, it is combined with *Codonopsis Radix* (dang shen) and *Atractylodis Macrocephalae Rhizoma* (bai zhu). In the treatment of heart qi insufficiency pattern manifested by palpitation and irregular pulse, it is combined with *Ginseng Radix et Raizoma* (ren shen), *Asini Corii Colla* (e jiao) and *Cinnamomi Ramulus* (gui zhi), to form up Honeyed Liquorice Decoction (Zhi Gan Cao Tang).

(1) 脾气虚,心气虚证。本品味甘性平,入心脾经,具补脾气、益心气之功。治脾虚倦怠,食少便溏,可与党参、白术等同用。治心气不足,心动悸、脉结代,可与人参、阿胶、桂枝等同用,如炙甘草汤。

(2) Cough with excessive sputum. The medici-

(2) 痰多咳嗽。本品功

nal herb acts to dissolve phlegm, moisturize lung, stop cough and soothe panting, applied to treat cough and panting due to various causes. In the treatment of cough due to wind-cold, it is combined with *Ephedrae Herba* (ma huang) and ku xing ren, to form up Three Disobediences Decoction (San Ao Tang). In the treatment of cough and panting due to heat in lung, it is combined with *Gypsum Fibrosum* (shi gao), *Ephedrae Herba* (ma huang) and ku xing ren, to form up Ephedra, Apricot, Gypsum and Liquorice Decoction (Ma Xing Shi Gan Tang). In the treatment of cough and panting due to cold-phlegm, it is combined with *Zingiberis Rhizoma* (gan jiang) and *Asari Radix et Rhizoma* (xi xin). In the treatment of cough and panting due to damp-phlegm, it is combined with *Pinelliae Rhizoma* (ban xia) and *Poria* (fu ling), to form up Double Vintage Decoction (Er Chen Tang).

能祛痰润肺、止咳平喘，可用于多种原因的咳喘证。治风寒咳嗽，可与麻黄、苦杏仁同用，即三拗汤。治肺热咳喘，可配伍石膏、麻黄、杏仁，即麻杏石甘汤。治寒痰咳喘，配伍干姜、细辛同用。治湿痰咳嗽，配伍半夏、茯苓同用，如二陈汤。

(3) Spasm and pain at epigastria, abdomen and four limbs. The medicinal herb acts to relieve spasm and stop pain. In the treatment of spasm and pain at epigastria, abdomen and four limbs, it is combined with *Paeoniae Radix Alba* (bai shao), to form up Peony Root and Liquorice Decoction (Shao Yao Gan Cao Tang).

（3）脘腹及四肢挛急作痛。本品甘缓止痛。治脘腹既四肢挛急疼痛，常与白芍同用，即芍药甘草汤。

(4) Carbuncle and furuncle due to heat-toxin, sore throat and herb poisoning or food poisoning. The medicinal herb acts to relieve toxin. In the treatment of carbuncle and furuncle due to heat-toxin and sore throat, it is combined with the heat-clearing and toxin-relieving herbs. In the treatment of herb poisoning or food poisoning, it is applied singly in decoction or combined with *Semen Phasedi Radiati* (lü dou).

（4）痈肿疮毒，咽喉肿痛，中药物食物毒。本品清热不足，解毒力佳。与清热解毒药同用，可治热毒疮疡、咽喉肿痛。本品还能解药物或食物毒，可单味煎汤，或与绿豆同煎。

Furthermore, the medicinal herb acts to moderate herb property and harmonize other herbs, often applied in the formula composed of herbs with fierce property.

此外，本品能缓和药性，调和诸药，常在药性峻猛的方剂中应用。

Usage and dosage Apply 2～10 g in decoction. The medicinal herb acts to reinforce spleen, harmonize stomach, benefit qi and regulate pulse in honey-baked form, and acts to treat other diseases in crude form.

用法用量 煎服，2～10克。蜜炙补脾和胃，益气复脉，余皆生用。

Precautions for use It is prohibited to apply for those with distension, fullness and edema due to excessive damp. The medicinal herb is incompatible with *Euphorbiae Pekinensis Radix* (jing da ji), *Genkwa Flos* (yuan hua), *Radix Eupyorbiae Kansui* (gan sui) and *Sargassum* (hai zao).

使用注意 湿盛胀满、浮肿者忌用。反大戟、芫花、甘遂、海藻。

Mel (feng mi)

蜂蜜

It is the product from the honey made by bees, *Apis cerma* Fabricius or *Apis mellifera* L., family Apidae. The medicinal herb is collected from spring to autumn, applied after filtration.

为蜜蜂科昆虫中华蜜蜂或意大利蜂所酿的蜜。春至秋季采收，滤过。

Features Flavor: sweet. Property: neutral. Meridian tropism: the Lung Meridian, the Spleen Meridian and the Large Intestine Meridian.

性味归经 甘，平。归肺、脾、大肠经。

Actions Reinforce middle energizer, moisturize body, stop pain and relieve toxin.

功效 补中，润燥，止痛，解毒。

Application

应用

(1) Epigastric and abdominal pain. The medicinal herb is sweet, neutral and moist in property and acts to benefit qi, reinforce middle energizer, relieve spasm and stop pain. In the treatment of epigastric and abdominal pain, it is combined with *Paeoniae Radix Alba* (bai shao) and *Glycyrrhizae Radix et Rhizoma* (gan cao).

（1）脘腹疼痛。本品甘平润养，能益气补中、缓急止痛。治脘腹虚痛常与芍药、甘草等同用。

(2) Dry cough due to lung deficiency and constipation due to dryness in intestines. The medicinal herb is neutral and moist in property and acts to moisturize lung and stop cough, and to moisturize intestines and promote defecation. In the treatment of dry cough or cough with bloody sputum due to lung deficiency, it is combined with *Ginseng Radix et Raizoma* (ren shen), *Poria* (fu ling) and *Rehmanniae Radix* (sheng di huang). In the treatment of constipation due to dryness in intestines, it is applied singly in dose of 30～60 g for oral administration, or combined with *Angelicae Sinensis Radix* (dang gui), *Semen Sesami* (hei zhi ma) and *Polygoni Multiflori Radix* (he shou wu). It acts to increase the lung-moisturizing function of the cough-stopping herbs if the medicinal herb is prepared with the cough-stopping herbs.

（2）肺虚燥咳，肠燥便秘。本品性平质润，能润肺燥止咳，润肠燥通便。治肺虚燥咳、干咳咯血，常配人参、茯苓、生地等同用。治肠燥便秘，单用 30～60 克冲服，或与当归、黑芝麻、何首乌等同用。本品与止咳药共同炮制，能增强止咳药的润肺作用。

Furthermore, the medicinal herb acts to relieve toxin similar to *Aconiti Radix* (wu tou).

此外，本品能解乌头类毒。

Usage and dosage Apply 15～30 g in decoction or infused in boiling water.

用法用量 煎服或冲服，15～30 克。

Precautions for use It is cautious to apply for those with damp blocking middle energizer, accumulation of phlegm, heat and damp, loose feces or diarrhea.

使用注意 湿阻中满，湿热痰滞，便溏或泄泻者宜慎用。

Section 2 Yang-reinforcing herbs

第 2 节 补阳药

Cervi Cornu Pantotrichum (lu rong)

鹿茸

It is the dried product from the non-ossified horn of male beast of *Cervus nippon* Temminck or

为鹿科动物梅花鹿或马鹿的雄鹿未骨化密生茸毛的

Cervus elaphus L., family Cervidae. The medicinal herb is collected in summer and autumn, applied in sliced form or powdered form.

幼角。夏、秋二季锯取鹿茸。用时炮制成鹿茸片，或研细粉用。

Features Flavor: sweet and salty. Property: warm. Meridian tropism: the Kidney Meridian and the Liver Meridian.

性味归经 甘、咸，温。归肾、肝经。

Actions Strengthen kidney yang, benefit essence and blood, strengthen tendons and bones, regulate Thoroughfare and Conception Vessels, and drain pus and toxin.

功效 壮肾阳，益精血，强筋骨，调冲任，托疮毒。

Application

应用

(1) Kidney yang insufficiency pattern. The medicinal herb is sweet, salty and warm in property and acts to strengthen kidney yang and benefit essence and blood. In the treatment of kidney yang insufficiency pattern manifested by impotence, premature ejaculation, infertility due to cold in uterus, aching and pain at low back and knees, dizziness and tinnitus, it is applied singly by grinding into fine powder for oral administration, or combined with *Ginseng Radix et Raizoma* (ren shen) and *Morindae Officinalis Radix* (ba ji tian).

(1) 肾阳不足证。本品甘咸性温，为壮肾阳、益精血的要药。治阳痿早泄、宫寒不孕、腰膝酸痛、头晕耳鸣等肾阳不足证，单用研末服。或与人参、巴戟天等配伍同用。

(2) Essence and blood deficiency pattern. The medicinal herb is attributive to the Liver and Kidney Meridians and acts to reinforce liver and kidney, benefit essence and blood and strengthen tendons and bones. In the treatment of liver and kidney insufficiency pattern or essence and blood deficiency pattern manifested by flaccidity and weakness of tendons and bones and retarded development of infants, it is combined with *Dioscoreae Rhizoma* (shan yao), *Corni Fructus* (shan zhu yu) and *Rehmanniae Radix Praeparata* (shu di huang).

(2) 精血亏虚证。本品能入肝肾经，能补肝肾、益精血、强筋骨。治肝肾不足、精血亏虚的筋骨痿软、小儿发育迟缓等，常与山药、山茱萸、熟地黄等同用。

(3) Metrorrhagia, metrostaxis and morbid leu-

(3) 崩漏，带下。本品性

corrhea. The medicinal herb is warm in property and acts to reinforce liver and kidney, and regulate Thoroughfare and Conception Vessels, applied to treat metrorrhagia, metrostaxis and morbid leucorrhea due to deficiency and cold. In the treatment of metrorrhagia and metrostaxis, it is combined with *Angelicae Sinensis Radix* (dang gui), *Asini Corii Colla* (e jiao) and *Artemisiae Argyi Folium* (ai ye). In the treatment of excessive leucorrhea, it is combined with *Angelicae Dahuricae Radix* (bai zhi) and *Euryales Semen* (qian shi).

温，功能补肝肾、调冲任、固崩止带，多用于虚寒性崩漏、带下诸证。治崩漏，可与当归、阿胶、艾叶等同用。治白带过多，可与白芷、芡实等同用。

(4) Chronic and unhealed ulcer in carbuncle and furuncle. The medicinal herb acts to warm and reinforce essence and blood, drain toxin and pus, engender muscle and heal wound. In the treatment of chronic and unhealed ulcer in carbuncle and furuncle, it is combined with *Astragali Radix* (huang qi), *Angelicae Sinensis Radix* (dang gui) and *Cinnamomi Cortex* (rou gui).

（4）疮疡久溃不敛。本品能温补精血，托毒外出、生肌收口。治疮疡久溃不敛，可与黄芪、当归、肉桂同用。

Usage and dosage Apply 1～2 g powder, or apply by liquor-saturating.

用法用量 研末冲服，1～2 克。亦可浸酒服。

Precautions for use It is not advisable to apply in large dose. It is prohibited to apply for those with heat in blood, damp-heat, excess heat pattern of zang-fu organs, or febrile disease due to exogenous pathogens.

使用注意 注意用量，不宜骤用大量。凡血热、湿热或脏腑实热证，外感热病等忌用。

Morindae Officinalis Radix (ba ji tian)

巴戟天

It is the dried product from the root of *Morinda officinalis* How, family Rubiceae. The medicinal herb is collected all over the year, applied in prepared form by steaming.

为茜草科植物巴戟天的干燥根。全年均可采挖。蒸制后用。

Features Flavor: sweet and pungent. Property: slightly warm. Meridian tropism: the Kidney

性味归经 甘、辛，微温。归肾、肝经。

Meridian and the Liver Meridian.

Actions Reinforce kidney yang, strengthen tendons and bones, and eliminate wind-damp.

Application

(1) Kidney yang deficiency pattern. The medicinal herb is sweet, moist and warm and acts to warm kidney yang and benefit essence and blood. In the treatment of impotence due to kidney deficiency or infertility due to cold in uterus, it is combined with *Ginseng Radix et Raizoma* (ren shen), *Dioscoreae Rhizoma* (shan yao). In the treatment of frequency of urination due to kidney deficiency, it is combined with shan yao and *Mantidis OÖTheca* (sang piao xiao).

(2) Bi (Obturation) Pattern due to wind-damp, and flaccidity and weakness of tendons and bones. The medicinal herb acts to eliminate wind-damp and reinforce kidney yang. In the treatment of kidney yang deficiency pattern with wind-damp manifested by flaccidity and weakness of tendons and bones, and pain at low back and knees, it is combined with *Eucommiae Cortex* (du zhong) and *Taxilli Herba* (sang ji sheng).

Usage and dosage Apply 3～15 g in decoction.

Precautions for use It is prohibited to apply for those with yin deficiency and fire hyperactivity or those with damp-heat.

Epimedii Folium (yin yang huo)

It is the dried product from the acrial part of *Epimedium brevicornu* Maxim., or *Epimedium sagittatum* (Sieb. et Zucc.) Maxim., *Epimedium pubescens Maxim.*, or *Epimedium korenum* Nakai,

功效 补肾阳,强筋骨,祛风湿。

应用

(1) 肾阳虚证。本品甘润性温而不燥,具温肾阳、益精血之功。治肾虚阳痿、宫冷不孕,常与人参、山药等同用。肾虚尿频,与山药、桑螵蛸等同用。

(2) 风湿痹痛,筋骨痿软。本品具祛风湿、补肾阳之功。常用于肾阳虚兼风湿之证,症见筋骨痿软、腰膝痹痛等,可与杜仲、桑寄生等同用。

用法用量 煎服,3～15克。

使用注意 阴虚火旺或有湿热者忌用。

淫羊藿

为小檗科植物淫羊藿、箭叶淫羊藿、柔毛淫羊藿或朝鲜淫羊藿的干燥地上部分。又名仙灵脾。夏、秋季

family Berberidaceae. The medicinal herb is also called xian ling pi, collected in summer and autumn when it is flourishing, applied in crude form or stir-baked form.

茎叶茂盛时采割。生用或炙用。

Features Flavor: pungent and sweet. Property: warm. Meridian tropism: the Liver Meridian and the Kidney Meridian.

性味归经 辛、甘，温。归肝、肾经。

Actions Reinforce kidney yang, strengthen tendons and bones and eliminate wind-damp.

功效 补肾阳，强筋骨，祛风湿。

Application

应用

(1) Kidney yang deficiency pattern. The medicinal herb acts to warm kidney, strengthen yang, benefit essence and treat flaccidity. In the treatment of impotence due to kidney deficiency, it is applied singly by liquor-saturating, or combined with *Rehmanniae Radix Praeparata* (shu di huang), *Lycii Fructus* (gou qi zi) and *Morindae Officinalis Radix* (ba ji tian).

（1）肾阳虚证。本品功善温肾壮阳、益精起痿，且效佳。治肾虚阳痿，可单味浸酒服，如淫羊藿酒，或与熟地黄、枸杞子、巴戟天等同用。

(2) Bi (Obturation) Pattern due to wind-damp, and flaccidity and weakness of tendons and bones. The medicinal herb acts to eliminate wind and dissolve damp, and also to reinforce liver and kidney and strengthen tendons and bones as well. In the treatment of Bi (Obturation) Pattern due to wind-damp, numbness and spasm of body and limbs, it is applied singly by liquor-saturating, or combined with *Clematidis Radix et Rhizoma* (wei ling xian), *Xanthii Fructus* (cang er zi) and *Cinnamomi Cortex* (gui xin). In the treatment of liver and kidney insufficiency pattern manifested by flaccidity and weakness of tendons and bones, and walking unsteadily, it is combined with *Eucommiae Cortex* (du zhong), ba ji tian and *Taxilli Herba* (sang ji sheng).

（2）风湿痹痛，筋骨痿软。本品既祛风除湿，又补肝肾、强筋骨。治风湿痹痛、肢体麻木拘挛，可单用浸酒服，或与威灵仙、苍耳子、桂心等同用。治肝肾不足的筋骨痿软、步履艰难，可配伍杜仲、巴戟天、桑寄生等同用。

Usage and dosage Apply 6～10 g in decoction. The medicinal herb is applied in crude form. It acts to reinforce kidney yang in mutton fat-baked form.

Precautions for use It is prohibited to apply for those with yin deficiency and fire hyperactivity.

Cistanchis Herba (rou cong rong)

It is the dried product from the fleshy stem of *Cistauche deserticola* Y. C. Ma, or *Cistanche tubulosa* (Wchrenk) wight, family Orobanchaceae. The medicinal herb is collected in spring before or just after the sprouts come up, applied in crude form or liquor-prepared form.

Features Flavor: sweet and salty. Property: warm. Meridian tropism: the Kidney Meridian and the Large Intestine Meridian.

Actions Reinforce kidney yang, benefit essence and blood, moisturize intestines and promote defecation.

Application

(1) Kidney yang insufficiency pattern and essence and blood deficiency pattern. The medicinal herb is salty and warm in property and acts to reinforce kidney yang and benefit essence and blood. In the treatment of impotence or infertility due to kidney deficiency, it is combined with *Rehmanniae Radix Praeparata* (shu di huang), *Cuscutae Semen* (tu si zi) and *Schisandrae Chinensis Fructus* (wu wei zi). In the treatment of infertility due to cold in uterus, it is combined with *Cervi Cornu Pantotrichum* (lu rong) and *Angelicae Sinensis Radix* (dang gui). In the treatment of essence and blood deficiency, aching and weakness at low back and knees,

用法用量 煎服，6～10克。一般生用，羊脂油炙可增补肾阳之功。

使用注意 阴虚火旺者忌服。

肉苁蓉

为列当科植物肉苁蓉或管花肉苁蓉的干燥带鳞叶的肉质茎。多于春季苗未出土或刚出土时采挖。生用或酒制用。

性味归经 甘、咸，温。归肾、大肠经。

功效 补肾阳，益精血，润肠通便。

应用

(1) 肾阳不足，精血亏虚证。本品甘咸性温，具补肾阳、益精血之功。治肾虚阳痿不育，常与熟地黄、菟丝子、五味子等同用。治宫冷不孕，常与鹿茸、当归等同用。治精血亏虚，腰膝酸软，筋骨无力，常与巴戟天、杜仲等同用。

flaccidity of tendons and bones, it is combined with *Morindae Officinalis Radix* (ba ji tian) and *Eucommiae Cortex* (du zhong).

(2) Constipation due to dryness in intestines. The medicinal herb acts to benefit essence and blood and moisturize intestines. In the treatment of constipation due to yang deficiency or essence deficiency, it is applied singly or combined with dang gui and *Aurantii Fructus* (zhi qiao).

（2）肠燥便秘。本品益精血、润肠燥，尤宜于阳虚精亏的便秘。可单用大剂量煎服，亦常与当归、枳壳等同用。

Usage and dosage Apply 6～10 g in decoction. The medicinal herb acts to moisturize intestines in crude form, and acts to reinforce kidney yang and benefit essence and blood in liquor-prepared form.

用法用量 煎服，6～10克。生用润肠，酒制补肾阳，益精血。

Precautions for use It is prohibited to apply for those with yin deficiency and fire hyperactivity, loose feces or constipation due to excess heat in stomach and intestines.

使用注意 阴虚火旺，大便溏泄及胃肠实热便秘者忌服。

Alpiniae Oxyphyllae Fructus (yi zhi)

益智

It is the dried product from the ripe fruit of *Alpinia oxyphylla* Miq., family Zingiberaceae. The medicinal herb is collected in summer and autumn when the fruits are changing from green to red, applied in crude form or stir-baked form.

为姜科植物益智的干燥成熟果实。又名益智仁。夏秋间果实由绿变红时采收。生用或炙用。

Features Flavor: pungent. Property: warm. Meridian tropism: the Spleen Meridian and the Kidney Meridian.

性味归经 辛，温。归脾、肾经。

Actions Warm kidney, hold essence and control urination, and warm spleen, stop diarrhea and control saliva.

功效 暖肾固精缩尿，温脾止泻摄唾。

Application

应用

(1) Kidney deficiency manifested by seminal emission, seminal leakage, enuresis and frequency

（1）肾虚遗精滑精，遗尿尿频。本品既补肾助阳，又

of urination. The medicinal herb acts to reinforce kidney and assist yang, and also to astringe essence and urination as well. In the treatment of seminal emission and seminal leakage, it is combined with *Psoraleae Fructus* (bu gu zhi), *Os Draconis* (long gu) and *Rosae Laevigatae Fructus* (jin ying zi). In the treatment of enuresis or frequency of urination at night, it is combined with *Dioscoreae Rhizoma* (shan yao) and *Linderae Radix* (wu yao), to form up Spring-Reducing Pills (Suo Quan Wan).

性兼收涩，尤善固精缩尿。治肾虚遗精滑精，可与补骨脂、龙骨、金樱子等同用。治遗尿或夜尿频多，可与山药、乌药同用，如缩泉丸。

(2) Cold in spleen manifested by diarrhea, cold pain at abdomen and salivation. The medicinal herb acts to warm spleen and stop diarrhea, and to improve stomach and control saliva. In the treatment of diarrhea due to deficiency and cold in spleen and stomach, it is combined with *Atractylodis Macrocephalae Rhizoma* (bai zhu) and *Zingiberis Rhizoma* (gan jiang). In the treatment of salivation or unceasing saliva leakage in infants, it is combined with *Codonopsis Radix* (dang shen), bai zhu and *Citri Reticulatae Pericarpium* (chen pi).

（2）脾寒泄泻，腹中冷痛，口多涎唾。本品有温脾止泻，开胃摄唾之效。治脾胃虚寒泄泻，常与白术、干姜等同用。治口多涎唾或小儿流涎不禁，可配伍党参、白术、陈皮等同用。

Usage and dosage Apply 3～10 g in decoction. The medicinal herb is applied in crude form, and it is attributive to the Kidney Meridian in stir-baked form with salt solution.

用法用量 煎服，3～10克。一般生用，盐水炙入肾经。

Precautions for use It is prohibited to apply for those with yin deficiency and fire hyperactivity, or seminal emission, frequency of urination, metrorrhagia and metrostaxis due to heat.

使用注意 阴虚火旺或因热遗精、尿频、崩漏等者均忌服。

Psoraleae Fructus (bu gu zhi)

补骨脂

It is the dried product from the ripe fruits of *Psoalea corylifolia* L., family Leguminosae. The medicinal herb is collected in autumn, applied in

为豆科植物补骨脂的干燥成熟果实。秋季采收。生用或盐水炙用。

crude form or stir-baked form with salt solution.

Features Flavor: pungent and bitter. Property: warm. Meridian tropism: the Kidney Meridian and the Spleen Meridian.

性味归经 辛、苦，温。归肾、脾经。

Actions Warm kidney, assist yang, warm spleen, stop diarrhea, accept qi and soothe panting.

功效 温肾助阳，暖脾止泻，纳气平喘。

Application

应用

(1) Kidney yang deficiency pattern. The medicinal herb acts to warm kidney, reinforce yang, control essence and hold urine. In the treatment of impotence due to kidney deficiency, it is combined with *Cuscutae Semen* (tu si zi) and *Semen Juglandis* (he tao ren). In the treatment of seminal emission, it is combined with *Mantidis OÖTheca* (sang piao xiao) and *Rosae Laevigatae Fructus* (jin ying zi). In the treatment of cold pain at low back and knees due to kidney deficiency, it is combined with *Eucommiae Cortex* (du zhong) and *Semen Juglandis* (he tao ren), to form up Black-Haired Girl's Pills (Qing E Wan). In the treatment of kidney deficiency manifested by chills, frequency of urination and enuresis, it is combined with *Foeniculi Fructus* (xiao hui xiang) in equal quantities, by making into pills for oral administration.

（1）肾阳虚证。本品能温肾补阳，固精缩尿。治肾虚阳痿，可与菟丝子、核桃仁等同用。治遗精，可与桑螵蛸、金樱子等同用。治肾虚腰膝冷痛，常与杜仲、胡桃肉同用，即青娥丸。治肾气虚冷，尿频遗尿，以之同茴香等份为丸服。

(2) Dawn diarrhea. The medicinal herb acts to reinforce kidney yang, warm spleen and stop diarrhea. In the treatment of dawn diarrhea due to spleen and kidney yang deficiency, it is combined with *Schisandrae Chinensis Fructus* (wu wei zi), *Myristicae Semen* (rou dou kou) and *Euodiae Fructus* (wu zhu yu), to form up Four Divinities Pills (Si Shen Wan).

（2）五更泄泻。本品能补肾阳以暖脾止泻。常与五味子、肉豆蔻、吴茱萸等同用，用治脾肾阳虚所致的五更泄泻，如四神丸。

(3) Panting of deficiency type. The medicinal herb acts to reinforce kidney yang, accept qi and

（3）虚喘。本品能补肾阳、纳气平喘。治肺肾两虚

soothe panting. In the treatment of panting of deficiency type due to lung and kidney deficiency, it is combined with he tao ren.

治虚喘，常与胡桃肉同用。

Furthermore, the medicinal herb acts to eliminate wind and remove speckles. In the treatment of vitiligo or alopecia areata, it is applied by grinding into powder or making into tincture for external use.

此外，本品外用能消风祛斑，研末用或制成酊剂，外涂局部，治白癜风或斑秃。

Usage and dosage Apply 6～10 g in decoction. Apply a proper amount for external use. The medicinal herb is applied for external use in crude form, and applied for oral administration in stir-baked form with salt solution.

用法用量 煎服，6～10克。外用适量。生用多作外用，盐水炙多作内服。

Precautions for use It is prohibited to apply for those with yin deficiency and fire hyperactivity or those with constipation.

使用注意 阴虚火旺及大便秘结者忌服。

Cuscutae Semen (tu si zi)

菟丝子

It is the dried product from the ripe seeds of *Cuscuta australis* R. Br. or *Cuscuta chinensis* Lam., family Convulvulaceae. The medicinal herb is collected in autumn, applied in crude form or in stir-baked form with salt solution.

为旋花科植物南方菟丝子或菟丝子的干燥成熟种子。秋季采收。生用或盐水炙用。

Features Flavor: pungent and sweet. Property: neutral. Meridian tropism: the Liver Meridian, the Kidney Meridian and the Spleen Meridian.

性味归经 辛，甘，平。归肝、肾、脾经。

Actions Reinforce and benefit liver and kidney, control essence, hold urination, brighten eyes, stop diarrhea and quiet fetus.

功效 补益肝肾，固精缩尿，明目，止泻，安胎。

Application

应用

(1) Liver and kidney insufficiency pattern. The medicinal herb is neutral in property and acts to reinforce kidney, benefit liver, harmonize and reinforce yin and yang, control essence or hold urine.

（1）肝肾不足证。本品性平，能补肾益肝、平补阴阳，固精缩尿。治肝肾不足的腰膝酸痛，常与杜仲、牛膝

In the treatment of liver and kidney insufficiency pattern manifested by aching and pain at low back and knees, it is combined with *Eucommiae Cortex* (du zhong) and *Achyranthis Bidentatae Radix* (niu xi). In the treatment of kidney yang deficiency pattern manifested by impotence and seminal emission, it is combined with *Lycii Fructus* (gou qi zi), wu wei zi and. In the treatment of kidney deficiency manifested by frequency of urination or incontinence of urination, it is combined with *Mantidis OÖTheca* (sang piao xiao), *Cervi Cornu Pantotrichum* (lu rong) and *Schisandrae Chinensis Fructus* (wu wei zi).

等同用。治肾虚阳痿遗精，常与枸杞子、五味子等同用。治肾虚尿频或小便不禁，常与桑螵蛸、鹿茸、五味子等同用。

(2) Blurring of vision and dim eyesight. The medicinal herb acts to benefit kidney, nourish liver and brighten eyes. In the treatment of blurring of vision and dim eyesight due to liver and kidney insufficiency, it is combined with *Rehmanniae Radix Praeparata* (shu di huang), *Lycii Fructus* (gou qi zi) and *Plantaginis Semen* (che qian zi).

(2) 目暗不明。本品能益肾养肝而明目。治肝肾不足之目暗不明，常与熟地黄、枸杞子、车前子等同用。

(3) Diarrhea due to spleen and kidney deficiency. The medicinal herb acts to warm kidney and reinforce spleen so as to stop diarrhea of deficiency type. In the treatment of diarrhea due to spleen and kidney deficiency, it is combined with *Ginseng Radix et Raizoma* (ren shen), *Atractylodis Macrocephalae Rhizoma* (bai zhu) and *Psoraleae Fructus* (bu gu zhi).

(3) 脾肾虚泻。本品能温肾补脾而止虚泻。常配伍人参、白术、补骨脂等同用，治脾肾两虚泄泻。

(4) Irritable fetus. The medicinal herb acts to reinforce liver and kidney and hold and quiet fetus. In the treatment of liver and kidney deficiency manifested by irritable fetus or threatened miscarriage, it is combined with *Dipsaci Radix* (xu duan), *Taxilli Herba* (sang ji sheng) and *Asini Corii Colla* (e jiao), to form up Well-Lived Fetus Pills (Shou Tai

(4) 胎动不安。本品能补肝肾、固胎元。治肝肾虚之胎动不安、胎漏下血，常与续断、桑寄生、阿胶等同用，如寿胎丸。

Wan).

Furthermore, the medicinal herb acts to treat vitiligo for external use.

此外，本品外用治白癜风。

Usage and dosage Apply 6～12 g in decoction. Apply a proper amount for external use. The medicinal herb is attributive to the Kidney Meridian after stir-baking with salt solution.

用法用量 煎服，6～12克。外用适量。盐水炙入肾。

Precautions for use It is prohibited to apply for those with yin deficiency and fire hyperactivity, or those with constipation, or those with scanty and dark urine.

使用注意 阴虚火旺，大便燥结及小便短赤者忌服。

Astragali Complanati Semen (sha yuan zi)

沙苑子

It is the dried product from the ripe seed of the herbage *Astragalus complanatus* R. Br, family Leguminosae, also called sha yuan ji li or tong ji li. The medicinal herb is collected in late autumn and early winter when the fruits are ripe but not open, applied in crude form or in stir-baked form with salt solution.

为豆科植物扁茎黄芪的干燥成熟种子。又名沙苑蒺藜、潼蒺藜。秋末冬初果实成熟尚未开裂时采收。生用或盐水炙用。

Features Flavor: sweet. Property: warm. Meridian tropism: the Liver Meridian and the Kidney Meridian.

性味归经 甘，温。归肝、肾经。

Actions Reinforce kidney, control essence, nourish liver and brighten eyes.

功效 补肾固精，养肝明目。

Application

应用

(1) Kidney deficiency pattern. The medicinal herb is sweet and warm in property and acts to reinforce kidney yang, benefit kidney yin, control essence and hold urine. In the treatment of impotence, seminal emission, frequency of urination and morbid leucorrhea, it is combined with *Os Draconis* (long gu), and *Euryales Semen* (qian shi), to form up Golden Lock Essence-Controlling Pills (Jin Suo

(1) 肾虚证。本品甘温不燥，具补肾阳、益肾阴、固精缩尿之效。治阳痿遗精，尿频带下，常与龙骨、芡实等同用，如金锁固精丸；治肾虚腰痛，可单用本品；或与杜仲、续断等同用。

Gu Jin Wan). In the treatment of low back pain due to kidney deficiency, it is applied singly or combined with *Eucommiae Cortex* (du zhong) and *Dipsaci Radix* (xu duan).

(2) Dizziness and blurring of vision. The medicinal herb acts to reinforce and benefit liver and kidney and brighten eyes. In the treatment of dizziness and blurring of vision due to liver and kidney deficiency, it is combined with *Lycii Fructus* (gou qi zi) and *Chrysanthemi Flos* (ju hua).

（2）眩晕目昏。本品能补益肝肾、明目，可与枸杞子、菊花等同用，治肝肾两虚的眩晕目昏等症。

Usage and dosage Apply 9～15 g in decoction.

用法用量 煎服，9～15克。

Precautions for use It is cautious to apply for those with yin deficiency and fire hyperactivity or those with difficult urination.

使用注意 阴虚火旺及小便不利者慎用。

Cordyceps (dong chong xia cao)

冬虫夏草

It is the dried product from the compound of the stroma formed by *Cordyceps sinensis* (Berk.) Sacc., parasitized on the larva of *Hepialus armoricanus* Oberthru and the larva. The medicinal herb is collected in the early summer when the stroma comes up out of the ground and the spores have not burst. It is partially dried in sun and the fibriform attachment and impurity are removed. Then it is dried in sun or in low temperature. It is applied in crude form.

为麦角菌科真菌冬虫夏草菌寄生在蝙蝠蛾科昆虫幼虫上的子座和幼虫尸体的干燥复合体。初夏子座出土、孢子未发散时挖取。晒至6～7成干，除去似纤维状的附着物及杂质，晒干或低温干燥。生用。

Features Flavor: sweet. Property: neutral. Meridian tropism: the Lung Meridian and the Kidney Meridian.

性味归经 甘，平。归肺、肾经。

Actions Reinforce kidney, benefit lung, stanch blood and dissolve phlegm.

功效 补肾益肺，止血化痰。

Application

应用

(1) Kidney deficiency pattern manifested by

（1）肾虚腰痛，阳痿遗

low back pain, impotence and seminal emission. The medicinal herb acts reinforce kidney, assist yang, benefit essence and promote erection. In the treatment of impotence or seminal emission, it is applied singly by soaking in liquor, or combined with *Epimedii Folium* (yin yang huo), *Morindae Officinalis Radix* (ba ji tian) and *Cuscutae Semen* (tu si zi).

精。本品有补肾助阳，益精起痿之效。可单用浸酒服，或配伍淫羊藿、巴戟天、菟丝子等同用。

(2) Chronic cough, panting of deficiency type, and cough with bloody sputum. The medicinal herb is sweet and neutral in property and acts to reinforce qi of lung and kidney, benefit yin of lung and kidney, soothe cough and panting, stanch blood and dissolve phlegm. In the treatment of cough with bloody sputum, it is combined with *Glehniae Radix* (bei sha shen), *Fritillariae Cirrhosae Bulbus* (chuan bei mu) and *Asini Corii Colla* (e jiao). In the treatment of panting, cough and shortness of breath, it is combined with *Ginseng Radix et Raizoma* (ren shen), *Semen Juglandis* (he tao ren).

(2) 久咳虚喘，劳嗽痰血。本品甘平，既补肺肾之气，又益肺肾之阴，能平定喘嗽，兼能止血化痰。治劳嗽痰血，常配伍北沙参、川贝母、阿胶等同用。治喘咳短气，常与人参、胡桃肉等同用。

Furthermore, in the treatment of weak body after serious disease, spontaneous sweating and chills, it is applied by steaming with duck, chicken or pork. The medicinal herb acts to reinforce body and bring back health from weakness.

此外，病后体虚不复，自汗畏寒等，可以与鸭、鸡、猪肉等炖服，有补虚扶弱之效。

Usage and dosage Apply 3～9 g in decoction or stewed with other materials.

用法用量 煎汤或炖服，3～9 克。

Precautions for use It is not advisable to apply singly for those with yin deficiency and fire hyperactivity.

使用注意 阴虚火旺者不宜单独应用。

Eucommiae Cortex (du zhong)

杜仲

It is the dried product from the bark of *Eucommia ulmoides* Oliv., family Eucommiaceae. The

为杜仲科植物杜仲的干燥树皮。4～6 月剥取，刮去

medicinal herb is collected from April to June by scraping its rough skin, applied in crude form or in stir-baked form with salt solution.

粗皮。生用或盐水炙用。

Features Flavor: sweet. Property: warm. Meridian tropism: the Liver Meridian and the Kidney Meridian.

性味归经 甘，温。归肝、肾经。

Actions Reinforce liver and kidney, strengthen tendons and bones and quiet fetus.

功效 补肝肾，强筋骨，安胎。

Application

应用

(1) Liver and kidney insufficiency pattern. The medicinal herb acts to reinforce liver and kidney, strengthen tendons and bones and warm lower energizer. In the treatment of liver and kidney insufficiency pattern manifested by aching and pain at low back and knees, and flaccidity and weakness of tendons and bones, it is applied singly by soaking in liquor for oral administration, or combined with *Psoraleae Fructus* (bu gu zhi) and *Semen Juglandis* (he tao ren). In the treatment of kidney yang deficiency pattern manifested by impotence and frequency of urination, it is combined with *Corni Fructus* (shan zhu yu), *Cuscutae Semen* (tu si zi).

（1）肝肾不足证。本品善补肝肾而强筋骨，暖下元。为治肝肾不足之腰膝酸痛、筋骨痿软的要药，单用浸酒服即效，或常配补骨脂、胡桃肉等同用。治肾虚阳痿尿频，可与山茱肉、菟丝子等同用。

(2) Threatened miscarriage, uterine bleeding and irritable fetus. The medicinal herb acts to reinforce liver and kidney, adjust Thoroughfare and Conception Vessels, regulate menstruation, and quiet fetus. In the treatment of liver and kidney deficiency pattern manifested by irritable fetus, and pain and weighty sensation at low back, it is applied singly by grinding into powder to make into pills with *Fructus Ziziphi Jujubae* (da zao), or combined with *Dipsaci Radix* (xu duan), tu si zi and *Asini Corii Colla* (e jiao).

（2）胎漏下血，胎动不安。本品有补肝肾，调冲任，固经安胎之功。治肝肾亏虚的胎动不安、腰痛如坠，可单味研末，枣肉为丸服用，亦可与续断、菟丝子、阿胶等同用。

Usage and dosage Apply 10～15 g in decoc-

用法用量 煎服，10～

tion. The medicinal herb is strong in reinforcing kidney in stir-baked form with salt solution.

15克。盐水炙补肾力强。

Precautions for use It is cautious to apply for those with yin deficiency and fire hyperactivity.

使用注意 阴虚火旺者慎用。

Dipsaci Radix (xu duan)

续断

It is the dried product from the root of Himalaya Teasel, *Dipsacus asper* Wall. ex Henry, family Dipsacaceae. The medicinal is collected in autumn, applied in crude form, or in stir-fried form with liquor, or in stir-baked form with salt solution.

为川续断科植物川续断的干燥根。秋季采挖。生用或酒炒、盐炙用。

Features Flavor: bitter and pungent. Property: slightly warm. Meridian tropism: the Liver Meridian and the Kidney Meridian.

性味归经 苦、辛，微温。归肝、肾经。

Actions Reinforce liver and kidney, strengthen tendons and bones, set broken bone, stanch blood and quiet fetus.

功效 补肝肾，强筋骨，续折伤，止血安胎。

Application

应用

(1) Liver and kidney insufficiency pattern. The medicinal herb acts to reinforce liver and kidney and strengthen tendons and bones. In the treatment of liver and kidney insufficiency pattern manifested by aching, pain, flaccidity and weakness at low back and knees, it is combined with *Eucommiae Cortex* (du zhong), *Achyranthis Bidentatae Radix* (niu xi) and *Psoraleae Fructus* (bu gu zhi).

（1）肝肾不足证。本品善补肝肾、强筋骨。治肝肾不足的腰膝酸痛，软弱无力，常配伍杜仲、牛膝、补骨脂等同用。

(2) Bi (Obturation) Pattern due to wind, cold and damp, traumatic injury, and broken tendons and bones. The medicinal herb acts to promote blood flow in vessels and set broken bone, as the major herb to treat broken tendons and bones. In the treatment of Bi (Obturation) Pattern due to wind, cold and damp with pain, it is combined with *Angelicae Pubescentis Radix* (du huo) and

（2）风寒湿痹，跌打损伤，筋伤骨折。本品能行血脉、续折伤，为筋伤骨折要药。治风寒湿痹疼痛，可与独活、羌活等同用。治跌仆损伤、骨折肿痛，常与活血止痛、消肿续折药同用。

Notopterygii Rhizoma et Radix (qiang huo). In the treatment of traumatic injury and pain due to fracture, it is combined with the blood-activating and pain-relieving herbs and the swell-dissipating and fracture-treating herbs.

(3) Threatened miscarriage with uterine bleeding, metrorrhagia and metrostaxis. The medicinal herb acts to reinforce liver and kidney, adjust Thoroughfare and Conception Vessels, stanch blood and quiet fetus. In the treatment of liver and kidney deficiency manifested by threatened miscarriage with uterine bleeding and irritable fetus, it is combined with *Taxilli Herba* (sang ji sheng), *Cuscutae Semen* (tu si zi) and *Asini Corii Colla* (e jiao). In the treatment of metrorrhagia and metrostaxis, it is combined with *Astragali Radix* (huang qi) and *Artemisiae Argyi Folium* (ai ye).

(3) 胎漏下血,崩漏不止。本品能补肝肾、调冲任,止血安胎。治肝肾虚所致的胎漏下血、胎动欲坠,常与桑寄生、菟丝子、阿胶等同用。治崩漏不止,可与黄芪、艾叶等同用。

Usage and dosage Apply 9～15 g in decoction. The medicine acts to promote blood flow in vessels and set broken bone in stir-fried form with liquor, and acts to reinforce liver and kidney in stir-baked form with salt solution.

用法用量 煎服,9～15克。酒炒增行血脉、续伤折之力,盐水炙补肝肾。

Section 3 Blood-reinforcing herbs

第3节 补血药

Angelicae Sinensis Radix (dang gui)

It is the dried product from the root of *Angelica sinensis* (Oliv.) Diels, family Umbelliferae. The medicinal herb is collected in late autumn, applied in crude form or in stir-baked form with liquor.

当归

为伞形科植物当归的干燥根。秋末采挖。生用或酒炙用。

Features Flavor: sweet and pungent. Proper-

性味归经 甘、辛,温。

ty: warm. Meridian tropism: the Liver Meridian, the Heart Meridian and the Spleen Meridian.

归肝、心、脾经。

Actions Reinforce blood, activate blood, regulate menstruation, relieve pain, moisturize intestines and promote defecation.

功效 补血活血，调经止痛，润肠通便。

Application

应用

(1) Blood deficiency pattern. The medicinal herb is sweet, warm and moist in property, and acts to reinforce blood and nourish blood, as the major herb to reinforce blood. In the treatment of blood deficiency pattern manifested by sallow-yellow complexion, dizziness, blurring of vision and palpitation, it is combined with *Rehmanniae Radix Praeparata* (shu di huang), *Chuanxiong Rhizoma* (chuan xiong) and *Paeoniae Radix Alba* (bai shao), to form up Four Agents Decoction (Si Wu Tang). In the treatment of qi and blood deficiency pattern, it is combined with *Astragali Radix* (huang qi) and *Ginseng Radix et Raizoma* (ren shen), to form up Angelica Blood-Nourishing Decoction (Dang Gui Bu Xue Tang).

(1) 血虚诸证。本品甘温质润，功善补血养血，为补血要药。治血虚萎黄、眩晕心悸，常与熟地黄、川芎、白芍同用，即四物汤。若气血两虚者，常与黄芪、人参等同用，如当归补血汤。

(2) Irregular menstruation, dysmenorrhea and amenorrhea. The medicinal herb acts to reinforce blood and activate blood, and to regulate menstruation and stop pain as well, as the major herb for gynecological diseases. In the treatment of irregular menstruation, dysmenorrhea and amenorrhea due to blood deficiency or blood stasis, it is combined with shu di huang, bai shao and chuan xiong, to form up Four Agents Decoction (Si Wu Tang). For those with severe blood stasis, it is advisable to add *Persicae Semen* (tao ren) and *Carthami Flos* (hong hua). For those with severe qi stagnation, it is advisable to add *Cyperi Rhizoma* (xiang fu) and *Corydalis*

(2) 月经不调，痛经经闭。本品既补血活血，又调经止痛，为妇科调经之要药，治血虚或血滞的月经不调、痛经经闭，常与熟地黄、白芍、川芎同用，即四物汤。瘀滞甚者，加桃仁、红花。兼气滞者，加香附、延胡索等。寒凝甚者，加肉桂、艾叶。

Rhizoma (yan hu suo). For those with severe cold coagulation, it is advisable to add *Cinnamomi Cortex* (rou gui) and *Artemisiae Argyi Folium* (ai ye).

(3) Traumatic injury and Bi (Obturation) Pattern due to wind and damp. The medicinal herb acts to reinforce blood and activate blood, and to eliminate cold and stop pain as well. In the treatment of traumatic injury, it is combined with *Olibanum* (ru xiang) and *Myrrha* (mo yao). In the treatment of Bi (Obturation) Pattern due to wind and damp with pain or numbness of body and limbs, it is combined with *Notopterygii Rhizoma et Radix* (qiang huo), *Cinnamomi Ramulus* (gui zhi) and *Gentianae Macrophyllae Radix* (qin jiao).

（3）跌打损伤，风湿痹痛。本品既补血活血、又散寒止痛。治跌打损伤，常配伍乳香、没药等同用。治风湿痹痛、肢体麻木，常与羌活、桂枝、秦艽等同用。

(4) Carbuncle and furuncle. The medicinal herb acts to activate blood and reinforce blood, and to subside swell and stop pain. In the treatment of carbuncle and furuncle in early stage, it is combined with *Lonicerae Japonicae Flos* (jin yin hua), *Forsythiae Fructus* (lian qiao). In the treatment of carbuncle and furuncle in diabrotic stage, it is combined with ren shen, huang qi and shu di huang.

（4）痈疽疮疡。本品能活血补血、消肿止痛。治疮疡初期，常与金银花、连翘等同用。痈疽溃后，可与人参、黄芪、熟地黄等同用。

(5) Constipation due to dryness in intestines. The medicinal herb acts to nourish blood, moisturize intestines and promote defecation. In the treatment of constipation due to blood deficiency or dryness in intestines, it is combined with *Cannabis Fructus* (huo ma ren) and *Cistanchis Herba* (rou cong rong).

（5）肠燥便秘。本品能养血润肠通便。治血虚肠燥便秘，常配伍火麻仁、肉苁蓉等同用。

Usage and dosage Apply 6～12 g in decoction. The medicinal herb is applied in crude form for most conditions, and it acts to activate blood and dredge meridians in stir-baked form with liquor. Furthermore, dang gui body acts to reinforce

用法用量 煎服，6～12克。一般生用，酒炙活血通经。当归身补血，当归尾活血，全当归和血(补血活血)。

blood, dang gui tail acts to activate blood, and whole dang gui acts to harmonize blood (i.e. to reinforce blood and activate blood).

Precautions for use It is prohibited to apply for those with excessive damp in middle energizer or those with loose feces.

使用注意 湿盛中满、大便溏泄者忌服。

Rehmanniae Radix Praeparata (shu di huang)

熟地黄

It is the dried product prepared from *Rehmanniae Radix* (sheng di huang). The medicinal herb is applied in prepared form by steaming.

为生地黄的炮制加工品。蒸制用。

Features Flavor: sweet. Property: slightly warm. Meridian tropism: the Liver Meridian and the Kidney Meridian.

性味归经 甘,微温。归肝、肾经。

Actions Reinforce blood, nourish yin, benefit essence and supplement marrows.

功效 补血滋阴,益精填髓。

Application

应用

(1) Blood deficiency pattern. The medicinal herb is the major herb to reinforce blood. In the treatment of blood deficiency pattern manifested by sallow-yellow complexion, palpitation, dizziness, irregular menstruation, metrorrhagia and metrostaxis, it is combined with *Angelicae Sinensis Radix* (dang gui), *Chuanxiong Rhizoma* (chuan xiong) and *Paeoniae Radix Alba* (bai shao), to form up Four Agents Decoction (Si Wu Tang).

(1) 血虚诸证。本品为补血要药。治血虚萎黄、心悸眩晕、月经不调、崩漏等证,常与当归、川芎、白芍同用,即四物汤。

(2) Kidney yin deficiency pattern. The medicinal herb is the major herb to nourish yin. In the treatment of kidney yin deficiency pattern manifested by tidal fever, nocturnal sweats, seminal emission and diabetes, it is combined with *Corni Fructus* (shan zhu yu) and *Dioscoreae Rhizoma* (shan yao), to form up Rehmannia Pills with Six Ingredients (Liu Wei Di Huang Wan).

(2) 肾阴虚证。本品又为滋阴主药。治肾阴虚的潮热、盗汗、遗精、消渴,常与山萸肉、山药等同用,如六味地黄丸。

(3) Essence and blood deficiency pattern. The medicinal acts to reinforce blood, benefit essence, nourish yin and supplement marrows. In the treatment of essence and blood deficiency pattern manifested by aching and weakness at low back and knees, dizziness, tinnitus and early grey hair, it is combined with *Polygoni Multiflori Radix* (he shou wu), *Lycii Fructus* (gou qi zi) and *Cuscutae Semen* (tu si zi), to form up Seven Jewels and Black Hair Elixir (Qi Bao Mei Ran Dan).

(3) 精血亏虚证。本品能补血益精、滋阴填髓。治精血亏虚的腰膝酸软，眩晕耳鸣，须发早白，常与制何首乌、枸杞子、菟丝子等同用，如七宝美髯丹。

Usage and dosage Apply 9～15 g in decoction.

用法用量 煎服，9～15克。

Precautions for use It is cautious to apply for those with spleen and stomach deficiency, or those with excessive phlegm in middle energizer or those with poor appetite and loose feces.

使用注意 脾胃虚弱，中满痰盛及食少便溏者慎用。

Remarks *Rehmanniae Radix* (sheng di huang) and *Rehmanniae Radix Praeparata* (shu di huang)

按语 生地黄与熟地黄

Both are the products from the root of *Rehmannia glutinosa* Libosch., family Scrophulariaceae and act to nourish yin. Sheng di huang is the fresh and dried product, and cold-cool in property, and acts to clear heat, cool blood, nourish yin and produce fluid. Shu di huang is the prepared product by steaming, and sweet and slightly warm in property, and acts to reinforce blood, benefit essence and supplement marrows.

二药均来源于玄参科地黄，均能滋阴。不同的是生地黄为地黄的干燥品，性偏寒凉，功偏清热凉血，且能养阴生津。熟地黄为蒸制后的加工品，味甘性微温，功偏补血益精填髓。

Polygoni Multiflori Radix (he shou wu)

何首乌

It is the dried product from the tuberous root of *Polygonum multiflorum* Thunb., family Polygonaceae. The medicinal herb is collected in autumn and winter when the leaves are withered, applied in

为蓼科植物何首乌的干燥块根。秋、冬二季叶枯萎时采挖。生用或蒸制用。

crude form or in prepared form by steaming.

Features Flavor: bitter, sweet and astringent. Property: slightly warm. Meridian tropism: the Liver Meridian, the Heart Meridian and the Kidney Meridian.

性味归经 苦、甘、涩，微温。归肝、心、肾经。

Actions Reinforce liver and kidney, benefit essence and blood, blacken hair, strengthen tendons and bones, treat malaria, relieve toxin, moisturize intestines and promote defecation.

功效 补肝肾益精血，乌须发，强筋骨，截疟解毒，润肠通便。

Application

(1) Blood and essence deficiency pattern. The medicinal herb, in neutral property without dryness, acts to reinforce blood, nourish liver, benefit essence, strengthen kidney, blacken hair and strengthen tendons and bones. In the treatment of blood deficiency pattern manifested by dizziness, blurring of vision, palpitation, insomnia, sallow-yellow complexion and fatigue, it is combined with *Angelicae Sinensis Radix* (dang gui), *Paeoniae Radix Alba* (bai shao) and *Rehmanniae Radix Praeparata* (shu di huang). In the treatment of essence deficiency pattern manifested by dizziness, tinnitus, aching and weakness at low back and knees, seminal emission, uterine bleeding, morbid leucorrhea and early grey hair, it is applied singly by soaking in liquor for oral administration, or combined with *Lycii Fructus* (gou qi zi), *Cuscutae Semen* (tu si zi) and *Ecliptae Herba* (mo han lian).

(2) Weak body, chronic malaria, constipation due to dryness in intestines, carbuncle and furuncle, and scrofula. The medicinal herb acts to treat malaria, moisturize intestines and relieve toxin. In the treatment of weak body, chronic malaria and qi and blood consumption, it is combined with *Ginseng*

应用

（1）血虚精亏证。本品能补血养肝，益精固肾，乌须发、强筋骨，且性平不燥。治血虚的头昏目眩，心悸失眠，萎黄乏力，常与当归、白芍、熟地黄等同用。治精亏眩晕耳鸣，腰膝酸软，遗精崩带，须发早白等，可单用浸酒常服，或与枸杞子、菟丝子、墨旱莲等同用。

（2）体虚久疟，肠燥便秘，痈疽、瘰疬。本品能截疟、润肠、解毒。治体虚久疟，气血耗伤者，常配人参、当归等同用，如何人饮。治肠燥便秘，血虚津亏者，与当

Radix et Raizoma (ren shen) and dang gui, to form up Polygoni Multiflori Drink (He Ren Yin). In the treatment of constipation due to dryness in intestines, blood deficiency and fluid deficiency, it is combined with dang gui and *Cannabis Fructus* (huo ma ren). In the treatment of carbuncle and furuncle, it is combined with *Lonicerae Japonicae Flos* (jin yin hua) and *Forsythiae Fructus* (lian qiao). In the treatment of scrofula and tuberculosis, it is combined with *Prunellae Spica* (xia ku cao), *Bulbus Fritillariae Thunbergii* (zhe bei mu) and *Cyperi Rhizoma* (xiang fu).

归、火麻仁等同用。治痈疽疮疡，配金银花、连翘等同用。治瘰疬结核，与夏枯草、浙贝母、香附等同用。

Usage and dosage Apply 6～15 g in decoction. The medicinal herb acts to treat malaria, relieve toxin, moisturize intestines and promote defecation in crude form, and acts to reinforce liver and kidney, benefit essence and blood, blacken hair and strengthen tendons and bones in prepared form.

用法用量 煎服，6～15克。生用截疟、解毒、润肠通便。制用补肝肾益精血，乌须发、强筋骨。

Precautions for use It is not advisable to apply for those with loose feces or those with severe damp-phlegm.

使用注意 大便溏泄及湿痰较重者不宜服。

Appendix *Polygoni Multiflori Caulis* (shou wu teng)

附药 首乌藤

It is the dried product from the stem of *Polygonum multiflorum* Thunb., family Polygonaceae, also called ye jiao teng. The medicinal herb is sweet in flavor, neutral in property and attributive to the Heart Meridian and the Liver Meridian. It acts to nourish blood, calm mind, eliminate wind and dredge collaterals, applied to treat insomnia and dream-disturbed sleep due to heart blood deficiency, aching of whole body, Bi (Obturation) Pattern due to wind and damp and skin itch. Apply 9～15 g in decoction, and apply a proper amount for external use.

为蓼科植物何首乌的干燥藤茎，又名夜交藤。性味甘平。归心、肝经。功能养血安神、祛风通络。适用于心血虚的失眠多梦、身痛，风湿痹痛，皮肤瘙痒。煎服，9～15克。外用适量。

Paeoniae Radix Alba (bai shao)

It is the dried product from the root of *Paeonia Lactiflora* Pall., family ranunculaceae. The medicinal herb is collected in summer and autumn, applied in crude form, or in stir-fried form or in stir-baked form with liquor.

Features Flavor: bitter and sour. Property: slightly cold. Meridian tropism: the Liver Meridian and the Spleen Meridian.

Actions Nourish blood, regulate menstruation, soften liver, stop pain, soothe and inhibit liver yang, hold yin and stop sweating.

Application

(1) Blood deficiency pattern. The medicinal herb acts to nourish blood and regulate menstruation. In the treatment of blood deficiency pattern manifested by sallow-yellow complexion and irregular menstruation, it is combined with *Angelicae Sinensis Radix* (dang gui), *Rehmanniae Radix Praeparata* (shu di huang) and *Chuanxiong Rhizoma* (chuan xiong), to form up Four Agents Decoction (Si Wu Tang).

(2) Headache, dizziness, hypochondriac pain, and spasm and pain at epigastria, abdomen and four limbs. The medicinal herb acts to nourish liver, soften liver, regulate liver, soothe liver, relieve spasm and stop pain. In the treatment of liver yang hyperactivity manifested by headache and dizziness, it is combined with *Rehmanniae Radix* (sheng di huang), *Achyranthis Bidentatae Radix* (niu xi) and *Haliotidis Concha* (shi jue ming). In the treatment of liver qi stagnation manifested by hypochondriac pain, it is combined with dang gui, *Atractylodis*

白芍

为毛茛科植物芍药的干燥根。夏、秋二季采挖。生用或炒用、酒炙用。

性味归经　苦、酸，微寒。归肝、脾经。

功效　养血调经，柔肝止痛，平抑肝阳，敛阴止汗。

应用

（1）血虚证。本品能养血调经。治血虚萎黄、月经不调，常与当归、熟地黄、川芎同用，即四物汤。

（2）头痛眩晕，胁肋疼痛，脘腹四肢拘挛作痛。本品有养肝柔肝，调肝平肝，缓急止痛之效。治肝阳上亢的头痛眩晕，常与生地黄、牛膝、石决明等同用。治肝郁胁痛，常与当归、白术、柴胡等同用，如逍遥散。治脘腹手足挛急疼痛，常配甘草同用，如芍药甘草汤。

Macrocephalae Rhizoma (bai zhu) and *Bupleuri Radix* (chai hu), to form up Free Wanderer Powder (Xiao Yao San). In the treatment of spasm and pain at epigastria, abdomen and four limbs, it is combined with *Glycyrrhizae Radix et Rhizoma* (gan cao), to form up Peony Root and Liquorice Decoction (Shao Yao Gan Cao Tang).

(3) Nocturnal sweats due to yin deficiency and spontaneous sweating due to exterior deficiency. The medicinal herb is sour in flavor and acts to hold yin and stop sweating. In the treatment of nocturnal sweats due to yin deficiency, it is combined with *Rehmanniae Radix* (sheng di huang) and *Ostreae Concha* (mu li). In the treatment of disharmony between Ying (Nutrient) and Wei (Defense) Phases and spontaneous sweating due to exterior deficiency, it is combined with *Cinnamomi Ramulus* (gui zhi), to form up Cinnamon-Twig Decoction (Gui Zhi Tang).

（3）阴虚盗汗，表虚自汗。本品味酸，能敛阴止汗。治阴虚盗汗，可与生地黄、牡蛎等同用。治营卫不和，表虚自汗，常与桂枝配伍，如桂枝汤。

Usage and dosage Apply 6～15 g in decoction. The medicinal herb acts to soothe liver and hold yin in crude form, and acts to nourish blood, soften liver and regulate menstruation in stir-fried form or in stir-baked form with liquor.

用法用量 煎服，6～15克。生用平肝、敛阴，炒用或酒炙养血柔肝、调经。

Precautions for use The medicinal herb is incompatible with *Radix et Rhizoma Veratri Nigri* (li lu).

使用注意 反藜芦。

Asini Corii Colla (e jiao)

阿胶

It is the dried or fresh product from the donkey hide stewed and concentrated as gelatinous mass of *Equus asinus* L., family Equidae. The medicinal herb is applied by smashing into small pieces or by stir-frying with *Gecko* (ge jie) powder.

为马科动物驴的干燥皮或鲜皮，经煎煮、浓缩制成的固体胶。捣碎或以蛤粉烫炒成珠用。

Features Flavor: sweet. Property: neutral. Meridian tropism: the Lung Meridian, the Liver Meridian and the Kidney Meridian.

性味归经 甘，平。归肺、肝、肾经。

Actions Reinforce blood, stanch blood, nourish yin and moisturize body.

功效 补血，止血，滋阴润燥。

Application

应用

(1) Blood deficiency pattern. The medicinal herb is sweet, neutral and moist in property and acts to reinforce blood, as the major herb to reinforce blood. In the treatment of blood deficiency pattern manifested by sallow-yellow complexion, dizziness and palpitation, it is applied singly by stewing with yellow millet wine, or combined with *Rehmanniae Radix Praeparata* (shu di huang), *Angelicae Sinensis Radix* (dang gui) and *Astragali Radix* (huang qi).

（1）血虚证。本品甘平质润，善能补血，为补血之佳品。治血虚萎黄，眩晕心悸，可单用黄酒炖服，或与熟地黄、当归、黄芪等同用。

(2) Bleeding pattern. The medicinal herb acts to stanch blood. In the treatment of bleeding pattern with yin deficiency or blood deficiency, it is applied singly or combined with other medicinal herbs according to patterns.

（2）出血证。本品又能止血，且效佳。尤宜于出血兼阴虚、血虚者，单用即可，或随证配伍其他药物同用。

(3) Yin deficiency pattern. The medicinal herb acts to nourish yin and moisturize body. In the treatment of lung yin deficiency with fire manifested by panting, cough, dry throat, scanty sputum or bloody sputum, it is combined with *Arctii Fructus* (niu bang zi) and *Armeniacae Amarum Semen* (ku xing ren), to form up Lung-Reinforcing Ass-Hide Glue Decoction (Bu Fei E Jiao Tang). In the treatment of dryness in lung manifested by dry cough without sputum, it is combined with *Ophiopogonis Radix* (mai dong) and ku xing ren. In the treatment of febrile disease consuming yin manifested by restlessness and insomnia, it is combined with *Coptidis Rhizoma* (huang lian), *Paeoniae*

（3）阴虚证。本品功善滋阴润燥。治肺虚火盛、喘咳咽干痰少或痰中带血，与牛蒡子、苦杏仁等同用，如补肺阿胶汤。治肺燥干咳无痰，可与麦冬、杏仁等同用。治热病伤阴，虚烦不眠，可与黄连、白芍、鸡子黄等同用，如黄连阿胶汤。治热病伤阴，虚风内动，手足瘈疭，可与龟甲、牡蛎、白芍等同用。

Radix Alba (bai shao) and *Egg Yolk* (ji zi huang), to form up Coptis and Ass-Hide Glue Decoction (Huang Lian E Jiao Tang). In the treatment of febrile disease consuming yin and producing endogenous wind manifested by twitching and spasm of hand and foot, it is combined with *Plastrum Testudinis* (gui jia), *Ostreae Concha* (mu li) and bai shao.

Usage and dosage Apply 3～9 g by melting for oral administration. The medicinal herb acts to moisturize lung in stirfried form with ge jie powder.

Precautions for use It is prohibited to apply for those with stomach weakness or those with loose feces.

用法用量 3～9克，烊化兑服。蛤粉炒阿胶用于润肺。

使用注意 胃弱便溏者忌服。

Section 4 Yin-reinforcing herbs

第4节 补阴药

Glehniae Radix (bei sha shen)

It is the dried product from the root of *Glehnia littoralis* Fr. Schmidt ex Miq., family Umbelliferae. The medicinal herb is collected in summer and autumn, applied in crude form.

Features Flavor: sweet and slightly bitter. Property: slightly cold. Meridian tropism: the Lung Meridian and the Stomach Meridian.

Actions Nourish yin, purify lung, benefit stomach and produce fluid.

Application

(1) Cough due to dryness in lung, cough with bloody sputum due to lung yin deficiency. The medicinal herb acts to nourish lung yin and eliminate dryness and heat. In the treatment of cough due to

北沙参

为伞形科植物珊瑚菜的干燥根。夏、秋两季采挖。生用。

性味归经 甘、微苦，微寒。归肺、胃经。

功效 养阴清肺，益胃生津。

应用

（1）肺燥咳嗽，劳嗽痰血。本品有养肺阴、清燥热之功。治肺燥咳嗽，常与麦冬、玉竹、冬桑叶等同用，如

dryness in lung, it is combined with *Ophiopogonis Radix* (mai dong), *Polygonati Odorati Rhizoma* (yu zhu) and *Mori Folium* (sang ye), to form up Glehnia and Ophiopogon Decoction (Sha Shen Mai Dong Tang). In the treatment of cough due to yin deficiency or chronic cough with bloody sputum, it is combined with *Anemarrhenae Rhizoma* (zhi mu), *Fritillariae Cirrhosae Bulbus* (chuan bei mu) and *Ophiopogonis Radix* (mai dong).

沙参麦冬汤。治阴虚劳嗽，久咳痰血，常知母、川贝母、麦冬等同用。

(2) Thirst due to fluid consumption. The medicinal herb acts to nourish stomach yin, reduce heat in stomach and produce fluid. In the treatment of thirst due to stomach yin deficiency, or thirst and dry throat due to febrile disease consuming fluid, it is applied singly by decocting for oral administration, or combined with mai dong and *Dendrobii Herba* (shi hu).

（2）津伤口渴。本品能养胃阴、清胃热、生津液。常用于胃阴虚之口渴，或热病伤津的口渴咽干，可单用水煎服用，或与麦冬、石斛等同用。

Usage and dosage Apply 5～12 g in decoction.

用法用量 煎服，5～12克。

Precautions for use The medicinal herb is incompatible with *Radix et Rhizoma Veratri Nigri* (li lu).

使用注意 反藜芦。

Appendix *Adenophorae Radix* (nan sha shen)

It is the dried product from the root of *Adenophora tetraphylla* (Thunb.) Fisch., or *Adenophora stricta* Miq., family Campanulaceae. The medicinal herb is sweet in flavor, slightly cold in property and attributive to the Lung Meridian and the Stomach Meridian. It acts to nourish yin, purify lung, benefit stomach, produce fluid, dissolve phlegm and benefit qi, applied to treat dry cough due to heat in lung, dry cough with scanty sputum due to yin deficiency, and thirst due to stomach yin deficiency or due to qi and yin deficiency. Apply 9～15 g in de-

附药 南沙参

为桔梗科植物轮叶沙参或沙参的干燥根，味甘性微寒。归肺、胃经。功能养阴清肺，益胃生津，化痰，益气。适用于肺热燥咳、阴虚劳嗽的干咳少痰，胃阴虚或气阴两虚的口渴。煎服，9～15克。反藜芦。

coction. The medicinal herb is incompatible with *Radix et Rhizoma Veratri Nigri* (li lu).

Ophiopogonis Radix (mai dong)

It is the dried product from the tuberous root of *Ophiopogon japonicus* (L. f.) Ker-Gawl., family Liliaceae, also called mai men dong. The medicinal herb is collected in summer, applied in crude form.

Features Flavor: sweet and slightly bitter. Property: slightly cold. Meridian tropism: the Heart Meridian, the Lung Meridian and the Stomach Meridian.

Actions Nourish yin, moisturize lung, benefit stomach, produce fluid, purify heart and relieve restlessness.

Application

(1) Cough due to dryness in lung and cough with bloody sputum due to lung yin deficiency. The medicinal herb acts to nourish lung yin, reduce heat in lung and moisturize lung. In the treatment of dry cough with sticky sputum and dry throat and nose, it is combined with *Mori Folium* (sang ye), *Armeniacae Amarum Semen* (ku xing ren) and *Asini Corii Colla* (e jiao), to form up Dryness-Eliminating and Lung-Rescuing Decoction (Qing Zao Jiu Fei Tang). In the treatment of cough with bloody sputum due to lung yin deficiency, it is combined with *Asparagi Radix* (tian dong), to form up Asparagus and Ophiopogon Ointment (Er Dong Gao).

(2) Thirst due to yin deficiency and constipation due to dryness in intestines. The medicinal herb acts to benefit stomach, produce fluid, reduce heat and moisturize intestines. In the treatment of stomach yin insufficiency pattern, it is combined with

麦冬

为百合科植物麦冬的干燥块根。又名麦门冬。夏季采挖。生用。

性味归经 甘、微苦，微寒。归心、肺、胃经。

功效 养阴润肺，益胃生津，清心除烦。

应用

（1）肺燥咳嗽，劳嗽咳血。本品有养肺阴、清肺热、润肺燥之功。治燥咳痰黏、咽干鼻燥，常与桑叶、杏仁、阿胶等配伍，如清燥救肺汤。治阴虚劳嗽咳血，常配天冬，即二冬膏。

（2）阴虚口渴，大便燥结。本品功善益胃生津、清热润燥，为治胃阴不足之佳品，常配玉竹、沙参等同用。若治津伤便秘，常与玄参、生

Polygonati Odorati Rhizoma (yu zhu) and *Glehniae Radix* (bei sha shen). In the treatment of constipation due to fluid consumption, it is combined with *Scrophulariae Radix* (xuan shen) and *Rehmanniae Radix* (sheng di huang), to form up Humor-Increasing Decoction (Zeng Ye Tang).

地黄等同用,如增液汤。

(3) Restlessness and insomnia. The medicinal herb acts to nourish yin, purify heart, relieve restlessness and calm mind. In the treatment of restlessness and insomnia due to yin deficiency with heat, it is combined with *Rehmanniae Radix* (sheng di huang) and *Ziziphi Spinosae Semen* (suan zao ren). In the treatment of pathogenic heat disturbing heart and Ying (Nutrient) Phase manifested by feverish sensation in body and restlessness, it is combined with *Coptidis Rhizoma* (huang lian), sheng di huang and *Lophatheri Herba* (dan zhu ye).

(3) 心烦不眠。本品能养阴清心、除烦安神。治阴虚有热的心烦不眠,常与生地黄、酸枣仁等同用。治邪扰心营,身热烦躁,常与黄连、生地黄、淡竹叶等同用。

Usage and dosage Apply 6～12 g in decoction.

用法用量 煎服,6～12克。

Precautions for use It is cautious to apply for those with spleen deficiency and loose feces.

使用注意 脾虚便溏者慎用。

Asparagi Radix (tian dong)

天冬

It is the dried product from the tuberous root of *Asparagus cochincchinensis* (Lour.) Merr., family Liliaceae, also called tian men dong. The medicinal herb is collected in autumn and winter, applied in crude form.

为百合科植物天冬的干燥块根。又名天门冬。秋、冬二季采挖。生用。

Features Flavor: sweet and bitter. Property: cold. Meridian tropism: the Lung Meridian and the Kidney Meridian.

性味归经 甘、苦,寒。归肺、肾经。

Actions Nourish yin, moisturize body, reduce fire and produce fluid.

功效 养阴润燥,清火,生津。

Application

(1) Cough due to dryness in lung and cough with bloody sputum due to lung yin deficiency. The medicinal herb is sweet, bitter, moist and cold in property and acts to reduce heat, nourish yin, purify lung, moisturize body and stop cough. In the treatment of cough due to dryness and heat, it is applied singly by making into ointment, or combined with *Ophiopogonis Radix* (mai dong), *Glehniae Radix* (bei sha shen) and *Fritillariae Cirrhosae Bulbus* (chuan bei mu). In the treatment of hemoptysis due to lung yin deficiency, or dry cough with sticky sputum or with bloody sputum, it is combined with mai dong, to form up Asparagus and Ophiopogon Ointment (Er Dong Gao), or combined with chuan bei mu, *Rehmanniae Radix* (sheng di huang) and *Asini Corii Colla* (e jiao).

(2) Kidney yin deficiency pattern. The medicinal herb acts to nourish kidney yin and reduce false fire. In the treatment of kidney yin deficiency and fire hyperactivity manifested by tidal fever, seminal emission, and aching and weakness at low back and knees, it is combined with *Rehmanniae Radix Praeparata* (shu di huang), *Anemarrhenae Rhizoma* (zhi mu) and *Phellodendri Cortex Chiensis* (huang bo).

(3) Diabetes and constipation due to dryness in intestines. The medicinal herb acts to nourish yin, reduce heat and produce fluid. In the treatment of diabetes due to yin deficiency or thirst due to febrile disease consuming fluid, it is combined with *Rehmanniae Radix* (sheng di huang) and *Ginseng Radix et Raizoma* (ren shen), to form up Three Talents Decoction (San Cai Tang). In the treatment of con-

应用

（1）肺燥咳嗽，劳嗽咳血。本品甘润苦泄，性寒清热，具养阴清肺，润燥止咳之功。治燥热咳嗽，单用熬膏，或与麦冬、沙参、川贝母等同用。治劳嗽咳血，或干咳痰黏，痰中带血，可与麦冬同用，如二冬膏，或配川贝母、生地黄、阿胶等同用。

（2）肾阴虚证。本品有滋肾阴、清虚火之功。治肾虚火旺，潮热遗精、腰膝酸软，常与熟地黄、知母、黄柏等同用。

（3）消渴证，肠燥便秘。本品具养阴、清热、生津之功。治阴虚消渴或热病伤津口渴，可与生地黄、人参等同用，如三才汤。治津伤便秘，可与生地黄、玄参等配伍。

stipation due to fluid consumption, it is combined with sheng di huang and *Scrophulariae Radix* (xuan shen).

Usage and dosage Apply 6～12 g in decoction.

Precautions for use It is cautious to apply for those with spleen deficiency and loose feces.

用法用量 煎服，6～12克。

使用注意 脾虚便溏者慎用。

Polygonati Rhizoma (huang jing)

黄精

It is the dried product from the rhizoma of *Polygonatum sibiricum* Red., or *Polygonatum kingianum* Coll. et Hemsl. or *Polygonatum cyrtonema* Hua, family Liliaceae. The medicinal herb is collected in spring and autumn, applied in crude form or in prepared form with liquor.

为百合科植物黄精、滇黄精或多花黄精的干燥根茎。春、秋二季采挖。生用或酒制用。

Features Flavor: sweet. Property: neutral. Meridian tropism: the Spleen Meridian, the Lung Meridian and the Kidney Meridian.

性味归经 甘，平。归脾、肺、肾经。

Actions Reinforce qi, nourish yin, moisturize lung, strengthen spleen and benefit kidney.

功效 补气养阴，润肺，健脾，益肾。

Application

应用

(1) Spleen and stomach deficiency pattern. The medicinal herb is sweet and neutral in property and acts to reinforce spleen qi and benefit spleen yin. In the treatment of spleen and stomach qi deficiency pattern manifested by fatigue, lassitude and poor appetite, it is combined with *Codonopsis Radix* (dang shen) and *Atractylodis Macrocephalae Rhizoma* (bai zhu). In the treatment of spleen and stomach yin deficiency pattern manifested by dry mouth and poor appetite, it is combined with *Dendrobii Herba* (shi hu), *Ophiopogonis Radix* (mai dong) and *Dioscoreae Rhizoma* (shan yao).

（1）脾胃虚弱证。本品甘补性平，能补脾气、益脾阴。治脾胃气虚的倦怠乏力、食欲不振，可与党参、白术等同用。治脾胃阴虚，口干食少，可与石斛、麦冬、山药等同用。

(2) Dry cough due to lung deficiency and cough

（2）肺虚燥咳，劳嗽咳

with bloody sputum due to lung yin deficiency. The medicinal herb acts to nourish yin of lung and kidney and moisturize lung and kidney. In the treatment of dry cough due to lung deficiency, it is applied singly by making into ointment, or combined with *Glehniae Radix* (bei sha shen), *Fritillariae Cirrhosae Bulbus* (chuan bei mu) and *Anemarrhenae Rhizoma* (zhi mu). In the treatment of chronic cough due to lung and kidney deficiency, it is combined with *Rehmanniae Radix Praeparata* (shu di huang), *Asparagi Radix* (tian dong) and *Stemonae Radix* (bai bu).

血。本品能滋肺肾阴，润肺肾之燥。治肺虚燥咳，可单用熬膏服，或配沙参、川贝母、知母等同用。治肺肾两虚，劳嗽久咳，可配伍熟地黄、天冬、百部等同用。

(3) Kidney deficiency and essence depletion pattern. The medicinal herb acts to reinforce kidney and benefit essence. In the treatment of kidney deficiency and essence depletion pattern manifested by aching and weakness at low back and knees, and early grey hair, it is combined with *Lycii Fructus* (gou qi zi) and prepared *Polygoni Multiflori Radix* (he shou wu).

(3) 肾虚精亏证。本品善补肾益精，为治肾虚精亏所常用。治肾虚精亏，症见腰膝酸软、须发早白，常与枸杞子、制何首乌等同用。

Furthermore, the medicinal herb also acts to treat diabetes.

此外，本品尚治消渴证。

Usage and dosage Apply 9～15 g in decoction. The medicinal herb is stronger in its reinforcing action in prepared form with liquor.

用法用量 煎服，9～15克。酒制补虚力强。

Precautions for use It is cautious to apply for those with spleen deficiency with dampness, or cough with excessive sputum, or loose feces.

使用注意 脾虚有湿，咳嗽痰多，大便溏薄者慎用。

Polygonati Odorati Rhizoma (yu zhu)

玉竹

It is the dried product from the rhizoma of *Polygonatum odoratum* (Mill.) Druce, family Liliaceae. The medicinal herb is collected in autumn, applied in crude form.

为百合科植物玉竹的干燥根茎。秋季采挖。生用。

Features Flavor: sweet. Property: slightly cold. Meridian tropism: the Lung Meridian and the Stomach Meridian.

性味归经 甘，微寒。归肺、胃经。

Actions Nourish yin, moisturize body, produce fluid and relieve thirst.

功效 养阴润燥，生津止渴。

Application

应用

(1) Yin deficiency and dryness in lung. The medicinal herb is sweet, moist and cool in property and acts to nourish lung yin, moisturize lung and stop cough. In the treatment of dry cough with scanty sputum due to yin deficiency, it is combined with *Glehniae Radix* (bei sha shen), *Ophiopogonis Radix* (mai dong) and *Mori Folium* (sang ye).

(1) 阴虚肺燥。本品甘润性凉，能养肺阴、润肺燥而止咳。治阴虚燥咳、干咳少痰，常与沙参、麦冬、桑叶等同用。

(2) Thirst due to fluid consumption and diabetes. The medicinal herb acts to nourish stomach yin, reduce heat, produce fluid and relieve thirst. In the treatment of febrile disease consuming fluid manifested by restlessness, feverish sensation and thirst, it is combined with *Rehmanniae Radix* (sheng di huang) and mai dong, to form up Stomach-Benefiting Decoction (Yi Wei Tang). In the treatment of diabetes, it is combined with sheng di huang and *Trichosanthis Radix* (tian hua fen).

(2) 伤津口渴，消渴。本品善能滋养胃阴、清热生津止渴。治热病伤津的烦热口渴，常配伍生地黄、麦冬等同用，如益胃汤。治消渴，可与生地黄、天花粉等同用。

Furthermore, the medicinal herb also acts to nourish yin without keeping pathogen inside, applied to treat yin deficiency with exogenous pathogen attack.

此外，还用治阴虚外感，具养阴不恋邪之特点。

Usage and dosage Apply 6～12 g in decoction.

用法用量 煎服，6～12克。

Precautions for use It is prohibited to apply for those with spleen deficiency and damp-phlegm.

使用注意 脾虚湿痰者忌服。

Dendrobii Herba (shi hu)

石斛

It is the fresh and dried product from the stem

为兰科植物金钗石斛、

of the perennial herbage *Dendrobium nobil* Lindll., or *Dendrobium chrysanthum* Lindl., or *Dendrobium fimbriatum* HooK., family Orchidaceae and other plants of the same genus. The medicinal herb is collected all over the year, better in period from late spring to early summer and in autumn, applied in crude form.

鼓槌石斛或流苏石斛的栽培品及其同属植物近似种的新鲜或干燥茎。全年均可采收,以春末夏初和秋季采收为佳。生用。

Features Flavor: sweet. Property: slightly cold. Meridian tropism: the Stomach Meridian and the Kidney Meridian.

性味归经 甘,微寒。归胃、肾经。

Actions Benefit stomach, produce fluid, nourish yin and clear heat.

功效 益胃生津,滋阴清热。

Application

应用

(1) Stomach yin insufficiency pattern, and febrile disease consuming fluid. The medicinal herb acts to nourish stomach yin, reduce heat in stomach and produce fluid. In the treatment of stomach yin deficiency pattern manifested by dry mouth and poor appetite, it is applied singly by making into tea for oral administration, or combined with *Ophiopogonis Radix* (mai dong) and *Rehmanniae Radix* (sheng di huang). In the treatment of thirst due to febrile disease consuming fluid, it is combined with *Trichosanthis Radix* (tian hua fen) and *Puerariae Lobatae Radix* (ge gen).

(1) 胃阴不足,热病伤津。本品善养胃阴、清胃热、生津液。治胃阴虚口干食少,可单用煎汤代茶,或与麦冬、生地黄等同用。治热病伤津口渴,可与天花粉、葛根等同用。

(2) Kidney yin deficiency pattern, or false heat pattern after severe disease. The medicinal herb acts to nourish kidney yin and reduce false heat. In the treatment of kidney yin insufficiency pattern or yin deficiency and fire hyperactivity pattern manifested by feverish sensation in body and tidal fever, it is combined with sheng di huang and *Anemarrhenae Rhizoma* (zhi mu). In the treatment of constant false heat after febrile disease, it is combined with

(2) 肾阴虚证,病后虚热。本品能滋肾阴、清虚热。治肾阴不足,阴虚火旺,骨蒸潮热,常与生地黄、知母等同用。治热病病后虚热不退,可与地骨皮、白薇等同用。

Lycii Cortex (di gu pi) and *Cynanchi Atrati Radix et Rhizoma* (bai wei).

Furthermore, the medicinal herb acts to reinforce kidney, nourish liver, brighten eyes and strengthen tendons and bones, applied to treat dim eyesight and blurring of vision, and flaccidity and weakness of tendons and bones.

此外，本品尚能补肾养肝明目、强筋骨作用，可用于目暗不明，筋骨痿软等证。

Usage and dosage Apply 6～12 g in decoction. Apply 15～30 g in fresh form.

用法用量 煎服，6～12 克。鲜用 15～30 克。

Precautions for use It is not advisable to apply for those with febrile disease in early stage. It is prohibited to apply for those with excess pattern of damp-heat.

使用注意 温热病初期不宜，湿热实证忌服。

Lycii Fructus (gou qi zi)

枸杞子

It is the dried product from the ripe fruit of *Lycium barbarum* L., family Solanaceae. The medicinal herb is collected in summer and autumn when the fruits are becoming red, applied in crude form.

为茄科植物宁夏枸杞干燥成熟果实。夏、秋二季果实呈红色时采收。生用。

Features Flavor: sweet. Property: neutral. Meridian tropism: the Liver Meridian and the Kidney Meridian.

性味归经 甘，平。归肝、肾经。

Actions Nourish and reinforce liver and kidney, benefit essence and brighten eyes.

功效 滋补肝肾，益精明目。

Application

Liver and kidney deficiency pattern. The medicinal herb is sweet and neutral in property and attributive to the Liver and Kidney Meridians, and acts to reinforce liver and kidney, benefit essence and blood, and brighten eyes the good herb to nourish and reinforce liver and kidney and to reinforce essence and brighten eyes. In the treatment of liver and kidney deficiency pattern, it is applied singly or combined with other medicinal herbs. In the treatment of kidney deficiency manifested by semi-

应用

肝肾亏虚证。本品味甘性平，入肝肾经，功善补肝肾、益精血、明目，为滋补肝肾、补精明目之良药。治肝肾亏虚证，可单用，或配伍其他药物同用。治肾虚遗精，腰膝酸软，常与生地黄、天冬等同用。治肝肾两虚，目暗不明，常配菊花、熟地黄等同

nal emission, aching and weakness at low back and knees, it is combined with *Rehmanniae Radix* (sheng di huang) and *Asparagi Radix* (tian dong). In the treatment of liver and kidney deficiency manifested by blurring of vision, it is combined with *Chrysanthemi Flos* (ju hua) and *Radix Rehmanniae preparata* (shu di huang), to form up Lycium, Chrysanthemun and Rehmannia Pills (Qi Ju Di Huang Wan). In the treatment of diabetes due to yin deficiency, it is combined with *Ophiopogonis Radix* (mai dong) and *Trichosanthis Radix* (tian hua fen).

用,如杞菊地黄丸。治阴虚消渴,可与麦冬、天花粉等同用。

Usage and dosage Apply 6～12 g in decoction.

用法用量 煎服,6～12克。

Remarks *Lycii Cortex* (di gu pi) and *Lycii Fructus* (gou qi zi)

按语 地骨皮与枸杞子

Both the herbs are the products from *Lycium barbarum* L., family Solanaceae. Di gu pi is the product from the root cortex, sweet and cold in property and attributive to the Lung, Liver and Kidney Meridians, acting to cool blood, reduce false heat and purify lung, as the false heat-clearing herb, and the true heat-clearing herb as well. Gou qi zi is the product from the fruit, sweet and neutral in property and attributive to the Liver and Kidney Meridians, acting to nourish and reinforce liver and kidney, and to brighten eyes, as a reinforcing herb.

二药均来源于茄科宁夏枸杞。不同的是地骨皮以根皮入药,性味甘寒,入肺肝肾经,功能凉血退蒸、清肺,为既清虚热、又清实热之品。枸杞子以成熟果实入药,性味甘平,入肝、肾经,功能滋补肝肾、明目,为滋补之品。

Ecliptae Herba (mo han lian)

墨旱莲

It is the dried product from the herb of *Eclipta prostrate* L., family Compositae, also called han lian cao. The medicinal herb is collected in summer and autumn when it is flowering, applied in crude form.

为菊科植物鳢肠的干燥地上部分。又称旱莲草。花开时采割。生用。

Features Flavor: sweet and sour. Property: cold. Meridian tropism: the Liver Meridian and the Kidney Meridian.

性味归经 甘、酸,寒。归肝、肾经。

Actions Nourish and reinforce liver and kidney, cool blood and stanch blood.

功效 滋补肝肾,凉血止血。

Application

应用

(1) Liver and kidney yin deficiency pattern. The medicinal herb is sweet, moist and cool in property and attributive to the Liver and Kidney Meridians, and acts to nourish kidney and reinforce liver. In the treatment of liver and kidney yin deficiency manifested by dizziness, blurring vision and early grey hair, it is combined with *Ligustri Lucidi Fructus* (nü zhen zi), to form up Double Supreme Pills (Er Zhi Wan).

(1) 肝肾阴虚证。本品甘润性凉,入肝肾经,具滋肾补肝之功。治肝肾阴虚、头晕目眩、须发早白,常与女贞子同用,即二至丸。

(2) Bleeding pattern due to yin deficiency and heat in blood. The medicinal herb acts to nourish yin, cool blood and stanch blood. In the treatment of yin deficiency and heat in blood manifested by spitting blood, epistaxis, bloody urine, blood feces, metrorrhagia and metrostaxis, it is applied singly or combined with *Rehmanniae Radix* (sheng di huang), *Asini Corii Colla* (e jiao) and *Typhae Pollen* (pu huang). It is advisable to smash the fresh product for external use to stanch blood due to traumatic injury.

(2) 阴虚血热的出血证。本品既滋阴,又凉血止血。治阴虚血热的吐衄、尿血、便血、崩漏,可单用,或与生地黄、阿胶、蒲黄等同用。鲜品捣烂外敷,可止外伤出血。

Usage and dosage Apply 6～12 g in decoction. Apply a proper amount for external use.

用法用量 煎服,6～12克。外用适量。

Precautions for use It is prohibited to apply for those with spleen and stomach deficiency and cold and those with loose feces.

使用注意 脾胃虚寒、大便泄泻者忌用。

Ligustri Lucidi Fructus (nü zhen zi)

女贞子

It is the dried product from the ripe fruit of *Ligustrum lucidum* Ait., family Oleaceae. The medicinal herb is collected in winter, applied in crude form or in liquor-prepared form.

为木犀科植物女贞的干燥成熟果实。冬季采收。生用或酒制用。

Features Flavor: sweet and bitter. Property: cool. Meridian tropism: the Liver Meridian and the Kidney Meridian.

性味归经 甘、苦,凉。归肝、肾经。

Actions Nourish and reinforce liver and kidney, brighten eyes and blacken hair.

功效 滋补肝肾,明目乌发。

Application

Liver and kidney yin deficiency pattern. The medicinal herb is sweet and cool in property and acts to nourish and reinforce yin of liver and kidney, brighten eyes, blacken hair and reduce false heat with its moderate nature. In the treatment of liver and kidney yin deficiency manifested by dizziness, tinnitus, aching and weakness at low back and knees, it is combined with *Rehmanniae Radix Praeparata* (shu di huang) and *Cuscutae Semen* (tu si zi). In the treatment of blurring of vision, it is combined with *Lycii Fructus* (gou qi zi) and *Chrysanthemi Flos* (ju hua). In the treatment of early grey hair, it is combined with *Ecliptae Herba* (mo han lian). In the treatment of fever due to yin deficiency, it is combined with *Lycii Cortex* (di gu pi) and *Rehmanniae Radix* (sheng di huang).

应用

肝肾阴虚证。本品甘补性凉,功善滋补肝肾之阴、明目乌发、清退虚热,惟药力平和。治肝肾阴虚、眩晕耳鸣、腰膝酸软,可与熟地黄、菟丝子等配伍。治目暗不明,常与枸杞子、菊花等同用。治须发早白,常配墨旱莲等同用。治阴虚发热,可与地骨皮、生地黄等同用。

Usage and dosage Apply 6～12 g in decoction. The medicinal herb has a stronger action to reinforce and benefit liver and kidney in liquor-prepared form.

用法用量 煎服,6～12克。酒制可增补益肝肾之力。

Precautions for use It is prohibited to apply for those with spleen and stomach deficiency and

使用注意 脾胃虚寒泄泻及阳虚者忌服。

cold, diarrhea and yang deficiency.

Testudinis Carapax et Plastrum (gui jia)

It is the dried product from the carapace and plastron of *Chinemys reevesii* (Gray), family Testudinidae. The medicinal herb is collected all over the year, more commonly in autumn and winter, applied in crude form, or in stir-fried form with sand in quenched form with vinegar.

Features Flavor: salty and sweet. Property: slightly cold. Meridian tropism: the Liver Meridian, the Kidney Meridian and the Heart Meridian.

Actions Nourish yin, subdue yang, benefit kidney, strengthen bones, regulate menstruation, stanch blood, nourish blood and reinforce heart.

Application

(1) Yin deficiency and internal heat pattern, yin deficiency and yang hyperactivity pattern and yin deficiency inducing wind pattern. The medicinal herb is sweet and salty in flavor and cool in property, and acts to nourish and reinforce yin of liver and kidney, soothe liver, subdue yang and eliminate wind. In the treatment of yin deficiency and internal heat pattern manifested by feverish sensation and nocturnal sweats, it is combined with *Rehmanniae Radix Praeparata* (shu di huang), *Anemarrhenae Rhizoma* (zhi mu) and *Phellodendri Cortex Chiensis* (huang bo), to form up Great Yin Supplementation Pills (Da Bu Yin Wan). In the treatment of yin deficiency and yang hyperactivity pattern manifested by dizziness and blurring of vision, it is combined with *Rehmanniae Radix* (sheng di huang), *Haliotidis Concha* (shi jue ming) and *Chrysanthemi Flos* (ju hua).

龟甲

为龟科动物乌龟的背甲及腹甲。全年均可捕捉，以秋、冬二季为多。剥取甲壳。生用或砂炒醋淬用。

性味归经 咸、甘，微寒。归肝、肾、心经。

功效 滋阴潜阳，益肾健骨，固经止血，养血补心。

应用

（1）阴虚内热，阴虚阳亢，阴虚风动等证。本品甘咸性凉，功善滋补肝肾之阴，平肝潜阳息风。治阴虚内热、骨蒸盗汗，常与熟地黄、知母、黄柏等同用，如大补阴丸。治阴虚阳亢、头晕目眩，可与生地黄、石决明、菊花等同用。

(2) Kidney deficiency pattern manifested by flaccidity and weakness of tendons and bones. The medicinal herb acts to reinforce blood, nourish yin, benefit kidney and strengthen bones. In the treatment of kidney deficiency pattern manifested by flaccidity and weakness of tendons and bones, and inclosure of infant's fontanel, it is combined with shu di huang, *Herba Cynomorli* (suo yang) and *Achyranthis Bidentatae Radix* (niu xi).

（2）肾虚筋骨痿软。本品能补血滋阴，益肾健骨。治肾虚筋骨痿软，小儿囟门不合等证，与熟地黄、锁阳、牛膝等同用。

(3) Metrorrhagia, metrostaxis and heavy blood flow in menstruation. The medicinal herb acts to reinforce liver and kidney, strengthen Thoroughfare and Conception Vessels, reduce heat and stanch blood. In the treatment of yin deficiency with heat pattern manifested by metrorrhagia, metrostaxis and heavy blood flow in menstruation, it is combined with huang bo and *Cyperi Rhizoma* (xiang fu).

（3）崩漏，月经过多。本品能补肝肾、固冲任，清热止血。治阴虚有热的崩漏下血，月经过多，可与黄柏、香附等同用。

(4) Fearful throbbing and insomnia. The medicinal herb acts to nourish blood and reinforce heart. In the treatment of fearful throbbing, insomnia, poor memory and dream-disturbed sleep, it is combined with *Os Draconis* (long gu) and *Polygalae Radix* (yuan zhi).

（4）惊悸失眠。本品能养血补心。治心虚惊悸失眠、健忘多梦，常与龙骨、远志等配伍。

Usage and dosage Apply 15～30 g in decoction. Apply it in crude form and decoct first.

用法用量 煎服，15～30克。生用宜先煎。

Precautions for use It is prohibited to apply for those with spleen and stomach deficiency and cold. It is cautious to apply for pregnant women.

使用注意 脾胃虚寒者忌服。孕妇慎用。

Trionycis Carapax (bie jia)

鳖甲

It is the dried product from the shell of *Trionyx sinensis* Wiegmann, family Trionychidae. The medicinal herb is collected all over the year, more

为鳖科动物鳖的背甲。全年均可捕捉。以秋、冬二季为多。剥取背甲。生用或

commonly in autumn and winter, applied in crude form, or in stir-fried form with sand in quenched form with vinegar.

砂炒后醋淬用。

Features Flavor: salty. Property: slightly cold. Meridian tropism: the Liver Meridian and the Kidney Meridian.

性味归经 咸,微寒。归肝、肾经。

Actions Nourish yin, subdue yang, reduce heat, relieve feverish sensation, soften the hard and relieve stasis.

功效 滋阴潜阳,退热除蒸,软坚散结。

Application

应用

(1) Yin deficiency and internal heat pattern, yin deficiency and yang hyperactivity pattern and yin deficiency inducing wind pattern. The medicinal herb acts to nourish yin, clear heat, subdue yang, eliminate wind, reduce heat and relieve feverish sensation. In the treatment of fever due to yin deficiency, it is combined with *Artemisiae Annuae Herba* (qing hao), *Gentianae Macrophyllae Radix* (qin jiao) and *Anemarrhenae Rhizoma* (zhi mu), to form up Sweet Wormwood and Turtle Shell Decoction (Qing Hao Bie Jia Tang) and Large-Leaved Gentian and Turtle Shell Powder (Qin Jiao Bie Jia San). In the treatment of yin deficiency and yang hyperactivity pattern manifested by dizziness and blurring of vision, it is combined with *Rehmanniae Radix* (sheng di huang), *Ostreae Concha* (mu li) and *Chrysanthemi Flos* (ju hua). In the treatment of yin deficiency inducing wind pattern due to febrile disease consuming yin manifested by twitching of hand and foot, it is combined with sheng di huang, *Testudinis Carapax et Plastrum* (gui jia) and *Ostreae Concha* (mu li).

(1) 阴虚发热,阴虚阳亢,阴虚风动等证。本品能滋阴清热,潜阳息风,退热除蒸。尤为治阴虚发热的要药,常与青蒿、秦艽、知母等,如青蒿鳖甲汤、秦艽鳖甲散等。治阴虚阳亢,头晕目眩,配生地黄、牡蛎、菊花等同用。治热病伤阴,阴虚风动,手足蠕动,常配伍生地黄、龟甲、牡蛎等同用。

(2) Abdominal masses. The medicinal herb acts to soften the hard and relieve stasis. In the treat-

(2) 癥瘕积聚。本品能软坚散结。治癥瘕积聚,常

ment of abdominal masses, it is combined with *Bupleuri Radix* (chai hu), *Moutan Cortex* (mu dan pi), to form up Turtle Shell Decoction Pills (Bie Jia Jian Wan).

与柴胡、牡丹皮等同用，如鳖甲煎丸。

Usage and dosage Apply 15～30 g in decoction. Apply it in crude form and decoct first.

用法用量 煎服，15～30克。生用宜先煎。

Precautions for use It is prohibited to apply for those with spleen and stomach deficiency and cold, poor appetite, loose feces and pregnant women.

使用注意 脾胃虚寒，食少便溏及孕妇均忌服。

Brief summary

小　结

1 Qi-reinforcing herbs

1 补气药

Both *Ginseng Radix et Raizoma* (ren shen) and *Codonopsis Radix* (dang shen) act to reinforce qi and produce fluid, applied to treat spleen qi deficiency pattern, lung qi deficiency pattern and thirst due to fluid consumption. Ren shen is stronger in reinforcing qi, as the major herb to reinforce Yuan (Primary) Qi, and acts to rescue life from collapse. It also acts to improve intelligence and calm mind, applied to treat irritability of heart mind manifested by palpitation, insomnia and poor memory. Dang shen is weaker in reinforcing qi, but acts to reinforce spleen qi, to reinforce lung qi and to reinforce blood, applied to treat blood deficiency pattern manifested by sallow-yellow complexion.

人参、党参，均能补气生津，治脾气虚、肺气虚证，津伤口渴。其中人参补气力佳，为大补元气之品，能挽救虚脱；且能增智安神，治心神不安的心悸、失眠、健忘等证。党参补气力弱，善补脾气、益肺气，兼能养血，治血虚萎黄。

Both *Panacis Quinquefolii Radix* (xi yang shen) and *Pseudostellariae Radix* (tai zi shen) act to reinforce qi and produce fluid, applied to treat thirst due to qi and fluid consumption. Xi yang shen is cool in property and stronger in reinforcing qi, and also acts to benefit yin and reduce fire, applied to treat qi and yin deficiency pattern with fire hyper-

西洋参、太子参，均能补气生津，治气津两伤的口渴。其中西洋参性凉，补气力强，且能益阴清火，故适用于气阴两伤兼火盛者。太子参性平，补气力弱，常用于气津两伤，火不盛者。

activity. Tai zi shen is neutral in property and weaker in reinforcing qi, applied to treat qi and yin deficiency pattern without fire.

Both *Astragali Radix* (huang qi) and *Atractylodis Macrocephalae Rhizoma* (bai zhu) are warm in property and act to reinforce qi, promote urination, strengthen body surface and stop sweating, applied to treat spleen and lung qi deficiency pattern manifested by spontaneous sweating, nocturnal sweats, edema and difficult urination. Huang qi is stronger in reinforcing qi and acts to reinforce qi and uplift yang, applied to treat sinking of Zhong (Middle Energizer) Qi with prolapse of internal organs. It acts to benefit qi and strengthen body surface, applied to treat spontaneous sweating due to exterior deficiency. It also acts to drain toxin and engender muscles, applied to treat deep pitting of carbuncle and furuncle due to qi and blood deficiency. Bai zhu is weaker in reinforcing qi, but acts to strengthen spleen. It is bitter in flavor and acts to desiccate damp, applied to treat spleen deificiency with damp. It also acts to quiet fetus, applied to treat irritable fetus due to spleen deficiency.

黄芪、白术，均性温，均能补气利尿、固表止汗，均治脾肺气虚证，自汗、盗汗，以及水肿、小便不利。其中黄芪补气力强，功善补气升阳，为治中气下陷、脏器下垂之要药；还能益气固表，治表虚自汗；且托毒生肌，治气血两虚之疮毒内陷。白术补气力弱，功善健脾，味苦燥湿，善治脾虚兼湿滞之证；又能安胎，治脾虚胎动不安。

Dioscoreae Rhizoma (shan yao) is sweet and neutral in property and attributive to the Lung, Spleen and Kidney Meridians, and acts to reinforce spleen and stomach, and benefit lung and kidney, applied to treat spleen and stomach deficiency pattern, false fire in lung and lung and kidney deficiency pattern. It acts to nourish yin and produce fluid, applied to treat diabetes due to yin deficiency. It also acts to benefit kidney and hold essence, applied to treat seminal emission due to kidney deficiency.

山药，味甘性平，入肺脾肾经，功善补脾胃、益肺肾，既治脾胃虚弱，又治肺虚火肺肾两虚之证；且能养阴生津，治阴虚消渴；还益肾涩精，治肾虚遗精等证。

Both *Glycyrrhizae Radix et Rhizoma* (gan cao)

甘草、蜂蜜，均味甘性

and *Mel* (feng mi) are sweet and neutral in property and act to reinforce middle energizer, benefit qi, moisturize lung, stop cough, relieve spasm and stop pain, applied to treat spleen deficiency pattern, cough due to dryness in lung and epigastric and abdominal pain. Gan cao acts to benefit heart qi, applied to treat palpitation and irregular pulse. It acts to dissolve phlegm, applied to treat cough with excessive sputum. It also acts to relieve toxin, applied to treat carbuncle and furuncle, and also to treat food poisoning and herb poisoning as well. Feng mi is moist in property and acts to moisturize intestines, applied to treat constipation due to dryness in intestines. It also acts to relieve toxin from *Aconiti Radix* (wu tou).

平，均能补中益气，润肺止咳、缓急止痛，治脾虚证、肺燥咳嗽，以及脘腹疼痛。其中甘草能益心气，治心动悸、脉结代；祛痰力强，为治咳嗽痰多所常用；且能解毒，既治疮痈，又治中食物、药物毒。蜂蜜质润，还能润肠燥，治肠燥便秘；亦解乌头毒。

2 Yang-reinforcing herbs

Both *Cervi Cornu Pantotrichum* (lu rong) and *Cistanchis Herba* (rou cong rong) are sweet and salty in flavor and warm in property, and act to reinforce kidney yang and benefit essence and blood, applied to treat kidney yang insufficiency pattern and essence and blood deficiency pattern. Lu rong, as the major herb to reinforce kidney yang and benefit essence and blood, acts to reinforce liver and kidney, strengthen tendons and bones, and regulate Thoroughfare and Conception Vessels, applied to treat liver and kidney insufficiency pattern manifested by flaccidity and weakness of tendons and bones, metrorrhagia, metrostaxis and heavy blood flow in menstruation. It also acts to benefit essence and blood and drain pus and toxin, applied to treat chronic and unhealed ulcers in carbuncle and furuncle. Rou cong rong is weaker than *Cervi Cornu*

2 补阳药

鹿茸、肉苁蓉，均味甘咸性温，均补肾阳、益精血，既治肾阳不足，又治精血亏虚。其中鹿茸为壮肾阳、益精血之要药；还能补肝肾、强筋骨、调冲任，治肝肾不足所致的筋骨痿软、崩漏下血等证；且能益精血、托疮毒，治疮疡久溃不敛。肉苁蓉性缓力弱，补肾阳、益精血之功逊于鹿茸，且能润肠通便，治阳虚便秘。

Pantotrichum (lu rong) in reinforcing kidney yang and benefit essence and blood, but it acts to moisturize intestines and promote defecation, applied to treat constipation due to yang deficiency.

Both *Morindae Officinalis Radix* (ba ji tian) and *Epimedii Folium* (yin yang huo) act to reinforce kidney yang and eliminate wind-damp, applied to treat kidney yang deficiency manifested by impotence and infertility, chronic Bi (Obturation) Pattern due to wind-damp, and flaccidity and weakness of tendons and bones. Ba ji tian is sweet, moist and warm in property with moderate action, while yin yang huo is warm and dry in property with strong action to strengthen yang and treat impotence.

巴戟天、淫羊藿,均能补肾阳、祛风湿,治肾虚阳痿、不孕,以及风湿久痹、筋骨痿软等证。其中巴戟天甘润性温而不燥,药力较缓。淫羊藿性温而燥,药力较强,具壮阳起痿之功。

Both *Psoraleae Fructus* (bu gu zhi) and *Alpiniae Oxyphyllae Fructus* (yi zhi) are attributive to the Spleen and Kidney Meridians. As the warming, reinforcing and astringing herbs, they act to warm spleen, benefit kidney, astringe essence and hold urine, applied to treat spleen and kidney deficiency pattern. Bu gu zhi is warm and acts to warm and reinforce kidney, applied to treat dawn diarrhea due to spleen and kidney yang deficiency. It also acts to accept qi and soothe panting, applied to treat panting due to kidney deficiency. Yi zhi acts to warm spleen, eliminate cold, improve appetite and hold saliva, applied to treat salivation.

补骨脂、益智,均入脾、肾经,同为温补固涩之品,能暖脾益肾,固精缩尿,均治脾肾两虚之证。其中补骨脂功偏温补肾阳而治脾肾两虚之五更泄泻;又纳气定喘,治肾虚气喘。益智功偏温脾散寒,且能开胃摄唾,治口多涎唾。

Both *Cuscutae Semen* (tu si zi) and *Astragali Complanati Semen* (sha yuan zi) act to reinforce kidney, assist yang, astringe essence, hold urine, nourish liver and brighten eyes, applied to treat kidney yang deficiency pattern manifested by impotence, seminal emission, frequency of urination,

菟丝子、沙苑子,均善补肾助阳,固精缩尿、养肝明目,治肾阳虚衰的阳痿遗精、尿频带下,以及目暗不明等证。其中菟丝子辛甘而平,不腻不燥,兼补肾阴,为平补

morbid leucorrhea and blurring of vision. Tu si zi is pungent, sweet and neutral, but not sticky and dry in property, and acts to reinforce kidney yin as well, as the major herb to reinforce both yin and yang. it acts to reinforce spleen and stop diarrhea, applied to treat diarrhea due to spleen deficiency. It also acts to reinforce liver and kidney and quiet fetus, applied to treat irritable fetus. Sha yuan zi is sweet and warm, but not dry in property, with strong astringing action.

阴阳之品，又善补脾止泻，治脾虚泄泻；且能补肝肾、安胎，治胎动不安。沙苑子甘温不燥，固涩力强，功唯温补固涩。

Cordyceps (dong chong xia cao) is sweet and neutral in property and attributive to the Lung and Kidney Meridians, and act to reinforce kidney, benefit lung, stanch blood and dissolve phlegm, especially acts to reinforce qi of lung and kidney, benefit yin of lung and kidney, and also acts to soothe lung and relieve panting, applied to treat chronic cough, panting of deficiency type, cough with bloody sputum due to lung yin deficiency. It also acts to reinforce and supplement body constitution, applied to cultivate and nourish the weak body.

冬虫夏草，味甘性平，入肺、肾经，为补益肺肾之品。功善补肾益肺，止血化痰，尤善补肺肾之气、益肺肾之阴，兼止血化痰，平定气喘，故为治久咳虚喘、劳嗽痰血所常用。还有补虚扶弱之功，可用于体虚调养。

Both *Eucommiae Cortex* (du zhong) and *Dipsaci Radix* (xu duan) are attributive to the Liver and Kidney Meridians and act to reinforce liver and kidney, strengthen tendons and bones and quiet fetus, applied to treat liver and kidney insufficiency pattern manifested by aching and pain at low back and knees, flaccidity and weakness of lower limbs, and to treat liver and kidney deficiency pattern manifested by irritable fetus, threatened miscarriage and uterine bleeding. Du zhong is warm in property and stronger in reinforcing liver and kidney and strengthening tendons and bones, applied to treat low back pain and foot flaccidity. Xu duan is slight-

杜仲、续断，均入肝、肾经，均能补肝肾、强筋骨、安胎，治肝肾不足之腰膝酸痛、下肢痿软，肝肾亏虚之胎动不安、胎漏下血等证。其中杜仲性温，补肝肾、强筋骨力强，为治腰痛足痿之要药。续断微温不热，补肝肾、强筋骨力弱，且善行血脉、续折伤，为治骨折筋伤所常用。

ly warm in property and weaker in reinforcing liver and kidney and strengthening tendons and bones, but acts to promote blood flow in vessels and set broken bones, applied to treat fracture of bone and injury of tendon.

3 Blood-reinforcing herbs

Both *Angelicae Sinensis Radix* (dang gui) and *Paeoniae Radix Alba* (bai shao) act to reinforce blood and regulate menstruation, applied to treat blood deficiency pattern and irregular menstruation. Dang gui is warm in property and acts to reinforce blood, as the major herb to reinforce blood. It acts to reinforce blood, activate blood and regulate menstruation, applied to treat irregular menstruation, dysmenorrheal and amenorrhea due to blood deficiency or cold coagulation or blood stasis. It is warm in property, and acts to eliminate cold, activate blood and stop pain, applied to treat traumatic injury and Bi (Obturation) Pattern due to wind and damp. It also acts to moisturize intestines and promote defecation, applied to treat constipation due to dryness in intestines. Bai shao is cool and sour in property, and acts to soften liver, stop pain, soothe liver, inhibit yang, astringe yin and stop sweating, applied to treat hypochondriac pain due to liver qi stagnation, epigastric and abdominal pain, dizziness due to liver yang hyperactivity, nocturnal sweats due to yin deficiency, and spontaneous sweating due to exterior deficiency.

Both *Rehmanniae Radix Praeparata* (shu di huang) and *Asini Corii Colla* (e jiao) act to reinforce blood and nourish yin, applied to treat blood deficiency pattern and yin deficiency pattern. Shu

3 补血药

当归、白芍，均能补血、调经，治血虚证及月经不调。其中当归性温，功善补血，为治血虚之要药；既补血又活血，又为调经之要药，血虚或寒凝血瘀所致的月经不调、痛经经闭皆可选用；性温散寒，活血止痛，可用治跌打损伤、风湿痹痛；并能润肠通便，治肠燥便秘。白芍性凉味酸，又能柔肝止痛、平抑肝阳、敛阴止汗，治肝郁胁痛，脘腹疼痛，阳亢眩晕，以及阴虚盗汗、表虚自汗。

熟地黄、阿胶，均能补血、滋阴，治血虚证、阴虚证所常用。其中熟地黄为补血、滋阴之要药，尤善治肾阴

di huang acts to reinforce blood and nourish yin, applied to treat kidney yin deficiency pattern. It also acts to benefit essence and supplement marraws, applied to treat essence and blood deficiency of liver and kidney manifested by aching and weakness at low back and knees, dizziness, tinnitus and early grey hair. E jiao acts to nourish yin, moisturize body and stanch blood, applied to treat bleeding pattern due to yin deficiency or blood deficiency.

虚证；并能益精填髓，用治肝肾精血亏虚之腰膝酸软、眩晕耳鸣、须发早白等证。阿胶功善滋阴润燥，且能止血，尤善治出血兼阴虚、血虚者。

Polygoni Multiflori Radix (he shou wu) has different actions in crude form and in prepared form. He shou wu in prepared form acts to reinforce liver and kidney, benefit essence and blood, blacken hair and strengthen tendons and bones, applied to treat blood deficiency and essence depletion pattern, as the major herb to treat early grey hair. He shou wu in crude form acts to treat malaria, relieve toxin, moisturize intestines and promote defecation, applied to treat chronic malaria, carbuncle and furuncle, and scrofula due to weak body constitution, and also to treat constipation due to dryness in intestines.

何首乌，生用、制用功效有别。制首乌长于补肝肾、益精血，乌须发、强筋骨，善治血虚精亏证，尤以乌须发之功见长，为治须发早白之要药。生首乌功偏截疟、解毒、润肠通便，可用治体虚久疟、痈疽、瘰疬，以及肠燥便秘等证。

4 Yin-reinforcing herbs

Both *Glehniae Radix* (bei sha shen) and *Ophiopogonis Radix* (mai dong) act to nourish yin, benefit stomach and produce fluid, applied to treat cough due to dryness in lung, cough with bloody sputum due to lung yin deficiency, and thirst due to fluid consumption. Bei sha shen acts to nourish lung yin and reduce heat in lung, applied to treat dry cough due to yin deficiency, cough due to lung yin deficiency and chronic cough. Mai dong acts to benefit stomach, produce fluid, reduce heat and moisturize body, ap-

4 补阴药

北沙参、麦冬，均能养阴、益胃生津，治肺燥咳嗽、劳嗽咳血，以及津伤口渴。其中北沙参长于养肺阴，且清肺热，为治阴虚燥咳、劳嗽久咳所常用。麦冬功善益胃生津、清热润燥，治津伤口渴或便秘；且能清心除烦，治阴虚有热的虚烦不眠。

plied to treat thirst or constipation due to fluid consumption. It also acts to purify heart and relieve restlessness, applied to treat yin deficiency with heat manifested by restlessness and insomnia.

All *Asparagi Radix* (tian dong), *Polygonati Odorati Rhizoma* (yu zhu) and *Dendrobii Herba* (shi hu) act to nourish yin and produce fluid, applied to treat diabetes due to fluid consumption. Tian dong is attributive to the Lung and Kidney Meridians and sweet, moist, bitter and dispersing in property, and acts to nourish yin of lung and kidney, reduce fire and moisturize body, applied to treat cough due to dryness in lung or lung yin deficiency, and to treat kidney yin deficiency pattern. Yu zhu is attributive to the Lung and Stomach Meridians and sweet and cool in property, and acts to nourish yin of lung and stomach, applied to treat lung and stomach yin deficiency pattern. It also acts to nourish yin without keeping pathogen inside, applied to treat yin deficiency with exogenous pathogen attack. Shi hu is attributive to the Stomach and Kidney Meridians, and acts to nourish yin of stomach and kidney, and reduce false heat, applied to treat prolonged low-grade fever after febrile disease. It also acts to reinforce kidney, nourish liver, brighten eyes and strengthen tendons and bones.

天冬、玉竹、石斛，均能养阴、生津，治津伤口渴证。其中天冬入肺、肾经，甘润苦泄，以滋养肺肾之阴为主，兼有清火、润燥之功，为肺燥或劳嗽，肾阴虚证所常用。玉竹入肺、胃经，甘凉不寒，以滋养肺胃之阴为主，多用治肺胃阴虚证；并具养阴不敛邪之特点，治阴虚外感。石斛入胃肾经，以滋养胃肾之阴为主，兼能清虚热，治热病后虚热不退；且能补肾养肝明目、强筋骨。

Polygonati Rhizoma (huang jing) is sweet and neutral in property and attributive to the Spleen, Lung and Kidney Meridians, and acts to reinforce and benefit spleen, lung and kidney, reinforce qi, nourish yin, moisturize lung and strengthen spleen, as the major herb to cultivate and regulate spleen, lung and kidney.

黄精，味甘性平，入脾肺肾经，具有补益脾肺肾之功，且既补气、养阴，又润肺、健脾，为调补脾肺肾各脏之良药。

All *Lycii Fructus* (gou qi zi), *Ecliptae Herba* (mo han lian) and *Ligustri Lucidi Fructus* (nü zhen

枸杞子、墨旱莲、女贞子，均入肝肾经，均能滋补肝

zi) are attributive to the Liver and Kidney Meridians, and act to nourish and reinforce liver and kidney, applied to treat liver and kidney insufficiency pattern. Gou qi zi is neutral in property, and acts to reinforce liver and kidney, benefit essence and blood and brighten eyes, the key herb to nourish and reinforce liver and kidney and to reinforce essence and brighten eyes. Mo han lian is cold in property, and acts to nourish yin of liver and kidney, cool blood and stanch blood, applied to treat bleeding pattern due to yin deficiency or heat in blood. Nü zhen zi is cool in property with moderate action, and acts to brighten eyes and blacken hair, applied to treat early grey hair.

肾，治肝肾不足证。其中枸杞子性平，功善补肝肾，益精血、明目，为滋补肝肾、补精明目之要药。墨旱莲性寒，既滋肝肾阴，又凉血止血，可治阴虚血热的出血证。女贞子性凉，药力平和，且能明目乌发，常用于须发早白。

Both *Testudinis Carapax et Plastrum* (gui jia) and *Trionycis Carapax* (bie jia) act to nourish yin and subdue yang. Gui jia is stronger in nourishing yin, applied to treat yin deficiency and yang hyperactivity pattern. It also acts to benefit kidney, strengthen bones, nourish blood, reinforce heart, regulate menstruation and stanch blood, applied to treat weakness of bones due to kidney deficiency, palpitation, insomnia, metrorrhagia and metrostaxisdue due to yin deficiency. Bie jia acts to reduce false heat, applied to treat fever due to yin deficiency. It also acts to soften the hard and relieve stasis, applied to treat abdominal masses.

龟甲、鳖甲，均能滋阴潜阳。其中龟甲滋阴力佳，善治阴虚阳亢之证；且能益肾健骨、养血补心、固经止血，治肾虚骨弱、心悸失眠、阴虚崩漏等证。鳖甲长于清虚热，善治阴虚发热；且能软坚散结，治癥瘕积聚等证。

Chapter 17 Astringing Herbs

第 17 章 收涩药

The medicinal herbs acting to astringe and hold body fluids are called the astringing herbs.

以收敛固涩为主要作用的药物，称为收涩药，又称固涩药。

The medicinal herbs are mostly sour and astringent in flavor and neutral or warm in property, and act to strengthen body surface to stop sweating, astringe lung to stop cough, astringe intestines to stop diarrhea, hold essence, control urine, stanch blood and control leucorrhea, applied to treat chronic disease causing weak body, decrease of checking function of Zheng (Anti-Pathogenic) Qi and functional decrease of zang-fu organs manifested by spontaneous sweating, nocturnal sweats, chronic cough, cough of deficiency type, chronic diarrhea, chronic dysentery, seminal emission, nocturnal emission, enuresis, frequency of urination, metrorrhagia, metrostaxis and morbid leucorrhea.

本类药味多酸涩，性平或温，具有固表止汗、敛肺止咳、涩肠止泻、固精缩尿、收敛止血、收涩止带等作用，主要用于久病体虚、正气不固、脏腑功能减退所致的自汗、盗汗、久咳虚喘、久泻、久痢、遗精滑精、遗尿尿频、崩带不止等滑脱证。

In the application of this type of medicinal herbs, it is necessary to pay attention to the herb actions. These medicinal herbs, as the herbs to treat the branch of disease, are applied by combining with other herbs according to the causes of leakage and collapse. Due to their astringing action, these medicinal herbs may keep the pathogens inside, it is not advisable to apply the medicinal herbs for those with excess Xie (Pathogenic) Qi pattern due to ex-

使用本类药需注意，本类药为治标之品，应根据滑脱的病因作适当配伍。本类药性涩易敛邪，凡外感、湿热、血热等邪实之证，不宜应用。

ogenous attack of pathogens, damp-heat or heat in blood.

Ephedrae Radix Et Rhizoma (ma huang gen)

It is the dried product from the root and rhizoma of *Ephedra sinica* Stapf. or *Ephedra intermedia* Schrenk et C. A. Mey., family ephedraceae. The medicinal herb is collected in late autumn, applied in crude form.

Features Flavor: sweet and astringent. Property: neutral. Meridian tropism: the Heart Meridian and the Lung Meridian.

Actions Strengthen body surface and stop sweating.

Application

Spontaneous sweating and nocturnal sweats. The medicinal herb is sweet and neutral in property and acts to astringe lung, strengthen body surface and stop sweating. In the treatment of spontaneous sweating due to qi deficiency, it is combined with *Astragali Radix* (huang qi) and *Atractylodis Macrocephalae Rhizoma* (bai zhu). In the treatment of nocturnal sweats due to yin deficiency, it is combined with *Rehmanniae Radix* (sheng di huang) and *Ostreae Concha* (mu li). In the treatment of constant sweating after delivery due to qi and blood insufficiency, it is combined with *Angelicae Sinensis Radix* (dang gui) and huang qi, to form up Ephedra Root Powder (Ma Huang Gen San).

Furthermore, The medicinal herb is applied by grinding into fine powder for external use to stop sweating.

Usage and dosage Apply 3～10 g in decoction. Apply a proper amount for external use.

麻黄根

为麻黄科植物草麻黄或中麻黄的干燥根及根茎。秋末采挖。生用。

性味归经 甘,涩,平。归心、肺经。

功效 固表止汗。

应用

自汗,盗汗。本品甘平,功专敛肺固表止汗。治气虚自汗,常配伍黄芪、白术等。治阴虚盗汗,常配伍生地黄、牡蛎等。治产后气血不足之虚汗不止,配伍当归、黄芪等同用,如麻黄根散。

此外,本品亦可研末撒扑,外用止汗。

用法用量 煎服,3～10克。外用适量。

Precautions for use It is prohibited to apply for those with exterior pathogens.

使用注意 有表邪者忌用。

Remarks *Ephedrae Herba* (ma huang) and *Ephedrae Radix Et Rhizoma* (ma huang gen)

按语 麻黄与麻黄根

Both the medicinal herbs are the products from *Ephedra sinica* stapf., *Ephedra Intermedia* Schrenk et C. A. Mey., or *Ephedra Equisetina* Bunge, family ephedraceae. Ma huang is the herbaceous stem, is pungent, slightly bitter and warm in property, and acts to make sweating and relieve the exterior, applied to treat exterior excess pattern without sweating due to wind-cold. It also acts to disperse lung, soothe panting and promote water flow. Ma huang gen is the root, sweet, astringent and neutral in property, and acts to strengthen body surface and stop sweating.

二药均来源于麻黄科植物草麻黄或中麻黄。不同的是麻黄以草质茎入药,味辛微苦性温,功偏发汗解表,善治风寒表证表实无汗,且能宣肺、平喘、利水。麻黄根以根入药,甘涩性平,功专固表止汗。

Tritici Levis Fructus (fu xiao mai)

浮小麦

It is the dried product from the blighted caryopsis of *Triticum aestivum* L., family Gramineae. The medicinal herb is produced all over the country, applied in crude form or in stir-fried form.

为禾本科植物小麦干燥的未成熟颖果。全国各地均产。生用或炒用。

Features Flavor: sweet. Property: cool. Meridian tropism: the Heart Meridian.

性味归经 甘,凉。归心经。

Actions Stop sweating, benefit qi and reduce heat.

功效 止汗,益气,除热。

Application

应用

(1) Spontaneous sweating and nocturnal sweating. The medicinal herb is sweet, cool, light and floating in property, and acts to benefit heart qi and astringe heart fluid. In the treatment of spontaneous sweating or nocturnal sweating, it is applied singly by stir-baking to brown and grinding into powder, for oral administration together with rice soup,

(1) 自汗,盗汗。本品甘凉轻浮,能益心气、敛心液。治自汗、盗汗,可单用炒焦研末,米汤调服,或与其他药物配伍同用。治自汗不止,常与煅牡蛎、麻黄根、黄芪等同用。治盗汗,可与五味子、麦

or combined with other medicinal herbs. In the treatment of spontaneous sweating, it is combined with baked *Ostreae Concha* (mu li), *Ephedrae Radix Et Rhizoma* (ma huang gen) and *Astragali Radix* (huang qi). In the treatment of nocturnal sweats, it is combined with *Schisandrae Chinensis Fructus* (wu wei zi), *Ophiopogonis Radix* (mai dong) and *Lycii Cortex* (di gu pi).

冬、地骨皮等合用。

(2) Feverish sensation and tidal fever due to yin deficiency. The medicinal herb is sweet and cool and acts to benefit qi and yin, astringe floating fire and reduce false heat. In the treatment of fever due to yin deficiency or tidal feverish sensation and tidal fever, it is combined with *Anemarrhenae Rhizoma* (zhi mu), *Ophiopogonis Radix* (mai dong) and *Rehmanniae Radix* (sheng di huang).

（2）骨蒸劳热。本品甘凉，能益气阴、敛浮火、除虚热，治阴虚发热，骨蒸劳热等证，常与知母、麦冬、生地黄等同用。

Usage and dosage Apply 15～30 g in decoction. Apply 3～5 g of fine powder.

用法用量 煎服，15～30 克。研末服，3～5 克。

Schisandrae Chinensis Fructus (wu wei zi)

五味子

It is the dried product from the ripe fruit of *Schisandra chinensis* (Tuecz.) Bail., family Magnoliaceae, also called "bei wu wei zi". The medicinal herb is collected in autumn, applied in crude form or in prepared form with vinegar.

为木兰科植物五味子的干燥成熟果实。习称“北五味子”。秋季采收。生用或醋制用。

Features Flavor: sour and sweet. Property: warm. Meridian tropism: the Lung Meridian, the Heart Meridian and the Kidney Meridian.

性味归经 酸、甘，温。归肺、心、肾经。

Actions Astringe and hold fluids, benefit qi, produce fluid, reinforce kidney and quiet heart.

功效 收敛固涩，益气生津，补肾宁心。

Application

应用

(1) Chronic cough and panting of deficiency type. The medicine herb is sour and astringent in property and attributive to the Lung and Kidney

（1）久咳虚喘。本品酸收，入肺肾经，能敛肺气，滋肾阴，为肺虚或肺肾两虚咳

Meridians, and acts to astringe lung qi and nourish kidney yin, as the major herb to treat cough and panting due to lung deficiency or due to lung and kidney deficiency. In the treatment of panting and cough due to lung deficiency, it is combined with *Ginseng Radix et Raizoma* (ren shen), *Astragali Radix* (huang qi) and *Aster Radix et Rhizoma* (zi wan). In the treatment of cough and panting due to lung and kidney deficiency, it is combined with *Corni Fructus* (shan zhu yu), *Rehmanniae Radix Praeparata* (shu di huang) and *Dioscoreae Rhizoma* (shan yao), to form up Major Qi Pills (Du Qi Wan).

喘所常用。治肺虚喘咳，可与人参、黄芪、紫菀等同用。治肺肾两虚之咳喘，可与山茱萸、熟地黄、山药等同用，如都气丸。

(2) Spontaneous sweating and nocturnal sweats. The medicinal herb acts to astringe lung and stop sweating. In the treatment of spontaneous sweating due to qi deficiency, it is combined with huang qi, *Atractylodis Macrocephalae Rhizoma* (bai zhu) and *Ostreae Concha* (mu li). In the treatment of nocturnal sweats due to yin deficiency, it is combined with *Scrophulariae Radix* (xuan shen), *Ophiopogonis Radix* (mai dong) and *Corni Fructus* (shan zhu yu).

(2) 自汗，盗汗。本品能敛肺止汗。治气虚自汗，常配伍黄芪、白术、牡蛎等。治阴虚盗汗，常配伍玄参、麦冬、山茱萸等。

(3) Seminal emission and seminal leakage. The medicinal herb is sour, sweet, astringent and tonic in property, and acts to reinforce kidney and astringe essence. In the treatment of seminal emission and nocturnal emission due to kidney deficiency, it is combined with *Mantidis OÖTheca* (sang piao xiao) and *Os Draconis* (long gu).

(3) 遗精，滑精。本品酸收甘补，具补肾、涩精之功。治肾虚遗精、滑精，常与桑螵蛸、龙骨等同用。

(4) Chronic diarrhea. The medicinal herb acts to astringe intestines and stop diarrhea. In the treatment of chronic diarrhea due to deficiency and cold of spleen and kidney, it is combined with *Psoraleae Fructus* (bu gu zhi), *Myristicae Semen* (rou dou

(4) 久泻不止。本品能涩肠止泻。治脾肾虚寒的久泻不止，可与补骨脂、肉豆蔻、吴茱萸等同用。

kou) and *Euodiae Fructus* (wu zhu yu).

(5) Thirst due to fluid consumption and diabetes. The medicinal herb is sour and sweet in flavor, and acts to benefit qi, produce fluid and relieve thirst. In the treatment of heat consuming qi and yin manifested by profuse sweating and thirst, it is combined with *Ginseng Radix et Raizoma* (ren shen) and *Ophiopogonis Radix* (mai dong), to form up Pulse-Engendering Powder (Sheng Mai San). In the treatment of diabetes due to yin deficiency, it is combined with shan yao, *Anemarrhenae Rhizoma* (zhi mu) and *Trichosanthis Radix* (tian hua fen).

(5) 津伤口渴，消渴。本品酸甘，能益气生津、止渴。治热伤气阴，汗多口渴，常配伍人参、麦冬，即生脉散。治阴虚消渴，可与山药、知母、天花粉等同用。

(6) Palpitation, insomnia and dream-disturbed sleep. The medicinal herb is attributive to the Heart and Kidney Meridians, and acts to benefit heart qi, calm heart and mind and nourish kidney yin. In the treatment of yin and blood deficiency, loss of nourishment in heart or heart and kidney disharmony manifested by palpitation, insomnia and dream-disturbed sleep, it is combined with *Ziziphi Spinosae Semen* (suan zao ren), mai dong and *Angelicae Sinensis Radix* (dang gui).

(6) 心悸，失眠，多梦。本品入心肾经，能益心气、安心神、滋肾阴。治阴血亏虚、心失所养或心肾不交所致的虚烦心悸、失眠多梦，常与酸枣仁、麦冬、当归等同用。

Usage and dosage Apply 2～6 g in decoction. The medicinal herb has a stronger astringing action in prepared form with vinegar.

用法用量 煎服，2～6克。醋制后收涩力强。

Precautions for use It is not advisable to apply for those with retaining of exterior pathogen, or those with internal excess heat, or those with cough in early stage, or those with measles in early stage.

使用注意 表邪未解，内有实热，咳嗽初起，麻疹初起，均不宜用。

Mume Fructus (wu mei)

乌梅

It is the dried product from the smoked unripe fruit of *Prunus mune (Sieb)* Sieb. et Zucc., family Rosaceae. The medicinal herb is collected in sum-

为蔷薇科植物梅的干燥近成熟果实。夏季果实近成熟时采收。生用或炒炭用。

mer when the fruit is nearly ripe, applied in crude form or in carbonized form.

Features Flavor: sour and astringent. Property: neutral. Meridian tropism: the Liver Meridian, the Spleen Meridian, the Lung Meridian and the Large Intestine Meridian.

性味归经 酸、涩,平。归肝、脾、肺、大肠经。

Actions Astringe lung to stop cough, astringe intestines to stop diarrhea, produce fluid, relieve thirst, quiet roundworm and stop pain.

功效 敛肺止咳,涩肠止泻,生津止渴,安蛔止痛。

Application

(1) Chronic cough due to lung deficiency. The medicinal herb is sour and astringent in property and attributive to the Lung Meridian, and acts to astringe lung and stop cough. In the treatment of lung deficiency manifested by chronic cough, or cough with scanty sputum or dry cough without sputum, it is combined with *Schisandrae Chinensis Fructus* (wu wei zi) and *Stemonae Radix* (bai bu).

(2) Chronic diarrhea and chronic dysentery. The medicinal herb is attributive to the Large Intestine, and acts to astringe intestines and stop diarrhea. In the treatment of chronic diarrhea or chronic dysentery, it is combined with *Myristicae Semen* (rou dou kou) and *Ginseng Radix et Raizoma* (ren shen).

(3) Restlessness and thirst due to false heat. The medicinal herb is sour in flavor and acts to produce fluid and relieve thirst. In the treatment of restlessness and thirst due to false heat, it is applied singly or combined with ren shen, *Trichosanthis Radix* (tian hua fen) and *Ophiopogonis Radix* (mai dong), to form up Jade Spring Pills (Yu Quan Wan).

(4) Abdominal pain due to roundworm. The

应用

(1) 肺虚久咳。本品酸涩收敛,入肺经,敛肺止咳。治肺虚久咳少痰或干咳无痰,常与五味子、百部等同用。

(2) 久泻久痢。本品入大肠经,涩肠止泻。治久泻久痢,常与肉豆蔻、人参等同用。

(3) 虚热消渴。本品味酸,善生津止渴。治虚热烦渴,可单用煎服,或配伍人参、天花粉、麦冬等同用,如玉泉丸。

(4) 蛔厥腹痛。本品味

medicinal herb is extremely sour in flavor and acts to quiet roundworm and stop pain. In the treatment of syncope pattern due to roundworm manifested by abdominal pain, vomiting and chills in four limbs, it is combined with *Zanthoxyli Pericarpium* (hua jiao), *Zingiberis Rhizoma* (gan jiang) and *Coptidis Rhizoma* (huang lian), to form up Black Plum Pills (Wu Mei Wan).

极酸,能安蛔、止痛。治蛔厥证,症见腹痛、呕吐、四肢厥冷,常与花椒、干姜、黄连等同用,如乌梅丸。

Usage and dosage Apply 6～12 g in decoction, applied in crude form. The medicinal herb in carbonized form acts to stop diarrhea.

用法用量 煎服,6～12克。一般生用,炒炭止泻。

Precautions for use It is not advisable to apply for those with exterior pathogen or those with internal excess heat.

使用注意 外有表邪或内有实热积滞者均不宜服。

Myristicae Semen (rou dou kou)

肉豆蔻

It is the dried product from ripe seed of the arbor *Myristica fragrans* Houtt., family Myristicacene. The medicinal herb is collected from April to June or from November to December, applied in prepared form by roasting.

为肉豆蔻科植物肉豆蔻的干燥种仁。4～6 月或11～12 月采收。煨制用。

Features Flavor: pungent. Property: warm. Meridian tropism: the Spleen Meridian, the Stomach Meridian and the Large Intestine Meridian.

性味归经 辛,温。归脾、胃、大肠经。

Actions Astringe intestines, stop diarrhea, warm middle energizer and move qi.

功效 涩肠止泻,温中行气。

Application

(1) Chronic diarrhea and chronic dysentery. The medicinal herb is pungent, warm and astringent in property, and attributive to the Large Intestine Meridian, and acts to astringe intestines and stop diarrhea. In the treatment of chronic diarrhea and chronic dysentery due to deficiency and cold of spleen and kidney, it is combined with *Ginseng*

应用

(1) 久泻久痢。本品辛温而涩,入大肠经,能涩肠止泻。治脾肾虚寒之久泻久痢,常与人参、肉桂等同用。治脾肾阳虚之五更泄泻,常与补骨脂、吴茱萸、五味子同用,即四神丸。

Radix et Raizoma (ren shen) and *Cinnamomi Cortex* (rou gui). In the treatment of dawn diarrhea due to spleen and kidney yang deficiency, it is combined with *Psoraleae Fructus* (bu gu zhi), *Euodiae Fructus* (wu zhu yu) and *Schisandrae Chinensis Fructus* (wu wei zi), to form up Four Divinities Pills (Si Shen Wan).

(2) Cold in stomach manifested by gastric distension and pain, poor appetite and vomiting. The medicinal herb is pungent, fragrant, warm and dry in property, and acts to warm middle energizer and spleen, move qi, stop pain, improve appetite and digest food. In the treatment of deficiency, cold or qi stagnation of spleen and stomach manifested by epigastric and abdominal distension and pain, poor appetite and vomiting, it is combined with *Aucklandiae Radix* (mu xiang), *Pinelliae Rhizoma* (ban xia) and *Zingiberis Rhizoma* (gan jiang).

（2）胃寒胀痛，食少呕吐。本品辛香温燥，有温中暖脾、行气止痛、开胃消食作用。治脾胃虚寒气滞的脘腹胀痛、食少呕吐等证，可与木香、半夏、干姜等同用。

Usage and dosage Apply 3～10 g in decoction. It is necessary to apply after roasting and deoiling for oral administration.

用法用量 煎服，3～10克。内服须煨熟去油用。

Precautions for use It is not advisable to apply for those with diarrhea or dysentery due to damp-heat.

使用注意 湿热泻痢者不宜服用。

Remarks *Semen Amomi Fructus Rotundus* (bai dou kou) and *Myristicae Semen* (rou dou kou)

按语 白豆蔻与肉豆蔻

Both the medicinal herbs act to warm middle energizer and move qi. Bai dou kou is the dried product from the ripe fruit of *Amomum kravanh* Pierre ex Gagnep or *Amonum compactum* Soland. ex Maton, family Zingiberaceae, and pungent and warm in property, acting to dissolve dam and move qi, as the major herb to treat damp blocking spleen and stomach pattern. Rou dou kou is the dried

均能温中行气。不同的是白豆蔻来源于姜科植物，味辛性温，功善化湿行气，为湿阻脾胃证多用。肉豆蔻来源于肉豆蔻科植物，性涩收敛，既能涩肠止泻，又能温中行气。

product from ripe seed of the arbor *Myristica fragrans* Houtt., family Myristicacene, and astringent in property, acting to astringe intestines and stop diarrhea, and also to warm middle energizer and move qi as well.

Halloysitum Rubrum (chi shi zhi)

赤石脂

It is the product from the mineral of silicate salt of polyhydrate kaolinate group, containing mainly hydrated Aluminum silicate [$Al_4(Si_4O_{10})(OH)_8 \cdot 4H_2O$]. The medicinal herb is collected all over the year, applied in powdered form or in calcined form.

为硅酸盐类矿物多水高岭石族多水高岭石。主要成分为含水硅酸铝。全年均可采挖。研细粉或煅后捣碎。

Features Flavor: sweet, sour and astringent. Property: warm. Meridian tropism: the Large Intestine Meridian and the Stomach Meridian.

性味归经 甘、酸、涩，温。归大肠、胃经。

Actions Astringe intestines, stop diarrhea, astringe and stanch blood, astringe sores and engender muscles.

功效 涩肠止泻，收敛止血，敛疮生肌。

Application

应用

(1) Chronic diarrhea and chronic dysentery. The medicinal herb is sour, astringent, warm, heavy and descending in property, and acts to astringe intestines and stop diarrhea. In the treatment of chronic diarrhea and chronic dysentery, it is combined with *Myristicae Semen* (rou dou kou) and *Schisandrae Chinensis Fructus* (wu wei zi).

(1) 久泻久痢。本品酸涩性温，质重下行，善走下焦，有涩肠止泻之功。治久泻久痢，常与肉豆蔻、五味子等同用。

(2) Metrorrhagia, metrostaxis and morbid leucorrhea. The medicinal herb acts to astringe and stanch blood. In the treatment of metrorrhagia, metrostaxis and uterine bleeding, it is combined with *Platyclaoi Cacumen* (ce bai ye). In the treatment of morbid or bloody leucorrhea, it is combined with *Paeoniae Radix Alba* (bai shao) and *Euryales*

(2) 崩漏带下。本品能固崩止带、收敛止血。治崩漏下血，常与侧柏叶等同用。治赤白带下，可与白芍、芡实等同用。

Semen (qian shi).

(3) Unhealed carbuncle and furuncle, eczema or ulcer. The medicinal herb acts to dissolve damp, astringe ulcer and engender muscle. In the treatment of unhealed carbuncle and furuncle, eczema or ulcer, it is combined with *Os Draconis* (long gu) and calcined *Gypsum Fibrosum* (shi gao) by grinding into fine powder for external use.

（3）疮疡不敛，湿疹，湿疮。本品外用能收湿敛疮、生肌收口。治疮疡不敛、湿疹、湿疮，可与煅龙骨、煅石膏等研末，撒敷患处。

Usage and dosage Appy 9～15 g in decoction. Apply a proper amount for external use. It is advisable to decoct first in crude form, and it acts to heal ulcer in calcined form.

用法用量 煎服，9～15克。外用适量。生用宜先煎，煅用敛疮。

Precautions for use It is not advisable to apply with *Cinnamomi Cortex* (rou gui).

使用注意 不宜与肉桂同用。

Corni Fructus (shan zhu yu)

山茱萸

It is the dried product from the ripe sarcocarp of the deciduous arbor *Cornus officinalis* Sieb. et Zucc., family Cornaceae. The medicinal herb is collected in late autumn and early winter, applied in crude form or in liquor-prepared form.

为山茱萸科植物山茱萸的干燥成熟果肉。秋末冬初时采收。生用或酒制用。

Features Flavor: sour and astringent. Property: slightly warm. Meridian tropism: the Liver Meridian and the Kidney Meridian.

性味归经 酸，涩，微温。归肝、肾经。

Actions Reinforce and benefit liver and kidney, and astringe and hold prolapse.

功效 补益肝肾，收敛固脱。

Application

应用

(1) Liver and kidney deficiency pattern. The medicinal herb is sour, astringent, warm and moist in property, and attributive to the Liver and Kidney Meridians, acting to nourish yin of liver and kidney, and to warm and reinforce and kidney yang, as the major herb to reinforce both yin and yang. In the treatment of liver and kidney yin deficiency pat-

（1）肝肾亏虚证。本品酸涩微温质润，入肝肾经，既滋养肝肾之阴，又温补肾阳，为平补阴阳之品。治肝肾阴亏的腰膝酸软、头晕耳鸣，常与熟地黄、山药、茯苓等同用，如六味地黄丸。治肾阳

tern manifested by aching and weakness at low back and knees, dizziness and tinnitus, it is combined with *Rehmanniae Radix Praeparata* (shu di huang), *Dioscoreae Rhizoma* (shan yao) and *Poria* (fu ling), to form up Rehmannia Pills with Six Ingredients (Liu Wei Di Huang Wan). In the treatment of kidney yang insufficiency pattern manifested by fear of cold, chills in limbs, edema in limbs and body and difficult urination, it is combined with *Aconiti Lateralis Radix Praeparata* (fu zi) and *Cinnamomi Ramulus* (gui zhi), to form up Kidney Qi Pills (Shen Qi Wan).

不足之畏寒肢冷、肢体水肿、小便不利,常与附子、桂枝等同用,如肾气丸。

(2) Seminal emission, seminal leakage, enuresis and frequency of urination. The medicinal herb is sour and astringent in property, and acts to hold essence and astringe urine. In the treatment of seminal emission and nocturnal emission due to kidney deficiency, it is combined with *Psoraleae Fructus* (bu gu zhi) and *Cuscutae Semen* (tu si zi). In the treatment of enuresis and frequency of urination due to kidney deficiency, it is combined with *Mantidis OÖTheca* (sang piao xiao), *Poria cum Radix pini* (fu shen) and *Linderae Radix* (wu yao).

(2) 遗精滑精,遗尿尿频。本品味酸收敛,能固精止遗、缩尿。治肾虚遗精、滑精,常与补骨脂、菟丝子等同用。治肾虚遗尿尿频,可与桑螵蛸、茯神、乌药等同用。

(3) Metrorrhagia, metrostaxis and heavy blood flow in menstruation. The medicinal herb acts to reinforce liver and kidney, strengthen Thoroughfare and Conception Vessels, and astringe and stanch blood. In the treatment of liver and kidney deficiency pattern or Thoroughfare and Conception dysfunction pattern manifested by metrorrhagia, metrostaxis and heavy blood flow in menstruation, it is combined with *Astragali Radix* (huang qi), *Atractylodis Macrocephalae Rhizoma* (bai zhu) and *Os Draconis* (long gu).

(3) 崩漏下血,月经过多。本品有补肝肾、固冲任、收敛止血作用。治肝肾亏虚、冲任不固之崩漏下血、月经过多,常配伍黄芪、白术、龙骨等同用。

(4) Incessant sweating and collapse due to weak body. The medicinal herb acts to astringe sweat and treat collapse. In the treatment of chronic disease, collapse, profuse sweating, incessant sweating due to mistreatment, chills in limbs and weak pulse, it is combined with *Ginseng Radix et Raizoma* (ren shen), *Aconiti Lateralis Radix Praeparata* (fu zi) and *Os Draconis* (long gu).

(4) 大汗不止，体虚欲脱证。本品能敛汗固脱。治久病虚脱或大汗、误汗之大汗淋漓、肢冷、脉微者，常与人参、附子、龙骨等同用。

Furthermore, the medicinal herb acts to treat diabetes.

此外，本品还可治消渴证。

Usage and dosage Apply 5～10 g in decoction. The medicinal herb acts to astringe and treat collapse in crude form, and acts to reinforce and benefit liver and kidney in liquor-prepared form.

用法用量 煎服，5～10克。生用收敛固脱，酒制补益肝肾。

Precautions for use It is not advisable to apply for those with fire and heat hyperactivity or those with strangury due to dampheat.

使用注意 火热炽盛，湿热淋证等不宜应用。

Remarks *Euodiae Fructus* (wu zhu yu) and *Corni Fructus* (shan zhu yu)

按语 吴茱萸与山茱萸

The two medicinal herbs are similar in names but different in actions. *Euodiae Fructus* (wu zhu yu) is the dried product from the nearly ripe fruit of *Evodia rutaecarpa* (Juss) Benth, *Felis bengalensis chinensis or Hydrophobic evodia rutacarpa*, while *Corni frucus* (shan zhu yu) is the dried product from the ripe sarcocarp of the deciduous arbor *Cornus officinalis* Sieb. et Zucc., family Cornaceae. Wu zhu yu is pungent, bitter and hot in property, and acts to eliminate cold, stop pain, subdue up-reverse flow of qi, relieve vomiting, assist yang and stop diarrhea, applied to treat interior cold pattern. Shan zhu yu is sour and astringent and acts to astringe and treat collapse, applied to treat leakage and collapse pattern, and also acts to reinforce and

二药药名相似，功效迥异。吴茱萸为芸香科植物，山茱萸为山茱萸科植物。吴茱萸辛苦性热，能散寒止痛、降逆止呕、助阳止泻，为里寒证多用；山茱萸酸涩，能收敛固脱，为滑脱证多用，还补益肝肾。

benefit liver and kidney as well.

Mantidis OÖTheca (sang piao xiao)

桑螵蛸

It is the dried product from the egg-case of Praying Mantis, *Tenodera sinensis* Saussure, *Statilia maculate* (Thunb.) or *Hierodula patellifera* (Serrille), family Mantidae. The medicinal herb is collected from late autumn to next spring, applied in steamed form.

为螳螂科昆虫大刀螂、小刀螂或巨斧螳螂的干燥卵鞘。深秋至次春采收。蒸制后用。

Features Flavor: sweet and salty. Property: neutral. Meridian tropism: the Liver Meridian and the Kidney Meridian.

性味归经 甘、咸，平。归肝、肾经。

Actions Astringe essence, hold urine, reinforce kidney and assist yang.

功效 固精缩尿，补肾助阳。

Application

应用

(1) Seminal emission, seminal leakage, enuresis and frequency of urination. The medicinal herb is sweet and salty in flavor and attributive to the Kidney Meridian, and acts to reinforce kidney, astringe essence and hold urine. In the treatment of kidney deficiency pattern manifested by seminal emission and seminal leakage, it is combined with *Os Draconis* (long gu) and *Schisandrae Chinensis Fructus* (wu wei zi), to form up Mantis Egg-case Pills (Sang Piao Xiao Wan). In the treatment of enuresis and frequency of urination, it is applied singly or combined with *Os Draconis* (long gu), *Acori Tatarinowii Rhizoma* (shi chang pu) and *Polygalae Radix* (yuan zhi).

（1）遗精滑精，遗尿尿频。本品甘咸入肾，能补肾固精缩尿。治肾虚之遗精滑精，常配伍龙骨、五味子等同用，如桑螵蛸丸。治遗尿尿频，可单用，亦可与龙骨、石菖蒲、远志等同用。

(2) Impotence due to kidney deficiency. The medicinal herb acts to reinforce kidney and assist yang. In the treatment of impotence due to kidney yang insufficiency, it is combined with *Cervi Cornu Pantotrichum* (lu rong), *Cistanchis Herba* (rou cong rong) and *Cuscutae Semen* (tu si zi).

（2）肾虚阳痿。本品又能补肾助阳，治肾阳不足之阳痿，常与鹿茸、肉苁蓉、菟丝子等同用。

Usage and dosage　Apply 5～10 g in decoction.

Precautions for use　It is prohibited to apply for those with seminal emission or frequency due to yin deficiency and fire hyperactivity or due to damp-heat in bladder.

用法用量　煎服，5～10克。

使用注意　阴虚火旺或膀胱湿热所致的遗精、尿频者忌用。

Rosae Laevigatae Fructus (jin ying zi)

It is the dried product from the ripe fruit of *Rosa laevigata* Michx., family Rosaceae. The medicinal herb is collected in autumn, applied in crude form by removing its core.

Features　Flavor: sour, sweet and astringent. Property: neutral. Meridian tropism: the Kidney Meridian, the Bladder Meridian and the Large Intestine Meridian.

Actions　Astringe essence, hold urine, astringe blood, treat morbid leucorrhea, astringe intestines and stop diarrhea.

Application

(1) Seminal emission, seminal leakage, enuresis and frequency of urination. The medicinal herb is sour and astringent in property and acts to astringe essence and hold urine. In the treatment of seminal emission, seminal leakage, enuresis and frequency of urination, it is applied singly by making into poultice, or combined with *Euryales Semen* (qian shi), to form up Land-Water Two Immortals Elixer (Shui Lu Er Xian Dan).

(2) Metrorrhagia, metrostaxis and morbid leucorrhea. The medicinal herb acts to astringe and stanch blood and treat morbid leucorrhea. In the treatment of metrorrhagia and metrostaxis, it is combined with *Zingiberis Rhizoma Praeparatum*

金樱子

为蔷薇科植物金樱子干燥成熟果实。10～11月果实成熟变红采收。生用。

性味归经　酸、甘，涩，平。归肾、膀胱、大肠经。

功效　固精缩尿，固崩止带，涩肠止泻。

应用

（1）遗精滑精，遗尿尿频。本品酸涩收敛，有固精缩尿之功。治遗精滑精、遗尿尿频，可单味熬膏服，或与芡实同用，即水陆二仙丹。

（2）崩漏带下。本品能固崩止漏、止带。治崩漏不止，可与炮姜、茜草炭等同用。治带下清稀，可与白芷、莲子等同用。

(pao jiang) and carbonized *Rubiae Radix Et Rhizoma* (qian cao). In the treatment of clear and thin leucorrhea, it is combined with *Angelicae Dahuricae Radix* (bai zhi) and *Nelumbinis Semen* (lian zi).

(3) Chronic diarrhea and chronic dysentery. The medicinal herb acts to astringe intestines and stop diarrhea. In the treatment of chronic diarrhea and chronic dysentery due to spleen deficiency, it is applied singly or combined with *Codonopsis Radix* (dang shen), *Atractylodis Macrocephalae Rhizoma* (bai zhu) and *Euryales Semen* (qian shi).

(3) 久泻久痢。本品又能涩肠止泻。治脾虚久泻、久痢，可单味煎服，或与党参、白术、芡实等同用。

Usage and dosage Apply 6～15 g in decoction.

用法用量 煎服，6～15克。

Nelumbinis Semen (lian zi)

莲子

It is the dried product from the ripe seed of *Nelumbo nucifera* Gaertn., family Nymphaeaceae. The medicinal herb is collected in autumn, applied in crude form by removing its core.

为睡莲科植物莲的干燥成熟种子。秋季采收。去心，生用。

Features Flavor: sweet and astringent. Property: neutral. Meridian tropism: the Spleen Meridian, the Kidney Meridian and the Heart Meridian.

性味归经 甘、涩，平。归脾、肾、心经。

Actions Reinforce spleen, stop diarrhea, treat morbid leucorrhea, benefit kidney, hold essence, nourish heart, and calm mind.

功效 补脾止泻，止带，益肾固精，养心安神。

Application

(1) Diarrhea due to spleen deficiency. The medicinal herb is sweet and astringent and acts to strengthen spleen, benefit qi, astringe intestines and stop diarrhea. In the treatment of diarrhea and poor sleep due to spleen deficiency, it is combined with *Ginseng Radix et Raizoma* (ren shen), *Poria* (fu ling) and *Atractylodis Macrocephalae Rhizoma* (bai zhu), to form up Ginseng, Poria and Atrac-

应用

(1) 脾虚泄泻。本品甘平补益，味涩收敛，功能健脾益气、涩肠止泻。治脾虚久泻，食欲不振，常与人参、茯苓、白术等同用，如参苓白术散。亦治脾肾两虚的久泻不止，可与补骨脂、肉豆蔻等同用。

tylodes Powder (Shen Ling Bai Zhu San). In the treatment of chronic diarrhea due to spleen and kidney deficiency, it is combined with *Psoraleae Fructus* (bu gu zhi) and *Myristicae Semen* (rou dou kou).

(2) Morbid leucorrhea. The medicinal herb is sweet and astringent in property and acts to reinforce spleen and kidney and treat morbid leucorrhea. In the treatment of leucorrhea due to spleen deficiency or due to spleen and kidney deficiency, it is combined with bai zhu, fu ling, *Dioscoreae Rhizoma* (shan yao) and *Euryales Semen* (qian shi).

(2) 带下证。本品甘补脾肾，性涩止带。治脾虚或脾肾两虚的带下，常与白术、茯苓、山药、芡实等同用。

(3) Seminal emission and seminal leakage. The medicinal herb is attributive to the Kidney Meridian and acts to benefit kidney, hold essence and stop emission. In the treatment of seminal emission and seminal leakage due to kidney deficiency and failure in holding essence, it is combined with *Astragali Complanati Semen* (sha yuan zi), *Euryales Semen* (qian shi) and *Os Draconis* (long gu), to form up Golden Lock Essence-Controlling Pills (Jin Suo Gu Jing Wan).

(3) 遗精，滑精。本品入肾经，能益肾固精止遗。治肾虚不固之遗精滑泄，常配伍沙苑子、芡实、龙骨等同用，如金锁固精丸。

(4) Insomnia and fearful throbbing. The medicinal herb acts to nourish heart, benefit kidney and harmonize heart and kidney. In the treatment of disharmony between heart and kidney manifested by restlessness, insomnia and fearful throbbing, it is combined with *Ziziphi Spinosae Semen* (suan zao ren), *Poria cum Radix pini* (fu shen) and *Polygalae Radix* (yuan zhi).

(4) 失眠惊悸。本品能养心益肾，交通心肾。治心肾不交之虚烦、失眠、惊悸，常与酸枣仁、茯神、远志等同用。

Usage and dosage Apply 6～15 g in decoction.

用法用量 煎服，6～15克。

Euryales Semen (qian shi)

It is the dried product from the ripe seed of Gordon Euryale, *Euryale ferox* Salisb., family Nymphaeaceae. The medicinal herb is collected in late autumn and early winter, applied in crude form or in bran-fried form.

Features Flavor: sweet and astringent. Property: neutral. Meridian tropism: the Spleen Meridian and the Kidney Meridian.

Actions Benefit kidney, hold essence, reinforce spleen, stop diarrhea, dissolve damp and treat morbid leucorrhea.

Application

(1) Seminal emission, seminal leakage, enuresis and frequency of urination. The medicinal herb is sweet and astringent in property and acts to reinforce kidney, hold essence and stop emission. In the treatment of seminal emission and seminal leakage due to kidney deficiency and failure in holding essence, it is combined with *Rosae Laevigatae Fructus* (jin ying zi), to form up Land-Water Two Immortals Elixer (Shui Lu Er Xian Dan), or combined with *Astragali Complanati Semen* (sha yuan zi), *Os Draconis* (long gu) and *Nelumbinis Semen* (lian zi), to form up Golden Lock Essence-Controlling Pills (Jin Suo Gu Jing Wan). In the treatment of incontinence of urine and infantile enuresis due to kidney deficiency, it is combined with *Cuscutae Semen* (tu si zi), *Alpiniae Oxyphyllae Fructus* (yi zhi) and *Mantidis OÖTheca* (sang piao xiao).

(2) Chronic diarrhea due to spleen deficiency. The medicinal herb is sweet in flavor and attributive to the Spleen Meridian, and acts to strengthen

芡实

为睡莲科植物芡的干燥成熟种仁。秋末冬初采收。生用或麸炒用。

性味归经 甘、涩，平。归脾、肾经。

功效 益肾固精，补脾止泻，除湿止带。

应用

（1）遗精滑精，遗尿尿频。本品甘涩收敛，功善补肾固精止遗。治肾虚不固之遗精滑精，常配伍金樱子同用，即水陆二仙丹；或与沙苑子、龙骨、莲子等同用，如金锁固精丸。治肾虚小便不禁、小儿遗尿，常与菟丝子、益智仁、桑螵蛸等同用。

（2）脾虚久泻。本品甘味入脾，善健脾除湿、涩肠止泻。治脾虚久泻，常与党参、

spleen, dissolve damp, astringe intestines and stop diarrhea. In the treatment of chronic diarrhea due to spleen deficiency, it is combined with *Codonopsis Radix* (dang shen), *Atractylodis Macrocephalae Rhizoma* (bai zhu) and *Poria* (fu ling).

白术、茯苓等同用。

(3) Morbid leucorrhea. The medicinal herb acts to benefit kidney, strengthen spleen, dissolve damp and treat morbid leucorrhea. In the treatment of excessive leucorrhea due to spleen and kidney deficiency, it is combined with *Corni Fructus* (shan zhu yu), *Cuscutae Semen* (tu si zi) and *Dioscoreae Rhizoma* (shan yao). In the treatment of morbid leucorrhea due to damp-heat, it is combined with *Phellodendri Cortex Chiensis* (huang bo) and *Plantaginis Semen* (che qian zi).

(3) 带下证。本品能益肾健脾、除湿止带。治脾肾两虚的白带过多，常与山茱萸、菟丝子、山药等配伍。治湿热带下，可与黄柏、车前子等同用。

Usage and dosage Apply 10～15 g in decoction.

用法用量 煎服，10～15 克。

Brief summary

小 结

Both *Ephedrae Radix Et Rhizoma* (ma huang gen) and *Tritici Levis Fructus* (fu xiao mai) act to stop sweating, applied to treat spontaneous sweating and nocturnal sweats. Ma huang gen is neutral in property and attributive to the Lung Meridian, and acts to astringe sweat and stop sweating, applied for oral administration or for external use by grinding into fine powder. Fu xiao mai is cool in property and attributive to the Heart Meridian, and acts to benefit heart qi, astringe heart fluid and reduce false heat, applied to treat spontaneous sweating and nocturnal sweats, and also to treat fever due to yin deficiency and feverish sensation due to yin deficiency.

麻黄根、浮小麦，均能止汗，治自汗、盗汗。其中麻黄根性平，专入肺经，功专于收敛止汗，内服或研末外扑皆可。浮小麦性凉，入心经，能益心气、敛心液、除虚热，既治自汗盗汗，又治阴虚发热、骨蒸劳热。

Both *Schisandrae Chinensis Fructus* (wu wei zi)

五味子、乌梅，均味酸性

and *Mume Fructus* (wu mei) are sour and astringent in property and act to astringe lung, astringe intestines and produce fluid, applied to treat chronic cough due to lung deficiency, chronic diarrhea, chronic dysentery, and thirst due to fluid consumption. Wu wei zi is sour, astringent and warm and acts to reinforce kidney, astringe lung and hold essence, and also acts to quiet heart and calm mind, applied to treat palpitation and insomnia due to yin deficiency or due to blood deficiency. Wu mei is sour, astringent and neutral in property and acts to produce fluid, relieve thirst and remove roundworm, as the major herb to treat diabetes due to false heat and abdominal pain due to roundworm.

涩，均能敛肺、涩肠、生津，治肺虚久咳，久泻久痢，津伤口渴。其中五味子酸收性温，补敛相兼，尚具补肾之功，能补肾敛肺、涩精；且能宁心安神，治阴虚血亏的心悸失眠。乌梅酸收性平，无补肾之功，但善生津止渴，且能安蛔，为治虚热消渴、蛔厥腹痛之要药。

Both *Myristicae Semen* (rou dou kou) and *Halloysitum Rubrum* (chi shi zhi) act to astringe intestines and stop diarrhea, applied to treat chronic diarrhea and chronic dysentery. Rou dou kou is pungent, warm and astringent and acts to warm middle energizer and move qi, applied to treat epigastric and abdominal distension and pain, poor appetite and vomiting due to cold or qi stagnation of stomach. Chi shi zhi is sweet, sour and astringent in property and acts to astringe intestines, stop diarrhea, heal ulcer, engender muscle, and astringe and stanch blood, applied to treat unhealed ulcer of carbuncle and furuncle, metrorrhagia, metrostaxis and morbid leucorrhea.

肉豆蔻、赤石脂，均能涩肠止泻，治久泻久痢。其中肉豆蔻辛温而涩，又能温中行气，可治胃寒气滞之脘腹胀痛、食少呕吐。赤石脂甘酸性涩，既涩肠止泻，又敛疮生肌、收敛止血，可治疮疡不敛，崩漏带下等证。

Corni Fructus (shan zhu yu) is sour, astringent and warm in property and attributive to the Liver and Kidney Meridians, and acts to reinforce liver and kidney and harmonize and reinforce yin and yang, applied to treat liver and kidney deficiency pattern. It also acts to astringe and control fluids,

山茱萸，酸涩性温，入肝肾经，补涩相兼，功善补肝肾、平补阴阳，为补肝肾之要药，善治肝肾亏虚之证；又善收敛固涩，用于各种滑脱证及体虚欲脱、虚汗不止。

applied to treat various types of leakage and collapse pattern, syncope due to weak body and incessant sweating due to deficiency.

Both *Mantidis OÖTheca* (sang piao xiao) and *Rosae Laevigatae Fructus* (jin ying zi) acts to astringe essence and hold urine, applied to treat kidney deficiency manifested by seminal emission, seminal leakage, enuresis and frequency of urination. Sang piao xiao acts to reinforce kidney, to astringe essence and hold urine, and also acts to reinforce kidney and assist yang, applied to treat impotence due to kidney yang deficiency. Jin ying zi acts to astringe intestines, stop diarrhea, astringe blood and treat morbid leucorrhea, applied to treat chronic diarrhea, chronic dysentery, metrorrhagia, metrostaxis and morbid leucorrhea.

桑螵蛸、金樱子，均能固精缩尿，治肾虚遗精滑精、遗尿尿频等证。其中桑螵蛸具补肾之功，既固精缩尿，又补肾助阳，还治肾虚阳痿等证。金樱子虽无补益作用，但长于收敛，还能涩肠止泻、固崩止带，用于久泻久痢、崩漏带下。

Both *Nelumbinis Semen* (lian zi) and *Euryales Semen* (qian shi) are sweet, astringent and neutral in property and attributive to the Spleen and Kidney Meridians, and act to benefit kidney, astringe essence, reinforce spleen and stop diarrhea, applied to treat seminal emission and seminal leakage due to kidney deficiency, and chronic diarrhea due to spleen deficiency. Lian zi is stronger in reinforcing spleen, and also acts to nourish heart and calm mind, applied to treat restlessness, palpitation and insomnia. Qian shi is weaker in reinforcing spleen, but acts to dissolve damp, applied to treat morbid leucorrhea of deficiency type or excess type.

莲子、芡实，均味甘涩性平，入脾肾经，均能益肾固精、补脾止泻，治肾虚遗精滑精、脾虚久泻等证。其中莲子补脾力较强，还能养心安神，治虚烦、心悸、失眠。芡实补脾力弱，善于祛湿，治带下病，虚实均宜。

Chapter 18 Herbs for External Application

第 18 章 外用药

The medicinal herbs acting to attack toxin, kill worms, desiccate damp and stop itching, applied for external use are called the herbs for external application.

以外用为主，具攻毒杀虫、燥湿止痒作用的药物，称为外用药。

The medicinal herbs are mainly applied for external use, and also applied for oral administration as well. The medicinal herbs applied for external use act to relieve toxin, kill worms, subside swell and stop pain, applied to treat scabies, eczema, carbuncle and furuncle, leprosy, syphilis and poisonous snake-bites. The methods for external use are as follows: topical application by spraying powder, wet compress, smearing method with ointment, fumigation with decoction, hot compress, etc. The medicinal herbs applied for oral administration act to purify lung, dissolve phlegm, reinforce fire, strengthen yang, promote defecation, eliminate wind and stop pain, applied to treat cough with sputum due to heat in lung, constipation due to kidney deficiency and Bi (Obturation) Pattern due to wind-damp.

本类药物以外用为主，兼可内服，外用主要具有解毒杀虫、消肿定痛等功效，适用于疥癣、湿疹、痈疮疔毒、麻风、梅毒、毒蛇咬伤等病证。外用方法有研末外撒、调敷，或制成软膏涂抹，或煎汤熏洗、热敷等。内服有清肺化痰、补火壮阳通便、祛风止痛等作用，主要用于肺热痰嗽、肾虚便秘、风湿痹痛等证。

In the application of this type of medicinal herbs, it should be noticed that these herbs are mostly poisonous. It is necessary to strictly control the dosage and usage in both external use and oral administration. It is not advisable to apply in over-

使用本类药需注意，大多有毒，无论外用、内服均应严格控制剂量和用法，不宜过量或持续使用。制剂时，应严格遵守炮制及制剂法

dose or for a long period of time. In the preparation of the herbs, it is necessary to follow the rules of preparation, so as to decrease their toxicity and to guarantee the safe medication.

度,以降低毒性,确保用药安全。

Sulfur (liu huang)

硫黄

It is the product from the refined product of the natural ore sulfur or sulfur minerals. The medicinal herb is collected all over the year, applied in prepared form.

为自然元素类矿物硫族自然硫或含硫矿物经加工制得。全年可采。制用。

Features Flavor: sour. Property: warm and poisonous. Meridian tropism: the Kidney Meridian and the Large Intestine Meridian.

性味归经 酸,温;有毒。归肾、大肠经。

Actions Relieve toxin, kill worms and stop itching in external use, and reinforce fire, strengthen yang and promote defecation in oral administration.

功效 外用解毒杀虫止痒;内服补火壮阳通便。

Application

(1) Scabies, eczema and skin itch. The medicinal herb acts to relieve toxin, kill worms and stop itching in external use. In the treatment of scabies, it is to grind the herb into fine powder and mix it with sesame oil to smear the sick area. In the treatment of stubborn tinea with itching, it is combined with *Borneolum Syntheticum* (bing pian), to grind them into fine powder and make into ointment for smearing sick area. In the treatment of eczema and skin itch, it is applied singly by grinding into fine powder for topical compress, or combined with *Cnidii Fructus* (she chuang zi) and dired *Alumen* (bai fan).

(2) Kidney yang deficiency pattern. The medicinal herb acts to reinforce fire, strengthen yang and promote defecation for oral administration. In

应用

(1) 疥癣,湿疹,皮肤瘙痒。本品外用有解毒杀虫止痒作用,尤善疗疥疮。治疥疮,可研末,用麻油调涂患处。治顽癣瘙痒,可与冰片等为末,调膏涂敷患处。治湿疹、皮肤瘙痒,可单用研末外撒,或配蛇床子、枯矾等同用。

(2) 肾阳虚证。本品内服能补火壮阳通便。治肾虚气喘,可与附子、肉桂、补骨

the treatment of panting due to kidney qi deficiency, it is combined with *Aconiti Lateralis Radix Praeparata* (fu zi), *Cinnamomi Cortex* (rou gui) and *Psoraleae Fructus* (bu gu zhi). In the treatment of impotence due to kidney deficiency, it is combined with *Cervi Cornu Pantotrichum* (lu rong) and *Epimedii Folium* (yin yang huo). In the treatment of constipation due to deficiency and cold, it is combined with *Pinelliae Rhizoma* (ban xia), to form up Pinellia and Sulfer Pills (Ban Liu Wan).

脂等同用。治肾虚阳痿，可与鹿茸、淫羊藿等同用。治虚冷便秘，常与半夏配伍，即半硫丸。

Usage and dosage Apply a proper amount for external use, by grinding the herb into fine powder for topical spray or combining the herb with sesame oil for topical compress. The medicinal herb in prepared form is applied for oral administration. Apply 1.5～3 g pills or powder.

用法用量 外用适量，研末撒敷或香油调涂。炮制后内服，入丸散，1.5～3 克。

Precautions for use It is prohibited to apply for those with yin deficiency and yang hyperactivity or for pregnant women. It is not advisable to apply with *Natrii Sulfas* (mang xiao).

使用注意 阴虚阳亢者及孕妇忌服。不宜与芒硝同用。

Alumen (bai fan)

白矾

It is the product from the refined product of the mineral Alunite of sulphate, mainly containing potassium aluminium sulfate [$KAl(SO_4)_2 \cdot 12H_2O$], applied in crude form or in calcined form.

为硫酸盐类矿物明矾石经加工提炼制成。主要成分为含水硫酸铝钾。生用或煅用。

Features Flavor: sour and atringent. Property: cold. Meridian tropism: the Lung Meridian, the Spleen Meridian, the Liver Meridian and the Large Intestine Meridian.

性味归经 酸、涩，寒。归肺、脾、肝、大肠经。

Actions Relieve toxin, kill worms, desiccate damp and stop itching in external use, and stanch blood, stop diarrhea, reduce heat and dissolve phlegm in oral administration.

功效 外用解毒杀虫，燥湿止痒；内服止血止泻，清热消痰。

Application

(1) Eczema, carbuncle and scabies. The medicinal herb acts to relieve toxin, kill worms, astringe damp and stop itching in external use. In the treatment of eczema and carbuncle, it is combined with *Phellodendri Cortex Chiensis* (huang bo) and calcined *Gypsum Fibrosum* (shi gao). In the treatment of skin itch due to scabies, it is combined with *Sulfur* (liu huang) and *Cnidii Fructus* (she chuang zi).

(2) Hematemesis, epistaxis, uterine bleeding, chronic diarrhea and chronic dysentery. The medicinal herb is astringent in property and acts to astringe and stanch blood, astringe intestines and stop diarrhea. In the treatment of hematemesis and epistaxis, it is combined with *Imperatae Rhizoma* (bai mao gen) and *Platyclaoi Cacumen* (ce bai ye). In the treatment of bloody feces, metrorrhagia and metrostaxis, it is combined with *Sanguisorbae Radix* (di yu) and *Rubiae Radix Et Rhizoma* (qian cao). In the treatment of chronic diarrhea and chronic dysentery, it is combined with *Mume Fructus* (wu mei) and *Halloysitum Rubrum* (chi shi zhi).

(3) Epilepsy and mania. The medicinal herb is cold in property and acts to dissolve phlegm, open aperture and reduce heat. In the treatment of epilepsy or mania due to wind-heat, it is combined with *Curcumae Radix* (yu jin), to form up White and Golden Pills (Bai Jin Wan).

Usage and dosage Apply a proper amount for external use, by grinding into fine powder for external compress or wash. Apply 0.5～1.5 g pills or powder for oral administration. The medicinal herb acts to relieve toxin, kill worms, stop diarrhea and dissolve phlegm in crude form, and acts to astringe

应用

（1）湿疹，湿疮，疥癣。本品外用能解毒杀虫、收湿止痒。治湿疹、湿疮，可与黄柏、煅石膏等同用。治疥癣所致的皮肤瘙痒，可与硫黄、蛇床子等同用。

（2）吐衄下血，久泻久痢。本品性涩收敛，能收敛止血、涩肠止泻。治吐血衄血，可与白茅根、侧柏叶等同用。治便血、崩漏，常与地榆、茜草等同用。治久泻、久痢，可与乌梅、赤石脂等同用。

（3）癫痫发狂。本品能祛痰开闭、性寒清热。治风痰所致的癫痫发狂，常与郁金同用，即白金丸。

用法用量 外用适量，研末调敷或化水洗；内服入丸散，0.5～1.5克。生用解毒杀虫、止泻、消痰；煅后称“枯矾”，收湿敛疮，止血。

damp, heal ulcer and stanch blood in calcined form, termed as "ku fan".

Precautions for use It is prohibited to apply for those with weak body, stomach deficiency and those without damp, heat, phlegm or fire.

使用注意 体虚胃弱及无湿热痰火者忌服。

Cnidii Fructus (she chuang zi)

蛇床子

It is the dried product from the ripe fruit of *Cnidium onnierii* (L.) Cusson, family Umbelliferae. The medicinal herb is collected in summer and autumn, applied in crude form.

为伞形科植物蛇床的干燥成熟果实。夏、秋二季采收。生用。

Features Flavor: pungent and bitter. Property: warm and slightly poisonous. Meridian tropism: the Kidney Meridian.

性味归经 辛、苦,温;有小毒。归肾经。

Actions Kill worms, stop itching, eliminate wind, desiccate damp, warm kidney and strengthen yang.

功效 杀虫止痒,祛风燥湿,温肾壮阳。

Application

应用

(1) Perineum pruritus, morbid leucorrhea, eczema and scabies. The medicinal herb is pungent, bitter and warm in property and acts to eliminate wind, desiccate damp, kill worms and stop itching. In the treatment of perineum pruritus and morbid leucorrhea, it is applied singly or combined with *Alumen* (bai fan), *Sophorae Flavescentis Radix* (ku shen) and *Phellodendri Cortex Chiensis* (huang bo) for external use by decocting and washing. In the treatment of eczema and scabies, it is combined with ku shen, *Cortex Meliae* (ku lian pi) and *Kochiae Fructus* (di fu zi) for external use by decocting and washing sick area.

(1) 阴痒带下,湿疹疥癣。本品辛散祛风,苦温燥湿,有祛风燥湿、杀虫止痒作用。治阴痒带下,可单用或配伍白矾、苦参、黄柏等煎汤外洗。治湿疹、疥癣,可配伍苦参、苦楝皮、地肤子等煎水敷洗患处。

(2) Bi (Obturation) Pattern due to damp and low back pain. The medicinal herb is bitter and warm in property, and acts to eliminate cold, re-

(2) 湿痹腰痛。本品苦温,能散寒祛风燥湿。治湿痹腰痛,常与杜仲、续断、桑

move wind and desiccate damp. In the treatment of Bi (Obturation) Pattern due to damp and low back pain, it is combined with *Eucommiae Cortex* (du zhong), *Dipsaci Radix* (xu duan) and *Taxilli Herba* (sang ji sheng).

寄生等同用。

(3) Impotence and infertility due to cold in uterus. The medicinal herb is attributive to the Kidney Meridian and acts to warm kidney and strengthen yang in oral administration. In the treatment of impotence and infertility due to kidney yang insufficiency, it is combined with *Schisandrae Chinensis Fructus* (wu wei zi) and *Cuscutae Semen* (tu si zi), or combined with *Rehmanniae Radix Praeparata* (shu di huang) and *Eucommiae Cortex* (du zhong).

（3）阳痿，宫冷不孕。本品入肾经，内服能温肾壮阳。治肾阳不足所致的阳痿、宫冷不孕，常与五味子、菟丝子同用，或配伍熟地黄、杜仲等同用。

Usage and dosage Apply 3～10 g in decoction. Apply a proper amount for external use.

Precautions for use It is not advisable to apply for oral administration for those with yin deficiency and fire hyperactivity or those with damp-heat in lower energizer.

用法用量 煎服，3～10克。外用适量。

使用注意 阴虚火旺或下焦有湿热者不宜内服。

Nidus Vespae (feng fang)

蜂房

It is the product from the honeycomb of *Polistes olivaceous* (Degeer), *Polistes japonicus* Saussure or *Parapolybia varia* Fabricius, family Vespidae. The medicinal herb is produced all over the country, more in the south. It is collected all over the year, applied in crude form.

为胡蜂科昆虫果马蜂、日本长脚胡蜂或异腹胡蜂的巢。全国各地均产，南方尤多。全年可采。生用。

Features Flavor: sweet. Property: neutral and poisonous. Meridian tropism: the Stomach Meridian.

性味归经 甘，平；有毒。归胃经。

Actions Relieve toxin, kill worms, eliminate wind and stop pain.

功效 攻毒杀虫，祛风止痛。

Application

应用

(1) Carbuncle, furuncle, scrofula and scabies.

（1）疮痈，瘰疬，癣疮。

The medicinal herb acts to relieve toxin and kill worms in both external use and oral administration. In the treatment of carbuncle, furuncle and acute mastitis, it is applied singly by grinding into fine powder for external compress or by baking into brownish for oral administration. In the treatment of scrofula, it is combined with *Scrophulariae Radix* (xuan shen) and *Prunellae Spica* (xia ku cao). In the treatment of scabies, it is applied singly by grinding into fine powder for external compress.

本品能攻毒杀虫，外用内服皆可。治疮痈、乳痈，可单用研末外敷，或焙黄研末内服。治瘰疬，可与玄参、夏枯草等同用。治癣疮，可外用研末调敷。

(2) Bi (Obturation) Pattern and toothache. The medicinal herb acts to eliminate wind and stop pain. In the treatment of Bi (Obturation) Pattern, it is combined with wind-eliminating and collateral-dredging herbs for oral administration. In the treatment of toothache, it is applied singly or combined with *Asari Radix et Rhizoma* (xi xin) and *Zanthoxyli Pericarpium* (hua jiao) by decocting and rinsing the mouth.

（2）风湿痹痛，牙痛。本品能祛风止痛。治风湿痹痛，可与祛风通络药配伍内服。治牙痛，可单用或配细辛、花椒煎水含漱。

Usage and dosage Apply a proper amount for external use by grinding into fine powder for topical compress or by decocting into water for local wash. Apply 3～5 g in decoction.

用法用量 外用适量，研末调敷或煎水漱洗患处。煎服，3～5 克。

Calamina (lu gan shi)

炉甘石

It is the product from the smithsonite of carbonate of calcite group, mainly containing zinc carbonate ($ZnCO_3$). The medicinal herb is applied in crude form or in powdered form.

为碳酸盐类矿物方解石族菱锌矿，主含碳酸锌。生用或煅后水飞用。

Features Flavor: sweet. Property: neutral. Meridian tropism: the Liver Meridian and the Stomach Meridian.

性味归经 甘，平。归肝、胃经。

Actions Relieve toxin, brighten eyes, treat cataract, desiccate damp, engender muscle and heal

功效 解毒明目退翳，收湿生肌敛疮。

ulcer.

Application

(1) Redness of eyes, cataract, swelling and ulceration of eyelids. The medicinal herb acts to relieve toxin, brighten eyes, treat cataract, desiccate damp, stop lacrimation and stop itching, as the major herb to treat eye diseases. In the treatment of redness of eyes and cataract, it is combined with *Natrii Sulfas* (mang xiao) by grinding into fine powder and melting in water for eye dropping. In the treatment of swelling and ulceration of eyelids, it is combined with *Borax* (peng sha) and *Borneolum Syntheticum* (bing pian) by grinding into fine powder for eye dropping.

(2) Unhealed ulcer and eczema. The medicinal herb acts to engender muscle, heal ulcer, desiccate damp and stop itching. In the treatment of unhealed ulcer, it is combined with *Os Draconis* (long gu) by grinding into fine powder for topical compress, or combined with *Indigo Naturalis* (qing dai), *Phellodendri Cortex Chiensis* (huang bo) and calcined *Gypsum Fibrosum* (shi gao) by grinding into fine powder for topical compress.

Usage and dosage Apply a proper amount for external use.

Precautions for use The medicinal herb is only applied for external use, never applied for oral administration.

应用

（1）目赤翳障，睑弦赤烂。本品能解毒明目退翳、收湿止泪止痒，为眼科要药。治目赤翳障，可与芒硝等份研末，化水点眼。治眼睑赤烂，常配伍硼砂、冰片等研细末点眼。

（2）溃疡不敛，皮肤湿疮。本品有生肌敛疮、收湿止痒作用。治诸疮久溃不敛，可配伍龙骨研细末，干掺患处，再用膏药外贴，或与青黛、黄柏、煅石膏等研末外用。

用法用量 外用适量。

使用注意 本品专作外用，不作内服。

Borax (peng sha)

It is the product from thecrystals prepared from the ore *Borax*. The medicinal herb is applied in crude form or in calcined form.

Features Flavor: sweet and salty. Property:

硼砂

为天然硼酸盐类硼砂族矿物硼砂经提炼精制而成的结晶体。生用或煅用。

性味归经 甘、咸，凉。

cool. Meridian tropism: the Lung Meridian and the Stomach Meridian.

归肺、胃经。

Actions Reduce heat and relieve toxin in external use, and purify lung and dissolve phlegm in oral administration.

功效 外用清热解毒，内服清肺化痰。

Application

应用

(1) Sore throat, mouth ulcer, redness of eyes and cataract. The medicinal herb acts to reduce heat, relieve toxin, subside swell and diminish inflammation, as the major herb to treat diseases of ophthalmology and otolaryngology. In the treatment of sore throat and mouth and tongue ulcer, it is combined with *Natrii Sulfas* Exsiccatus (xuan ming fen), *Cinnabaris* (zhu sha) and *Borneolum Syntheticum* (bing pian) by grinding into fine powder for spraying at sick area, to form up Borneol and *Borax* Powder (Bing Peng San). In the treatment of redness, swelling and pain of eyes, and cataract, it is applied singly in water solution for eye dropping, or combined with *Calamina* (lu gan shi), *Borneolum Syntheticum* (bing pian) and *Natrii Sulfas* Exsiccatus (xuan ming fen) by making into eye drops for eye dropping.

（1）咽喉肿痛，口舌生疮，目赤翳障。本品外用有清热解毒、消肿、防腐作用，为五官科疾患的常用药。治咽喉肿痛、口舌生疮，常与玄明粉、朱砂、冰片研末吹敷患处，如冰硼散。治目赤肿痛，目生翳障，可以本品水溶液洗眼，或与炉甘石、冰片、玄明粉等制成点眼剂点眼。

(2) Cough due to phlegm-heat. The medicinal herb acts to purify lung and dissolve phlegm in oral administration. In the treatment of cough due to phlegm-heat with yellow-thick sputum or with difficult spitting of sputum, it is applied singly as mouth lozenge, or combined with *Fritillariae Cirrhosae Bulbus* (chuan bei mu) and *Trichosanthis Fructus* (gua lou).

（2）痰热咳嗽。本品内服有清肺化痰作用。治痰热咯痰黄稠、咯吐不爽，可单用含化咽津，或与贝母、瓜蒌等同用。

Usage and dosage Apply a proper amount for external use. Apply 1.5～3 g pills or powder for oral administration.

用法用量 外用适量。入丸散服，每次 1.5～3 克。

Brief summary

Both *Sulfur* (liu huang) and *Alumen* (bai fan) act to relieve toxin, kill worms and stop itching, applied to treat scabies, eczema and skin itch. Both of them are applied for both external use and oral administration. Liu huang is warm and poisonous in property, and acts to reinforce fire, strengthen yang and promote defecation in oral administration, applied to treat kidney yang deficiency pattern and constipation due to deficiency and cold. Bai fan is cold and astringent in property, and acts to desiccate damp, applied to treat eczema and carbuncle in external use. It has a stronger astringing action in calcined form. It acts to stanch blood, stop diarrhea, reduce heat and dissolve phlegm in oral administration, applied to treat hemetemesis, epistaxis, uterine bleeding, chronic diarrhea, chronic dysentery, epilepsy and mania.

Cnidii Fructus (she chuang zi) is pungent, bitter and warm in property, and acts to kill worms, stop itching, eliminate wind, desiccate damp, warm kidney and strengthen yang. It is applied to treat perineum pruritus, morbid leucorrhea, eczema and scabies in external use, and to treat Bi (Obturation) Pattern, low back pain and impotence due to kidney deficiency in oral administration.

Nidus Vespae (feng fang) is sweet, neutral and poisonous in property, and acts to relieve toxin, kill worms, eliminate wind and stop pain, applied for both external use and oral administration. It is applied to treat carbuncle, furuncle, scrofula, Bi (Obturation) Pattern due to wind-damp, and tooth-

小　结

硫黄、白矾，均能解毒杀虫止痒，治疥癣、湿疹、皮肤瘙痒；均既可外用，又能内服。其中硫黄性温有毒，内服功能补火壮阳通便，可治肾阳虚证及虚冷便秘。白矾性寒且涩，外用还能燥湿，善治湿疹湿疮，煅用收涩之功更佳；内服止血止泻、清热化痰，治吐衄下血，久泻久痢，癫痫发狂。

蛇床子，辛苦性温，既杀虫止痒、祛风燥湿，又温肾壮阳。外用善治阴痒带下、湿疹疥癣；内服既治湿痹腰痛，又治肾虚阳痿。

蜂房，甘平有毒，功能攻毒杀虫、祛风止痛；既可外用，又能内服。善治疮痈瘰疬，以及风湿痹痛、牙痛等证。

ache.

Calamina (lu gan shi) is sweet and neutral in property, and acts to relieve toxin, brighten eyes and treat cataract, and also to desiccate damp, engender muscles and heal ulcer, only applied in external use as the major herb for eye diseases. It is also applied to treat unhealed ulcer.

炉甘石,味甘性平,功能解毒明目退翳、收湿生肌敛疮,专为外用,尤为眼科要药;且治疮疡不敛。

Borax (peng sha) is sweet, salty and cool in property, applied in both external use and oral administration. The medicinal herb acts to reduce heat, relieve toxin, subside swell and diminish inflammation, as the major herb to treat diseases of ophthalmology and otolaryngology. It is applied to treat sore throat and mouth ulcer. It acts to purify lung and dissolve phlegm in oral administration, applied to treat cough with yellow sputum due to heat in lung.

硼砂,甘咸性凉,外用、内服皆可。外用清热解毒、消肿、防腐,为五官科常用,治咽痛口疮等证;内服清肺化痰,治肺热痰黄。

Index I Chinese Materia Medica in Chinese

索引 I 中药中文名索引

Index Ⅱ Chinese Materia Medica in Latin Names

索引Ⅱ 中药拉丁名索引

A

C

X

Z

Shanghai Pujiang Education Press(Shanghai University of Traditional Chinese Medicine Press)
1550 Haigang Haigang Ave, Shanghai, P.R.China 201306

图书在版编目(CIP)数据

中药学:英汉对照/郭忻主编. —上海: 上海浦江教育出版社有限公司,2018.4
(精编实用中医文库/陈凯先,李其忠,何星海总主编)
ISBN 978-7-81121-545-8

Ⅰ.①中…　Ⅱ.①郭…　Ⅲ.①中药学—英、汉　Ⅳ.①R28

中国版本图书馆 CIP 数据核字(2018)第 050165 号

上海浦江教育出版社出版
社址:上海海港大道 1550 号上海海事大学校内　　邮政编码:201306
分社:上海蔡伦路 1200 号上海中医药大学内　　邮政编码:201203
电话:(021)38284910(12)(发行)　38284923(总编室)　38284916(传真)
E-mail: cbs@shmtu. edu. cn　URL: http://www. pujiangpress. cn
上海盛通时代印刷有限公司印装　上海浦江教育出版社发行
幅面尺寸:170 mm×240 mm　印张:34. 5　字数:657 千字
2018 年 4 月第 1 版　2018 年 6 月第 1 次印刷
责任编辑:黄　健　封面设计:赵宏义
定价:118. 00 元